SEX AND SEXUALITY IN
STUART
BRITAIN

This book is dedicated to Mr Rink and the staff at Royal Shrewsbury Hospital, Shrewsbury, England, who saved my life when I suffered from acute pancreatitis in 2016 shortly after giving birth. Had I lived in the Stuart period, I would almost certainly have died.

Also by Andrea Zuvich

Nonfiction
The Stuarts in 100 Facts
A Year in the Life of Stuart Britain

Fiction
His Last Mistress: The Duke of Monmouth & Lady Henrietta
Wentworth
The Stuart Vampire

Anthology
The Chambermaid (Steel & Lace Anthology)

SEX AND SEXUALITY IN
STUART BRITAIN

ANDREA ZUVICH

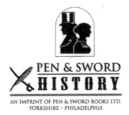

PEN & SWORD **HISTORY**

AN IMPRINT OF PEN & SWORD BOOKS LTD.
YORKSHIRE – PHILADELPHIA

First published in Great Britain in 2020 by
PEN AND SWORD HISTORY
An imprint of
Pen & Sword Books Ltd
Yorkshire – Philadelphia

ISBN 978 1 52675 307 6

Typeset in Times New Roman 11.5/14 by
Aura Technology and Software Services, India.
Printed and bound in the UK by TJ International Ltd.

Pen & Sword Books Limited incorporates the imprints of Atlas, Archaeology,
Aviation, Discovery, Family History, Fiction, History, Maritime, Military, Military
Classics, Politics, Select, Transport, True Crime, Air World, Frontline Publishing,
Leo Cooper, Remember When, Seaforth Publishing, The Praetorian Press,
Wharncliffe Local History, Wharncliffe Transport, Wharncliffe True Crime and
White Owl.

For a complete list of Pen & Sword titles please contact
PEN & SWORD BOOKS LIMITED
47 Church Street, Barnsley, South Yorkshire, S70 2AS, England
E-mail: enquiries@pen-and-sword.co.uk
Website: www.pen-and-sword.co.uk

Or

PEN AND SWORD BOOKS
1950 Lawrence Rd, Havertown, PA 19083, USA
E-mail: Uspen-and-sword@casematepublishers.com
Website: www.penandswordbooks.com

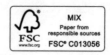

Contents

Acknowledgements

It would have been impossible for me to write a book like this without the help and support I received from many learned people—historians, teachers, independent researchers, archivists—throughout the world. Firstly, many thanks to my editors at Pen & Sword History, Claire Hopkins, Laura Hirst, and Alan Murphy, the Commissioning Editor at P&S, who approached me regarding the *Sex and Sexuality* history series back in June 2018.

Irish historian Liam Maloney at University College Dublin has been of immeasurable help—even staying up late on Skype to discuss parts of my book with me. He was indefatigable, promptly responded to my queries, and went through the whole first proof raising questions and offering suggestions for improvement. He is the creator of the #KeepItStuart hashtag and you can follow him on Twitter @cheapsellotape.

Author Melika Dannese Hick also took the time to provide me with valuable feedback on the first proof and inspired me to add explanations about the O.S/N.S. calendars.

Professor Steve Murdoch of the University of St. Andrews was extremely helpful and very generous with his time during the early stages of my research for this book. You can follow him on Twitter @ Prof_Murdoch.

I would also like to thank the archivists throughout the UK and USA who have been exceptionally helpful, including Sarah Davis and Nathaniel Stevens at Shropshire Archives, Katie Angus at Suffolk Archives, Jonathan Blaney at British History Online, Jonathan Barker at Kent Archives, David Tisley at Lancashire Archives, Frederick Alexander at the National Library of Scotland, Catherine Sutherland at Cambridge University, Eisha Neely at the Division of Rare and Manuscript Collections at Cornell University, Sandra Powlette at the British Library, and Sara Palmer at Emory University.

Many thanks also to Dr Nadine Akkerman, Cryssa Bazos, Anna Belfrage, Lucinda Brant, Professor Elaine Chalus, Melanie Clegg, Susan Margaret Cooper, Catherine Curzon, Leanda De Lisle, Dr David Davies, Jonathan Gordon, Leif Grahamsson, Jules Harper, Theodore Harvey, Dr Jonathan Healey, Julian Hick, James Hoare, Claire Hobson, Professor Laurie Johnson, Chris Jordan, Pete Langman, Professor Lloyd Llewellyn-Jones, Dr Kate Lister, Professor John McCafferty, Emma and James Monckton, Sarah Murden, Tracy Newberry, Fiona Orr, Margaret Porter, Laura Powell, Josh Provan, Liz Ramirez, Dr Sara Read, Dr Jacqueline Reiter, Robin Rowles, Dr Alana Skuse, Anita Seymour, Carly Silver, Mark Simner, Malinda Skorupa, Dr Leslie Smith, Charles Spencer, Elizabeth St. John, Deborah Swift, Aurora von Goeth, Jane Walton of *Hats Period,* and Dr Josephine Wilkinson.

Many thanks to Antonia Keaney, author and researcher at Blenheim Palace, who kindly spent a snowy afternoon taking me around the palace and discussing the major figures associated with Queen Anne's court.

Also thanks to the producers and crew of BBC Four's *Charles I: Downfall of a King,* in which I had the honour of participating while writing this book.

I am grateful also to those of you who follow me on Twitter (@17thCenturyLady), Instagram (17thCenturyLady), and Facebook (17thCenturyLady) for your constant support and encouragement, and for interacting with my hashtag #StuartsSaturday.

Some websites have been proved to be particularly helpful, for example:

Archive.org: an amazing, rich source of fascinating books now in the public domain.

EEBO (Early English Books Online): a veritable treasure-trove of literary goodness. I want to thank Paul Schaffner of the Text Creation Partnership and Text Creation Unit Digital Content & Collections, University of Michigan Library, in particular.

British History Online: This is an absolutely brilliant resource and well worth the subscription fee.

Green's Dictionary of Slang: https://greensdictofslang.com/

Rare Books and Manuscripts Section (RBMS) of the Association of College and Research Libraries, particularly their very helpful *Latin Place Names* File: http://rbms.info

On a more personal note, I wish to thank my parents, Edelmira and Ivan, my sisters, Millie and Vivian, and my in-laws, David and Yvonne, for their support.

Next, I owe a huge debt of gratitude to my husband, Gavin, who meticulously edited and proofread the manuscript before submission. This was, by far, the most demanding book I've written to date, not solely because of the content, but also because it proved extremely challenging—as a full-time mum and home-school teacher—to get sufficient opportunity to actually sit down and write it! This, combined with a stomach ulcer, a partially necrotic pancreas, and being grumpy due to little sleep, probably didn't always make me a joy to be around—so thank you for your continuing love and support.

Lastly, to my beloved daughter Juliet: although the content of this book is not appropriate for you at the moment, I hope that someday you'll read it and find it interesting.

A.Z.

Author's Note

Gentle Reader, for the purposes of this book, we will be looking at the period 1603 to 1714, which is often referred to as 'Stuart Britain' or 'the Stuart era' and is named after King James I of England & VI of Scotland. (Although there is a long line of *Stewart (Stiùbhairt)* monarchs who preceded King James, I specialise in this particular part of Stewart history—from the time James VI became heir to Elizabeth Tudor's English throne and unified these kingdoms under the Stuart dynasty in 1603 with the Union of Crowns.)

James's decision to move the royal court from Scotland to England inevitably makes this work more 'Anglocentric' than it might otherwise have been, but I have endeavoured—with the help of my friends and contacts in academia throughout the United Kingdom—to include Stuart-era histories from the great constituent countries as well, in order to give the reader a broad understanding of sexuality across these isles at this time.

I pondered over the situation regarding regnal numbers—or the roman numerals which follow a sovereign's name. Following the death of Elizabeth I, subsequent rulers had regnal numbers associated with the Scottish throne AND the English throne, so which takes precedence? After deliberation, I have decided that, after James VI of Scotland & I of England, to then have the English regnal numbers first, followed by the Scottish regnal numbers because again, the monarchs are primarily associated with the country in which they mainly lived: England. Hence, James II (of England) is also James VII (of Scotland), and so on and so forth.

During the Stuart period (1603–1714), two calendars were used. Although Scotland had already adopted the Gregorian Calendar or *New Style* (New Year beginning on 1 January) as many of the countries on the Continent had, England still used the Julian Calendar, or *Old Style* (with the New Year beginning on 24 March). Throughout this book, you'll find some dates written with two years (i.e. 1677/1678), for that is how the months from January to March were written due to this conflict between the two calendars. I understand this can seem confusing, but the more you are exposed to this, the easier it becomes. There is also a difference of ten days between them, which affected the whole year, meaning November 4 in one calendar is also November 14 in the other.

This work features quotations from a wide variety of documents that were published during the Stuart period, so you will often find words spelled differently than how we spell them today. Sometimes, spelling even differs between sources, since there were no standard rules at the time. You'll also sometimes encounter Words Capitalised Like This— initial letters of words were more commonly capitalised during the Stuart Age than they are today. This book is written in British English.

Readers familiar with my previous books, *The Stuarts in 100 Facts* and *A Year in the Life of Stuart Britain*, will have already had a foretaste of the topics which are expanded upon here. As will be seen, from the average man and woman on the streets of all Three Kingdoms of Stuart Britain—Scotland, England (which included Wales), and Ireland—right up to the privileged members of the highest echelons of Stuart society, matters of sex and sexuality influenced them all, and in turn influenced Stuart-era law, culture, and literature.

Just as I believe we should not judge past peoples based on popular modern standards of morality and virtue, I also believe it is not our place to label historical people using contemporary sexual terms. Accordingly, this book avoids terms such as 'transsexual', 'genderfluid', 'transgender', 'queer', and 'intersex'[1] (I shall, however, be covering hermaphroditism and cross-dressing, both of which were known about during the seventeenth and early eighteenth centuries). Not even the word 'gay' is used for same-sex relationships, since during the Stuart period that word was used exclusively to describe something or someone as bright, mirthful, or happy (e.g. 'See that gay Lady, that laughs aloud'[2]). The words 'lesbian' and 'homosexual' were also not used in Stuart Britain (they came into use during the nineteenth century[3]). Instead, terms used in the Stuart-era such as 'sodomite' and 'catamite' for men involved in male-male sexual activity and 'tribade' for women engaged in female-female sexual activity. Other modern terms such as 'hypersexuality' and 'sex addiction' are also avoided, in favour of the closest seventeenth-century terms for these subjects—namely 'satyriasis' and 'frenzie of the womb'. Although some of these terms might be less acceptable in the modern age, they are used here because they are were used during the Stuart period, and the goal of this book is to understand and accurately represent the people of this period—how they thought, spoke, and acted—whatever we might think of them today.

I found the subject matter for *Sex and Sexuality in Stuart Britain* somewhat daunting, since I knew that several of the topics mentioned and examples cited would be controversial and upsetting for some readers. Although my publisher and I agreed that I would avoid being 'pornographic, prurient, or inappropriate' in the writing of this work, the necessity of quoting from some of the texts of the period sometimes made that a challenge!

Most of my readers know that I am not an author who uses explicit language; however, in this work I felt that the inclusion of some of the crasser language and literature of the time was necessary to the reader being able to form a broad and full understanding of sexual attitudes during the Stuart period.

As with my previous books, I appeal to readers to set aside their modern perspectives to at least some degree, and to attempt to understand the world of the people we shall be covering from their point of view.

With this said, hold on to your periwigs and enjoy the ride, as we explore sex and sexuality in Stuart Britain!

Andrea Zuvich
Croydon, London
March 2019

Introduction

Scottish historian and Bishop of Salisbury, Gilbert Burnet—a man who lived from 1643 to 1715 and personally witnessed some of the major events of the late Stuart era—once opined that 'there is no instinct that is stronger and more universal, than the desire of happiness'.[1] Closely related to this, arguably, is the sexual instinct: one of the most powerful urges in human existence. The biological drive towards mating and reproduction, the carnal pleasure involved in sexual acts (rare in the animal world), and the social and moral views about sex and sexuality have been one of the most important aspects of human civilisations. Sex often goes hand-in-hand with human emotions, especially those of love and desire.

Love, sex, and the consequences of both—especially children—have brought peoples together and driven them apart and inspired humans throughout the world to compose music, pen great literature, and create amazing artwork. Effectively they have shaped the world's civilisations—but they have also had negative effects, such as sexually-transmitted diseases and the mistreatment of those whose preferences deviated from socially-accepted norms.

The Stuart era was one (among many) in which an individual's private sexual transgressions could, and often would, be followed by very public humiliation and punishment. Some sexual deeds were punishable by death, and some forms of love were hidden away and suppressed for fear of this fatal consequence.

This period saw some of the most tumultuous events in British history: the end of the Tudor era and the rise of the Stuart, the joining together of Scotland and England, the Irish Uprising of 1641, the Civil Wars of the 1640s and early 1650s, the Anglo-Dutch Wars which began in 1652, the Great Plague of 1665, the Great Fire of London in 1666, the Popish Plot of the late 1670s and early 1680s, Monmouth's Rebellion of 1685, the 'Glorious Revolution' of 1688, the Salem Witch Trials of 1692, the War of the Spanish Succession from 1701 to 1714, and the end of the Protestant Stuart dynastic line with Queen Anne in 1714.

Perhaps most controversial, however, remains the unification of Scotland and England which occurred during this time. This began with King James VI of Scotland (later James I of England) with the Union of Crowns in 1603, which he likened to a marriage,[2] but was formalised under Queen Anne with the Acts of Union in 1707. Indeed, to this day there are still strong feelings (and parliamentary and constitutional tensions) about this situation.

It is important to remember that the reach of Stuart Britain went far beyond the shores of the British Isles, for the makings of Britain's powerful empire were underway. Accordingly, this book includes histories of Stuart people in their sexual and romantic adventures and misadventures around the world—from the New World to Persia and Africa.

With great scientific advances being made in a hitherto deeply superstitious society, it's of little surprise that this period also witnessed changes in the sexual sphere. Nonetheless, the Post-Reformation Christian religion and its associated morality played a crucial part in Stuart-age life, so the considerable wealth of religious literature of the period has been heavily utilised in this work. Fear of incurring the wrath of the Almighty was not only of spiritual importance, but was also arguably a useful mechanism for controlling a population; the sometimes rigid moral tones were seen as a positive influence on humans, who are often apt to succumb to temptation.

One example of this moral severity can be seen in the Preface to Thomas Beard and Thomas Taylor's *The Theatre of God's Judgements* (1648):

> '...to the end that the most wicked, dissolute, and disordered sinners, that with loose reins run fiercely after their lust, if the manifest tokens of God's severity presented before their eyes do not touch them, yet the cloud and multitude of examples, through the sight of the inevitable anger and vengeance of God upon evil livers, might terrify and somewhat curb them: ... whoremongers, adulterers, ravishers, & tyrants, shall here see by the mischief that hath fallen upon their likes, that which hangeth before their eyes, and is ready to lay hold of them also'.[3]

In short, the most devoutly religious people hoped that those inclined towards sinfulness would be frightened from this course, which was one that could only end in their doom, and would instead aspire towards a godlier existence.

By drawing mainly from a wide variety of primary sources, this book aims to provide the reader with an insight into the sexual attitudes and behaviour of Stuart-era British people from various walks of life. We will explore the relationships between sex and power and will also look at an array of sex scandals throughout this fascinating period from 1603 to 1714.

Adultery and incest were both considered very serious crimes in Stuart Britain. Their moral equivalence at the time was such that legal literature would often mention both in the same line. We see this throughout the parliamentary journals of 1624 under King James VI & I, one example being: 'exception of adultery, simony, incest, schism and heresy; all other spiritual offences pardoned'. I have nevertheless separated these two crimes and added incest to the chapter devoted to 'deviant sexual practices'.

Even in the present age, when we are constantly bombarded with highly sexualised images in film, television and advertising, and when hardcore pornographic videos are easily accessible to anyone with an Internet connection, some of the sexual literature from the Stuart period still—remarkably—retains the capacity to titillate and offend.

Some may argue that humans in the West, particularly following the so-called 'sexual revolution' of the 1960s, have allowed sex to dominate our lives—and perhaps there is some truth to this. Nonetheless, with the exception of new, more effective, methods of contraception and more open attitudes towards sexual preferences once deemed immoral and illegal, matters of sex and sexuality have in some respects remained the same.

In other ways, however, things have changed remarkably. For example, during the seventeenth century, people didn't make their sexuality their identity as many do today: a man might engage in a sexual act with another man but not think of himself as a sodomite, just as a woman might engage in tribadism without thinking herself a tribade. The sexes were divided in some respects: women tended to be very close to other women, and men with men. Men slept in the same beds as other men, and women with other women—but not necessarily for the purpose of sexual activity.[4] Families and friends often shared beds, for various reasons: warmth, practicality, poverty, etc.

It's probable that while every kind of conceivable sexual act was performed during the Stuart period, most people were not exposed to much sexual variety. Certainly, some might get their hands on some erotica and become aroused by the images—if there were any—but the average person wasn't literate enough to read erotic literature, so wouldn't be able to learn about different kinds of sex in that manner. Perhaps some people learned a new sexual position from their visit to the local whorehouse, but most had more important things to think about—such as where their next meal or shelter would come from, and in what ways they could protect their kith and kin.

Although the majority of this work concerns itself with sex and sexuality in Stuart Britain on a 'macro' level (this forms the content of Part One), the latter chapters of the book (Part Two) present some 'micro' histories of each consecutive Stuart sovereign's sex life. Naturally, these are only overviews—whole books can be written about the romances of the Stuart monarchs!

Next, it would surely be wrong for us to assume that where there is love between two people there must always be sex. After all, there is—and certainly was in the Early Modern age—such a thing as platonic love. The style of correspondence during the Stuart period was much more effusive than is typical today and, as a result, modern readers are often inclined to interpret gushing and extravagant sentimentality as being something more than friendship. But this was not necessarily the case, as I will explain further in the course of this work.

There is also today a modern trend which seeks to focus, sometimes exclusively, on the narratives of 'strong' women. In my opinion this can disparage and disrespect the women (a majority) who tended to conform to the role expected of their sex at the time. When we glorify women from previous periods whom we find shared our modern values, but denigrate those who were content with a less dominant role, this is itself potentially a form of misogyny, which historians and casual readers alike should try to avoid. Are so-called 'weak' women somehow less worthy of our interest than their 'stronger' counterparts? Do women need to adopt traditionally-male-gendered qualities in order to seem strong? A typical Stuart-era person could reasonably argue that a woman could acquire great power over men merely by utilising her feminine charms.

Compared with the current age, in which radical notions of gender and sexuality are often vigorously promoted by academia and the media, it turns out that Stuart-era beliefs about sex and sexuality were relatively conventional.

This book isn't just about sexual acts; it also touches upon a great many of the pre-ambles to, and consequences of, those acts: childbirth, sexually transmitted diseases, pre-marital sex, marriage, wedding customs, adultery, bereavement, infertility, abortion, infanticide, and what the Stuarts found sexually alluring.

So, get your tankard of cock ale, sit back in your cane chair by the crackling fire, and as the smells of wood smoke and tobacco from a nearby pipe mingle with the hearty scent of freshly baked pigeon pie wafting in from next door, let us go back in time to the Stuart period...

PART ONE

Sex & Sexuality in Stuart Britain

'In men, desire begets love; in women, love begets desire'
Attributed to Barbara, Viscountess
Fitzharding (c.1654–1708)

Chapter 1

The Anatomy of a Stuart-Age Person

'Love has strange habits, various Effects upon the Bodies of Men and Women, sometimes casting a pale Shroud over them, at other times a rosy Blush'.[1]
– The Ladies Dictionary (1694)

While the anatomy of a Stuart-era man and woman differed little from ours today, trends in hygiene, body hair, and body modification have altered considerably and it is in our interest to touch upon these subjects before we proceed with the other topics. First, however, we need to think like a Stuart.

The Stuart-age person held that there are only two sexes—male and female.[2] Genitalia was sometimes referred to as the 'genitalles'[3] or 'privities', 'secret parts', or simply 'secrets'.[4]

Stuart-era peoples believed in the *humoral* theory, which dates back to Ancient Greece and was based on the four 'corporal humours', or bodily fluids: black bile (melancholy), phlegm, yellow bile (choler), and blood.[5] A healthy human being would have all four humours in balance. An imbalance would cause problems: too much black bile would, for example, lead to a depressive and melancholic emotional state ('heaviness and sadness of minde'[6]) whereas too much blood/sanguine would cause an aggressive and fiery temper.

Furthermore, it was believed that if foods or drinks were too hot or cold, this could be fatal. For example, Alice Thornton (1627–1707) believed her uncle died because he ate too many melons[7] and that the 'fruit was too cold for him'.[8] English diarist Samuel Pepys was concerned about drinking orange juice (which was new for the Stuart-age consumer), fearing that it might cause him some harm.[9] In Stuart Britain, another newly-introduced and exotic hot beverage, coffee, was rumoured to cause impotence—in 1674, a pamphlet, *The Women's Petition Against Coffee*, was purportedly written by angry, sexually-unsatisfied wives.[10]

2

It was also commonly believed during the Stuart period that the physical attributes of a given body gave outward indication of what lay within—especially in terms of sexuality. Giovanni Benedetto Sinibaldi's notorious book *The Cabinet of Venus Unlocked*, which was translated into English and published for the English market in 1658, stated many of these. Small ears, for example, were considered to signify 'aptness to venery'.[11] Shorter men were thought to have a greater sex drive than tall, lanky men,[12] and the body of a thinner man or woman was believed to be capable of experiencing 'far more delight than a fat, corpulent one'.[13]

The Stuart man

The male sex organ, the penis, was also referred to as a 'yard', a 'prick', a 'pillicock', a 'cock',[14] a 'phallus',[15] 'staff of love',[16] 'dandilolly', etc. The testicles were often referred to as 'the stones'—the vast majority of men had 'two stones' while, rarely, some were reported as having 'one, three, or even four'.[17] The foreskin on the penis would cover the glans, or what Stuart-era people sometimes called the 'nut'.[18]

Speaking of the foreskin, the external male sexual organ was generally left alone: circumcision was not a cultural norm in Stuart Britain. Indeed, the contemporary erotic literature confirms as much:

> 'The head of the Prick is compounded of fine Red flesh, much like a large Heart Cherry....over this Head is a Cup of Skin which slips backwards when the Prick stands...now when a Prick is thrust into a Cunt, the cap of skin which I before spoke of, and is called a repute slips backwards. This Skin some nations as the Jews and Turks cut off (calling it Circumcision)'.[19]

Nonetheless, artistic depictions of circumcision—particularly associated with Biblical scenes—were popular during this time, and can be seen on artworks such as tapestries and paintings. In literature, Richard Head's *The Miss Display'd* (1675) includes a character who has his foreskin removed with a razor.[20] Sinibaldi warned against such practices as 'it is a dangerous thing if the prepuce be cut, because it cannot be rejoyn'd'.[21]

Upon arousal, the penis fills with blood, causing a stiffening and lengthening, known as an erection. Stuart-era people, however, believed an erection was due to 'wind and spirits'.[22]

Some men during Stuart times worried about the length of their penis. Sinibaldi responded that a penis whose length is average is best; for while too long a penis was unlikely to maintain an erection, having one that was too short was worse, because 'it reaches not so far as sufficiently to provoke a woman's lust and seed'.[23] It's interesting to note that Stuart people believed women also contained 'seed'—today we can connect this notion to the woman's eggs.

The Stuart woman

Stuart-era girls reached *menarche* (or had their first menstruation) between the ages of twelve and fourteen,[24] but this was not the age at which most girls became pregnant. Indeed, the common wisdom of the time was that 'it would be much better both for themselves and their Children, if they married not till eighteen or twenty'.[25] There was concern that having sexual intercourse and bearing children at too young an age would be damaging to a young couple's health. Although child marriage did occur during the Stuart period, particularly amongst the aristocracy and royalty, it was not the norm, and the increasing consensus in Stuart society was that marriage was best left for people in their twenties, or late teens at the earliest—and most people did marry in their mid-twenties.

Various terms were used to refer to the female genitals, including the colloquial 'Tuzzy-Muzzy',[26] 'cunny burrow',[27] 'flapdoodle',[28] 'quim', 'garden of delight', 'cut',[29] and 'commodity'.[30] The Fallopian Tubes had been discovered in the sixteenth century by the Italian anatomist Gabriele Falloppio,[31] and were called the *Tuba Fallopiana* in some medical books and documents.[32]

Menstruation—often referred to as 'terms'[33] or 'flowers'—was treated as a mysterious aspect of womanhood. The medical writers of the Stuart period did not fully understand the biology behind women's monthly bleeding, and a missed period was not automatically associated with pregnancy.[34] The definition of 'Menstruous' in *The English Dictionarie* of 1623 is: 'having her sicknesse, foule, filthy'.[35] This clearly indicates that menstruation was seen—at least by the opposite sex—as a monstrous and dirty condition. As sanitary pads and tampons had yet to be invented, menstruating women would use rags to absorb their menstrual blood.

Just as some women in our time suffer from painful periods (Stuarts sometimes referred to this as 'strangulation of the mother'[36]), so it was with Stuart-age women—this was the case with Elisabeth Pepys, the wife of Samuel.[37] Women who had excessive amounts of menstrual bleeding, such as Lady Brilliana Harley, would be bled prior to their menstruation in the hopes that this would decrease the amount of menstrual blood.[38] The Menopause usually began around age forty-nine.[39]

Although women at the time had less autonomy than most of their descendants now enjoy, you may be surprised to discover that the Stuart era was one in which the woman's clitoris was rather venerated: 'For in lasses that begin to be amorous, the Clitoris does first discover itself'.[40] Several health books of the time indicate that medical scholars believed that the clitoris—when aroused—became erect in a similar way to the man's penis.[41]

Again, *Aristotle's Complete Master-Piece* goes into detail about the importance of the clitoris:

> 'The Clytoris, which is a sinewy and hard part of the womb, repleat with spungy and black Matter within, in the same manner as the Side-ligaments of the Yard (penis); and indeed resembles it in Form; suffers Erection, and Falling in the same Manner, and it both stirs up Lust, and gives Delight in Copulation: for without this, the Fair Sex neither desire marital Embraces, nor have Pleasure in 'em, nor conceive by 'em. They are more or less fond of Men's Embraces so that it may properly be stil'd the Seat of Lust'.[42]

From this text we see that the clitoris was considered integral to sexual enjoyment for the wife during copulation (and so the best means of producing children)—therefore deserving of respect. Again:

> '...as the Glans is in the Men, the Seat of the greatest Pleasure in the Act of Copulation, so is this of the Clitoris in Women, and therefore called the Sweetness of Love, and the Fury of Venery'.[43]

Given this, it's hardly surprising to learn that female genital mutilation (the cutting off of the clitoris)—which occurs in Britain today[44]—was virtually unheard of during the Stuart period.

Stuart-era hermaphroditism

> 'Sir, or Madam, choose you whether,
> Nature twists you both together'[45]
>> —'Upon a Hermaphrodite' by
>> John Cleveland (1613–1658)

Although most people are either male or female, in rare cases people throughout history were (and are), born with mixed sexes. The word 'hermaphrodite' was used in Stuart Britain to refer to these people and can be found listed in Cockeram's *The English Dictionarie of 1623*. It comes from Greek mythology, and is derived from the names of two Greek gods: Hermes, who is best known as a messenger, and Aphrodite, the goddess of love and beauty. According to the story, these two had a very handsome son together named Hermaphroditus who, when he was a teenager, became the object of desire for the nymph Salmacis. When Hermaphroditus rejected her sexual advances, Salmacis begged the gods to let her be with him forever. Her wish was granted... but the gods mixed Salmacis and Hermaphroditus together into one being with both sexes.[46] Artists and sculptors have subsequently made exquisite works of art based on these, such as Giovanni Francesco Susini's 1639 sculpture, *Hermaphrodite*.

According to Dr John Wallis (1616–1703), '...when God gives both Sexes to the same person, (such there are, and have been; and I think there is one yet living, who was first as a Woman married to a Man, and is since as a Man married to a Woman) and what hinders then, but that God, if he please may mingle the Effects of both these Sexes in the same Body?'.[47] Wallis continues by stating that plants are like this and are able to propagate by themselves, though he admitted that this is not the case with animals. Further, in terms of human sex, 'here is nothing impossible, nothing incredible'.[48] In another letter, however, Wallis states that there are only two sexes, and therefore was probably of the mind that, in most cases, a human being is distinctly one sex or the other.[49]

The most famous Stuart-era hermaphrodite was Thomas/Thomasine Hall, an English servant in the North American colony of Virginia whose cross-dressing and relationship with a maid led to Hall's trial in 1629. Another was Daniel Burghammer, who lived as a man, worked as a soldier and a blacksmith and was married to a woman, but could not impregnate his wife. Following sexual intercourse with a man, however, Burghammer conceived and in 1601 gave birth to a girl, whom he named Elizabeth (and breastfed from his breast)—thus proving that he had the full reproductive tract of a woman.[50]

Pubic hair

Pubic hair is hair that appears on the external sexual organs and groin of humans during puberty. In the seventeenth and early eighteenth centuries, people would sometimes lose their pubic hair as a consequence of having a sexually transmitted disease such as syphilis, or they might be obliged to shave all of it off following an infestation of pubic lice. Some women would resort to using a *merkin*, or pubic wig, to hide this abnormality. In *Sodom, Or, the Quintessence of Debauchery,* an explicitly sexual play often attributed to John Wilmot, two characters, Bolloximian and Pockenello have the following exchange:

> **Bolloximian:**
> 'My pleasures for new cunts I will uphold,
> And have reserves of kindness for the old.
> I grant in absence dildo may be used
> With milk of goats, when once our seed's infused
> My prick no more to bald cunt shall resort-
> Merkins rub off, and often spoil the sport.
>
> **Pockenello:**
> Let merkin, sir, be banished from the court.'[51]

In the same play, there is even a character named Virtuoso who is a 'dildo and merkin maker'.[52] This leads one to conclude that there was a preference for natural pubic hair during the Stuart period.[53] Nonetheless, there is an instance of a woman shaving the hair from her lady's area in Stuart-era literature—this is to be found in the novel *Eve Revived, or The Fair One Stark-Naked* from 1684.[54]

The artwork of the period, however, usually depicts a woman's pudendum as being bare. This was probably for aesthetic reasons and not a realistic representation of the state of most women's pudenda. The growth of pubic hair during menarche was considered indicative of a girl's physical capability to conceive a child (usually hand-in-hand with the commencement of menstruation).[55] It is probable, therefore, that most adult women of this time would have been inclined towards embarrassment if they lacked sufficient pubic hair, since it would suggest they were infertile.[56]

Body modification

What about genital piercings, you may ask? There is little documentation of this practice, but according to one account by a European traveller to the East Indies, male genital modification was performed in an effort to stop sodomy: 'One of the Queens of Pegu ordain'd that every man should carry in his Yard [penis] a little Bell, which would make it swell and he should not be able to do Nature any violence…These little bells are put in betwixt the skin and the flesh'.[57] This sort of procedure, however, appears to have declined in the region due to a surge of interest in new religions.[58] Perhaps some Stuart-era sailors had their members pierced? It's possible, but there is no evidence for there having been any genital piercings in Britain at this time. At any rate, it's safe to assume that genital piercings were certainly not a fashion in Stuart Britain.

Tattoos, during the Stuart period, were the preserve principally of criminals and/or seafarers. Captain John Smith (1580–1631) was intrigued by the tattoos on the Native American women whom he encountered in Virginia, enough to warrant writing about them: 'Their women some have their legs, hands, breasts, and face cunningly embroidered with diverse works such as beasts, serpents, artificially wrought into their flesh with black spots'.[59]

Castrati

During the seventeenth century, Baroque music increasingly celebrated the voice of *castrati*: men who had been castrated as youths (generally between the ages of seven and twelve) in order to retain an angelic, pre-pubescent singing voice. Depending on when the procedure was performed, a castrato could sometimes still have sex and ejaculate—but without sperm. This kind of castration differed from that of eunuchs in other parts of the world, who for the most part had the entirety of their external sexual organs removed following puberty; castrati only had their testicles removed, while their penis remained intact.[60]

Hortense Mancini, an Italian aristocrat who became one of King Charles II's mistresses, had a young page named Dery who is reputed to have had a beautiful singing voice. Upon the realisation that his voice had begun to break, Dery himself expressed his wish to be castrated in order to preserve his angelic tone.[61] At the tail end of the Stuart period, aristocrats increasingly attended performances in which castrati sang; and King William III and Queen Mary II were recorded as having attended, in 1681, an opera in which at least one castrato performed.[62] In Britain, the castrato voice would reach its zenith of popularity in the eighteenth century, particularly with the compositions of George Frideric Handel (1685–1759).

Castrati enjoyed more socialisation with women than did intact men, since there was no danger of a married woman becoming pregnant by the castrato and then passing off the illegitimate child as having been fathered by her husband.

Besides the issue of the mutilation of genitalia inherent in the making of castrati, there was further controversy surrounding them, and other eunuchs. For example, during the Stuart era, the purpose of marriage was held to be the propagation of children and, since men lacking testicles were unable to impregnate women, the subject of their marrying at all was debated. Some people wondered whether they were 'capable of Marriage, and if they ought to be suffer'd to enter into that State'.[63]

The Stuart child

Those unfamiliar with the culture of *breeching* often assume that a child seen wearing a dress in an Early Modern portrait is female. In fact, boys and girls wore very similar clothing until the boys were breeched—*viz.* ceremoniously given their first pair of breeches or trousers around the ages of six and eight.[64] There are many examples of aristocratic or royal portraiture which depict young boys in full dresses, including paintings of Charles, Prince of Wales (later Charles II), James, Duke of York (later James II & VII) and William of Orange (later William III & II). This was a custom practiced not only in Stuart Britain, but also elsewhere in Europe, as we can see from the portraits of toddlers Willem van Loon and Prince Federigo of Urbino (Dutch and Italian, respectively).[65]

Chapter 2

How to be a Sexy Stuart!

What was considered sexually appealing in Stuart Britain? Every age has its particular sense of what is deemed attractive or unattractive. Some people in Stuart Britain were downright sexy, others were *literally* Sexey (such as Andrew Sexey,[1] who died in 1698), while others happened to have 'Sex' as their surname, for example John Sex and Mary Sex – who were plaintiffs in a property dispute case in 1660.[2] There was also Colonel Edward Sexby (c. 1616–1658), the Leveller who unsuccessfully plotted to assassinate Oliver Cromwell![3] But, of course, not everyone had such alluring names, and almost everyone was interested in attracting a potential lover or spouse.

As a general rule, for women, very pale skin was much sought after, especially in the earlier half of the seventeenth century, with some ladies going to extreme lengths to attain this standard of beauty. A slight double chin was also considered attractive, going hand-in-hand with the physical plumpness associated with wealth. This is an inversion of today's Western society, where people from a lower socio-economic background are more likely to be obese than are the wealthy.[4] As William Austin, an English barrister, wrote in *Haec Homo* (1639): 'The beauty of a Woman cherisheth the face, and a Man loveth nothing better. And indeed well may her beauty be compared to a flower; and her self to a garden'.[5]

The description of one of the main characters in Gabriel de Brémond's *The Amorous Abbess* (1684), for example, is typical of what was generally considered attractive in women during the Stuart period: 'her Hair fair and thick; her Eyes blue and sparkling; her Mouth admirably well; her Nose very handsome, and her Teeth passable, with the shape of her Face so round and charming, that to say Truth, it was more fit to inspire Love than Devotion'.[6]

As was the case with many aspects of life in Stuart Britain, there was sometimes a moralising tone regarding beauty. In *Advice to a Daughter* (1688) George Savile, Marquis of Halifax, wrote:

> 'Very great Beauty may perhaps so dazzle for a time, that Men may not so clearly see the Deformity of those Affections: But when the Brightness goeth off, and that the Lover's Eyes are by that mean set at liberty to see things as they are, he will natural return to his lost senses, and recover the mistake into which the Lady's good looks had at first engag'd him; and being once undeceived, ceaseth to worship that as a Goddess…such women please only like the first opening of a scene, that hath nothing to recommend it but the being New'.[7]

In other words, don't let a woman's beauty make you fall in love with her; once the initial novelty of comeliness wears off, you're just left with the woman—so make sure she has other qualities, too.

Yet, at the same time, Thomas Brown and Edward Ward wrote: 'A Woman that neglects her Beauty, is in a fair way to neglect her soul'.[8] Exterior beauty was generally seen as an indicator of interior beauty—which, of course, is not necessarily the case.

With so much emphasis placed on what made a woman attractive—what about men? Surprisingly little time was spent considering which characteristics made for an attractive man. In the Elizabethan period, for example, a 'good leg'[9] was a feature of an attractive male. This continued into the subsequent Jacobean, and then Caroline periods, with tight hose emphasising a man's legs.

Age

> 'When Age with furrows shall have plow'd her Face,
> And all her Body o'er thick wrinkles place;
> Her Breasts turn black, her sparkling Eyes sink in,
> Fearfull to see the bristles on her Chin,
> Her painted Face grown swarthy, wan, and thin'.[10]
>   - In Praise of a Deformed, but Virtuous,
>   Lady; Or, A Satyr on Beauty

In Stuart Britain, age was considered to be detrimental to one's physical beauty, and both youth and beauty were regarded as indicators of fertility, especially in women. Although exaggerated for effect, the following from *A Comical View of London and Westminster* (1705) nevertheless indicates what Stuart era people thought of age and beauty: 'When you have once seen Twenty, that impudent underminder, Time, daily steals a charm from you...in short, Ladies, Love follows Beauty, as the Shadow follows the Body'.[11] John Wilmot, 2nd Earl of Rochester, opined that 'Here in England, look a Horse in the Mouth, and a Woman in the Face, you presently know both their Ages to a Year',[12] while Queen Mary II (1662–1694) complained of feeling old and of having the physical ailments of an aged person—when she was only thirty-one![13]

Fashion

Fashions change rapidly and a garment which represents the height of fashion at its time will often appear ridiculous only a decade later. Joseph Addison, one of the creators of the bestselling Late-Stuart-era periodical, *The Spectator*, knew this full well: in 1711, he wrote, 'Great Masters in Painting never care for drawing People in the Fashion; as very well knowing that the Headdress, or Periwig, that now prevails, and gives a Grace to their Portraitures at present, will make a very odd Figure, and perhaps look monstrous in the Eyes of Posterity'.[14]

The Frenchman François Maximilien Misson, a Huguenot refugee who settled in Stuart Britain in the late seventeenth century, made many fascinating observations concerning the peoples of his adoptive homeland in his 1698 work *Mémoires et observations faites par un voyageur en Angleterre*. He commented that the 'fops' and 'beaux'—who were men at the forefront of fashion—wore wigs and clothes covered in powder 'like millers with flour' and were often seen frequenting theatres, chocolate houses, or promenading ostentatiously in parks.

From Hammond's *The Whole Duty of Man* (1657), a popular book of the time: 'Men and women should content themselves with that sort of clothing which agrees to their sex and condition, not striving to exceed, and equal that of a higher rank...let every Man clothe himself in such sober attire as befits his place and calling, and not think himself disparaged, if another of his Neighbours have better than he'.[15] We might contrast this attitude with the deliberate 'dressing down' practiced by some rich, famous, and influential people of today who can afford to do otherwise!

Some intrepid people chose to wear very unusual outfits—but this didn't always work out well for them. In 1711, 'C' wrote to *The Spectator* and described a woman, recently arrived from London, who had entered the church for service wearing a strange headdress and a big, hooped skirt. 'Some stared at the prodigious Bottom, and some at the little Top of this strange Dress'.[16] No doubt the congregation remembered this fashion *faux pas* more than they remembered the contents of the sermon that day!

In Jacobean portraiture, women are often depicted wearing extremely low-cut gowns, with their breasts bulging out. Arguably the most famous of these portraits is that of Frances Howard, c. 1615, by William Larkin. Another example is the now-lost portrait of Lady Anne Clifford which was painted around 1610 and depicted her wearing a dress which completely revealed her breasts.[17]

French fashions became particularly popular following the Restoration of the monarchy in 1660. Charles II's mother, Henrietta Maria, was French, and—during his exile following his defeat at the Battle of Worcester in 1651—Charles lived at various courts, including that of France. It was during his reign that certain items of clothing came into use, some of which (including the three-piece suit) became a mainstay of men's fashion for centuries to come.

Occasionally, Stuart-era fashions would cross the line and blur gender roles, and cross-dressing (transvestism) occurred—which was seen by some as outrageous. Androgyny was not generally regarded as something to be celebrated or admired.[18] During the late Stuart period, aristocratic ladies began to wear men's hunting attire during hunts. Notable women who adopted this style include Mary of Modena and Frances 'La Belle' Stuart—the latter was painted thus attired in 1664 by Jacob Huysmans.[19] In literature, the character of Angelica in *Eve Revived* (1684) also dons men's clothing during her time with a prince.[20] Samuel Pepys, unimpressed with this trend, commented:

> 'walking in the galleries at White Hall, I find the Ladies of Honour dressed in their riding garbs, with coats and doublets with deep skirts, just for all the world like mine, and buttoned their doublets up the breast, with periwigs and

with hats; so that, only for a long petticoat dragging under their men's coats, nobody could take them for women in any point whatever; which was an odd sight, and a sight, [which] did not please me.[21]

Oxford antiquarian Anthony Wood also disapproved, writing: 'a strange effeminate age when men strive to imitate women in their apparel, viz. long periwigs, patches in their faces, painting, short wide breeches like petticoats, muffs, and their clothes highly scented, bedecked with ribbons of all colours'.[22] The women, Wood continued, 'would strive to be like men, viz. when they rode on horseback or in coaches wear plush caps like *monteros*, either full of ribbons or feathers, long periwigs which men use to wear'.[23]

The Quakers, who were one of many radical groups to emerge in the seventeenth century, had their own particular views on fashion. According to leading Quaker, and founder of Pennsylvania, William Penn in his *Reflections and Maxims* (1683), 'Excess in apparel is another costly folly. The very trimming of the vain world would clothe all the naked one'.[24] Clothing, he added, should be simple and plain, and 'if thou art clean and warm, it is sufficient; for more doth but rob the poor, and please the wanton'.[25] In a similar vein, the English politician Edward Coke believed that few wise people were taken in by sumptuous clothing, and wrote approvingly of attire that was 'plain and frugal'.[26]

There is no evidence that women of this period wore underwear such as knickers, or panties.[27] A woman's shift or smock seems to have been regarded as just as sexy as modern lingerie is today, for these garments would be closest to the wearer's naked flesh. Accordingly, in 1662, Samuel Pepys received quite a thrill when he came across underclothes belonging to Barbara Palmer, Lady Castlemaine, hanging out to dry: 'And in the Privy-garden saw the finest smocks and linen petticoats of my Lady Castlemaine's, laced with rich lace at the bottom, that ever I saw: and did me good to look at them'.[28]

After the shift, would come the stays, or what we would call a corset. One of the most frequently asked questions about Stuart-era stays is, 'How could women wear such tight and uncomfortable garments?' In fact, most clothing historians agree that a pair of stays was more comfortable than we might assume, since garments were not off-the-peg but were tailored for an individual's unique form.[29] An exquisite pair of pink silk stays trimmed with taffeta ribbons from the mid-seventeenth-century can be seen today at the Victoria & Albert Museum in London. The sleeves were optional and the boning is made of whalebone.[30]

Makeup

'God hath given you one face,
And you make your selves another.'[31]
— The Tragicall Historie of Hamlet, Prince of Denmark.
Act III, Scene I. William Shakespeare

During the Stuart period, white skin and a smooth complexion were very much sought-after, and those who had not been bestowed with these qualities by nature often resorted to artifice in order to achieve them. But the use of makeup, or 'paint', as it was then known, was controversial, as it was often associated with prostitutes. The diarist John Evelyn lamented this growing trend in his entry of May 1654: 'I now observed how the women began to paint themselves, formerly a most ignominious thing, and used only by prostitutes'.[32] This sentiment is also expressed in a Late Stuart-era song, *'A Hue and Cry after Beauty and Virtue'*: 'Whoring and Painting flourish so well, We hardly know where Honest Women dwell'.[33]

Makeup was almost exclusively worn by women until the late seventeenth century, when it began to be applied by both sexes (male usage, however, was generally associated with Restoration fops!). Cosmetics often contained toxic ingredients, which sometimes proved to be fatal.[34] That said, Stuart people were exposed to other toxins on a daily basis, too, such as pewter, which contained lead.[35]

Kenelm Digby (1603–1665), was a distinguished English diplomat and natural philosopher who took a keen interest in recipes and pharmacology. In his recipe for a 'more precious Cosmetick', Digby advised the use of a variety of harmless ingredients including flowers and beans, but also suggested dangerous additions such as ceruse (white lead), to create a cosmetic water that *'smooths, whitens, beautifies & preserves the Complexions of Ladies'*.[36]

Digby's wife, Lady Venetia Stanley (1600–1633), was—perhaps unsurprisingly—one of the most admired beauties of her time. Her life was cut short, though, by an apparent overdose of viper wine—a concoction which used lethal viper venom to create a beautifying elixir. The grieving Digby considered his wife to be still so gorgeous—even after death—that he had her death-bed portrait painted by Anthony van Dyck.

Patches arrived on the Stuart fashion scene towards the latter half of the seventeenth century. What were these, you might ask? Also known by the French word *mouches*, they were facial decorations made from black cloth, cut out into attractive shapes, such as circles, stars, half-moons, and more and were popular with ladies who wished to cover up smallpox scars, pimples, warts, or other facial blemishes. Smallpox was often fatal, and was notorious for ruining the beauty of those who survived. The disease caused pustules of pus to develop over the skin and eventually these turned into unsightly pits, and there are several notable examples of how smallpox ruined beauty.

Lady Frances Stuart, *'La Belle Stuart'*, was a woman so renowned for her good looks that she was not only the model for Britannia but was also pursued by a besotted King Charles II. After catching smallpox, however, she was never again called a great beauty. In 1619, Lady Katherine Howard, Countess of Suffolk (1564–1638), also lost her famed loveliness to smallpox[37]—had she lived later in the century, she might well have used patches. Lady Mary Wortley-Montague (1689–1762) was yet another famed beauty who lost her looks after her bout with smallpox. She later became a champion for smallpox inoculation, which saved countless future lives—and looks.[38]

Many of the books intended for homemakers included beauty recipes, and it's no wonder that a good complexion was regarded as essential for Stuart-era beauty considering the prevalence of disfiguring diseases at the time. *The Queen's Royal Cookery* (1709), for example, contained information on 'several Cosmetick or Beautifying Waters',[39] while *The English Housewife* (1623) stated that 'Rosemary water (the face washed therein both morning and night) causeth a fair and clear countenance'.[40] Samuel Pepys was rather put-out when his wife, Elisabeth, mentioned that she had bought some 'puppy-dog water', which was used by some women to improve their facial skin.[41] This might sound like an endearing product; however, the term referred either to a puppy's urine or—in most beauty recipes—meant the end result of killing and then roasting or boiling puppies! As stated in the recipe from Nicholas Culpeper's 'Oyl of Whelps': 'Take Sallet Oyl four pound, two Puppy-dogs newly whelped…

boyl the Whelps till they fall in pieces'.[42] Of course, a good, clear complexion is still much sought-after today, but we—mercifully—do not resort to concoctions such as puppy-dog water to try to achieve it.

John Evelyn was not alone in his dislike of makeup. An unnamed gentleman whose letter appeared in the 17 April 1712 edition of *The Spectator* went further: 'There are women who do not let their Husbands see their Faces till they are married…I mean plainly, that Part of the Sex who paint'.[43] This fellow was taken by his wife's good looks, but upon seeing her true, makeup-free, appearance in the morning following their wedding, he declared: 'she scarce seems young enough to be the Mother of her whom I carried to Bed the Night before'.[44]

Hair

In order to fully understand Stuart-era hairstyles, we should begin by discussing the matter of personal hygiene, and the attendant fact that parasites—in particular, lice, fleas, intestinal worms—were a very common problem at the time, and they had no regard for whether their hosts were rich or poor.[45] Keeping one's hair clean meant combing through it thoroughly to remove lice and nits.[46] There was no shampoo, as we know it today, but some people used a variety of herbs and water to rinse their hair—though this was done very rarely, as wetting one's hair was believed to endanger health!

During the Caroline period (1625–1649), it was fashionable for men to wear one lock of hair longer than the rest; this was known as a *lovelock*. King Charles I and George Villiers, Duke of Buckingham, are just two of the most well-known figures from this period who sat for portraits which clearly show them sporting lovelocks.

Men began to wear periwigs during the early 1660s, mainly for aesthetic reasons, with many opting to shave their own hair entirely. These wigs were comprised of cascading curls with three segments that fell below the shoulders: one section fell down the back, while the other two dangled down the chest like the floppy ears of a spaniel dog. Periwigs were worn only by more affluent men, however, for they were quite costly. In 1663, Pepys wrote of his periwig buying: 'two periwigs, one whereof costs me 3l. and the other 40s. I have worn neither yet, but will begin next week, God willing'.[47] Pepys also demonstrated the fire hazard dangers that wig-wearing entailed when he accidentally lit his periwig on fire by leaning too close to a lighted candle![48] Some men resorted to wigs not only for reasons of fashion, but because they were self-conscious about their physical attributes. In 1711, Richard Steele writing in *The Spectator*, confessed, 'I have been often put out of Countenance by the Shortness of my Face, and was formerly at great Pains in concealing it by wearing a Periwig with an high Foretop, and letting my Beard grow'.[49]

Women's hair was generally long, unless cut for religious purposes or because of illness, but some fashionable hairstyles also required hair to be cut, and this didn't meet with everyone's approval. From William Prynne's *Histrio-Mastix* (1633): 'Whores and adulteresses punished heretofore by cutting their hair, which our women now make a fashion'. Here, Prynne was referring to the cutting of hair to make a fringe, or bangs, which were then curled to frame a woman's face— Queen Henrietta Maria's early 1630s hairstyle is a good example of this. Prynne had strong opinions about men's hair-dos, too! For example: 'Men's wearing of long, false, curled hair and lovelocks, condemned by Deuteronomy 22.5, Ezekial 44.20'.

During late 1679, one of King Louis XIV of France's mistresses, the teenaged, doomed Marie-Angélique de Scorailles, Mlle des Fontanges,[50] was credited with having inadvertly created the *à la Fontanges* hairstyle[51]—one which became more and more elaborate, until it peaked as a tall headdress made of lace and wire, with copious false curls! By the 1690s, this hairstyle was all the rage in Stuart Britain—even adorning the heads of the *crème de la crème* of royalty and other fashion-conscious, wealthy persons. This style, along with the increasingly ostentatious periwigs worn by gentlemen, are two of the most well-known and immediately recognisable hair fashions of the Late Stuart period. Occasionally these striking coiffures proved useful if a patient suffered from bleeding from a skin ulcer or injury upon their scalp, as we gather from *A Description of Bandages and Dressings* (1701): 'the Periwig in Men, and the Coif in Women, hides all this Bandage'.[52]

By 1713, however, haircutting had become more socially acceptable for both sexes and all ages, as indicated by an advert in *The Guardian*: 'Bat. Pidgeon, the Hair-cutter, in the Strand, cuts Gentleman's, Ladies, and Children's hair on Mondays, Wednesdays, and Saturdays at his house exactly against Surry-Street near the Maypole'.[53]

18

Bathing & scent

'...with abundance of Rubbing, Scrubbing, Washing and Combing, we had made our selves tolerable Figures'[54]
– The London Spy Compleat (1703)

When one considers that people in Stuart Britain believed foul smells could spread disease, the fact most people didn't bathe as regularly as we do today can be surprising. It is true that—with the exception of hands and faces—full-body bathing between 1603 and 1714 wasn't very high on the list of priorities for the average Stuart man or woman. For one thing, most people didn't have running water (never mind *hot* running water)—so it could get pretty chilly! During this period the 'Little Ice Age' was in full blast, too—particularly in the latter part of the Stuart period. This made normally cold winters even colder due to global cooling.[55] John Evelyn was convinced that going to a *bagnio* in Italy, where he washed with both hot and cold water, had 'cost me one of the greatest colds I ever had in my life'.[56]

Nevertheless, when weather permitted, people during this time *did* bathe. Sometimes, this was while swimming. As John Evelyn recounted in his diary entry for 2 August 1651: 'I went with my wife to Conflans, where were abundance of ladies and others bathing in the river; the ladies had their tents spread on the water for privacy'.[57]

By the latter part of the century, King William III had bath-rooms installed in his residence, Paleis Het Loo, in the Dutch Republic.[58] He enjoyed regular bathing and applied lavender powder to smell nice.

Scented powder was also associated with famed Stuart bawd, Damaris Page, who is said to have uttered on her deathbed: 'To all the rotten pockified Whores (of which there is a great many) I give four-pence apiece, to buy them sweet powder, to keep them from stinking'.[59] The Stuart physician, Nicholas Culpeper, recommended an infusion of thistles to 'amend the rank smell of the Armpits'.[60]

With malodorous smells a part of daily life, Stuart-era man was 'forc'd with strong perfumes to guard his Nose from poys'nous Whiffs of Breath, Armpits, and Toes'.[61] This being the case, the ordinary Stuart-era housewife would have had the skills to make her own perfumes to help keep nasty stenches at bay. In Gervase Markham's *The English Housewife* (1631), one of the many recipes is 'to make an excellent sweet water for perfume',[62] which was comprised of basil, mints, marjoram, corne-flagge roots, hyssop, savory, sage, balm, lavender, rosemary, cloves, cinnamon, nutmeg, musk, civet, and ambergris. This would have produced a scent that was fairly typical of perfume recipes since Tudor times, but some of these ingredients—especially the exotic nutmeg—would have been quite costly, and therefore beyond the means of most people.

Scent wasn't only made into perfumes to be used as body fragrances; it was also incorporated into washing balls, home incense, pomanders, and other items. Jerkins and gloves were just two popular accessories that were often perfumed during this time. In short, with a plethora of foul smells everywhere, most Stuart-era people were keen to encounter a pleasant scent!

Masks

Vizards—or 'visards', as the word was usually spelled at the time—were masks which became fashionable during the seventeenth century, especially with those who wished to conceal their identities in public, (they were often used by courtesans, for example).[63] They made the wearer exude an air of mystery—which may have aided flirtatious behaviour. These masks were not only used for the purpose of anonymity, but also to protect the face from sunlight.[64]

Criminals also sometimes wore these: 'highwaymen, that rarely rob without vizards',[65] were one such problem. Across the Channel in France, the popularity of such masks became so troublesome that the wearing of them was eventually forbidden in an attempt to reduce criminal activity; but some French ladies ignored this law and continued to wear them nonetheless.[66]

In England, Quaker William Penn stated that 'women that rarely go abroad without vizard masks have none of the best reputation'.[67] The English diarist, Samuel Pepys, observed of Lady Mary Cromwell: 'when the House began to fill she put on her vizard, and so kept it on all the play; which of late is become a great fashion among the ladies, which hides their whole face'.[68] After this, he went out to the Great Exchange and bought a vizard for his wife, Elisabeth. The following year, he attended a court entertainment in which all twelve dancers, comprised of six members of both sexes, each wore vizards.[69] Yet, in *A Comical View of London* (1705), the author pokes fun at the kind of person who wears this accessory: 'Vizor-masque is very busy in the Pit [of the theatre] by seven'.[70]

The Bohemian engraver and artist, Wenceslas Hollar, was known for his striking etchings, including *The Winter habit of an English Gentlewoman* (1644), which depicts a gentlewoman attired in warm clothing to keep out the winter chill—she also wears a half-mask.[71]

Accessories

Accessories were vital to achieving peak Stuart sexiness! Those pesky, bitterly cold *Little Ice Age* winters meant that some accessories were *de rigeur*—for example, the ever-useful muff which was used by both sexes.

Pearls, whether in the form of earrings, necklaces, or sewn into one's clothing, were a prized fashion accessory amongst the few who could afford them: throughout the Stuart period there are countless portraits of the aristocracy in which the sitter wears these costly items of jewellery.

Snuffboxes were a popular gift; again, mainly among the wealthier of the population—Nell Gwynn received one from Charles II in 1668. Hers was made from silver, in the shape of a book, and engraved with the Latin words 'Ouid de arte amada' or, 'Ovid The Art of Love'.[72] A few years later, Nell returned the favour and gifted her royal lover a beautifully engraved silver snuffbox, with a Chinese scene on the lid.[73]

Teeth

Yellow teeth, though the norm, were considered unattractive. People used many recipes to improve the shade of their teeth and get that ultimate dazzling Stuart smile! In fact, the first recorded use of the word 'toothbrush' dates to 1651.[74] In order to make their teeth white, *The English Housewife* (1623) advised Stuart-era people to:

'Take a saucer of strong vinegar, and two spoonfuls of the powder of rock alum, a spoonful of white salt, and a spoonful of honey, seeth all these till it be thin as water, then put it into a close vial and keep it, and when occasion serves wash your teeth therewith, with a rough cloth, and rub them soundly, but not to bleed'.[75]

Another recipe for 'teeth that are yellow', was to crush equal parts of sage and salt until this formed a powdery consistency, then this combination would be rubbed onto the yellow teeth twice daily, once in the morning and again in the evening.[76]

Stuart people cared about their teeth for a greater reason than mere vanity: infections from rotten teeth could lead to more serious complications—one of the recorded principal causes of death in London was listed as 'teeth'.[77]

Tobacco usage

By the end of the Elizabethan period, the practice of smoking tobacco using long clay pipes had already become quite popular,[78] and the Stuarts continued with this nevertheless controversial habit. The new trend was considered loathsome by some—including the new king himself—who, in 1604, published *A Counterblast to Tobacco*—one of the earliest anti-smoking and anti-tobacco works. In this, he refers to tobacco usage as 'this Savage custom' which was harmful to health, for 'this stinking smoke being sucked up by the nose, and imprisoned in the cold and moist brains'.[79] So opposed to tobacco was King James, that he raised taxes on it by 4,000%,[80] but that did little to affect the popularity of the habit.

Dried tobacco leaves were smoked not only recreationally, but also for medicinal reasons, as doing so was generally believed to be beneficial to one's health! During the Great Plague of 1665, even children would smoke, because it was thought to protect them from the pestilential airs that many believed caused the plague. Indeed, children were sometimes subjected to corporal punishment if they failed to smoke during this time.[81]

Wealthier citizens sometimes preferred chewing tobacco—as was the case with Samuel Pepys[82]—and snuff, which is made from ground tobacco leaves, was another popular way that Stuart people took tobacco. A French publication from 1677, entitled *Histoire du tabac, Ou, Il est traite' particulierement du Tabac en Poudre*, goes into some detail about snuff-taking,[83] and occasionally, Stuart periodicals would list snuff products in their advertisement section, as was the case in *The Post Boy*, October 1709: 'Plain Spanish snuff, right and fine, in tin pots, at 4s. per Pound Finest Brazil snuff at 3s. 6d. an Ounce, to be sold by Mr Francis Zouch, in Thames-Street, at the corner of Garlick-Hill, near Queenhith'.[84]

In Sir John Chardin's *Voyages du Chevalier Chardin en Perse et autres lieux de l'Orient*, he mentions that the Persians enjoyed smoking a milder variety of tobacco and disliked *Tombacou Inglesi* (English tobacco), 'because the first European takers of Tobacco, with whom they had any commerce, were the English. The English us'd to bring this Tobacco from Brazil, and sell it in Persia…but the Persians finding it both too strong and too dear, they made use of it no longer'.[85]

Stuart supermodels

Perhaps there was no direct equivalent of today's supermodels during the Stuart era, but there were certainly some women who were so celebrated for their beauty that they were immortalised in works of art. People could buy cheap engravings and prints of the most popular beauties and Samuel Pepys, for one, was very pleased with his print of Barbara Palmer, which he proudly had framed.[86]

Just after the Restoration of the monarchy in 1660, Anne, Duchess of York, commissioned the talented artist Peter Lely to create a series of portraits of the most strikingly beautiful women at court. These portraits came to be known as the *Windsor Beauties*, for they hung in Windsor Castle until the early nineteenth century.[87] The paintings, created between 1662 and 1665, give us a good idea of what was considered physically attractive during this period, but some of the facial features are so similar that we can tell they were not entirely accurate depictions of the sitters. Samuel Pepys, who looked upon these portraits himself when they were recently completed, said they were 'good, but not like'.[88]

Many of these paintings are now on display at Hampton Court Palace. They have a dreamy, languid feel, and convey a sensuality and beauty without resorting to nudity. Notable among the sitters was Frances Stuart as Diana, holding that goddess's bow, her body clad in a golden dress with pearls at her neck and ears. Barbara Palmer, Countess Castlemaine and Duchess of Cleveland, is almost haughty as Pallas Athene, as she stands tall, her head adorned with feathers and with loose-fitting garments enveloping her body. Elizabeth Hamilton, another Restoration beauty, was Irish-born but French-raised, and Lely depicted her as the Christian martyr Saint Catherine.

During the reign of William and Mary in the 1690s, Queen Mary II continued in the Duchess of York's footsteps (after all, Anne had been her mother) and commissioned a series of paintings of court women who were not only beautiful on the outside, but good and virtuous on the inside. This series, known as the *Hampton Court Beauties*, was more formal in style and was painted by Godfrey Kneller, beginning in 1691.

Taking inspiration from these two series of portraits, the artist Michael Dahl was commissioned to create a similar range at Petworth House for the 'Proud Duke' Charles Seymour, 6th Duke of Somerset. These paintings, made around 1700, depicted not only Queen Anne, but also her ladies-in-waiting, including Sarah, Duchess of Marlborough. The painting of Sarah was the only portrait in the series that was not painted by Dahl (it was by Godfrey Kneller).[89] Also at Petworth is a smaller, lesser-known series of four portraits of 'Beauties', painted by Anthony Van Dyck in London in 1671.

Chapter 3

Pornography & Erotic Literature

'May lust incite your prick with flame and sprite,
Ever to fuck with safety and delight'[1]
—The Farce of Sodom, Or, The Quintessence of
Debauchery

The sexual language of the Stuart era was often breathtakingly graphic—even by the standards of the twenty-first-century—so prepare thyself! The literature of the period ranged from total smut (Hello, John Wilmot!) to the subtler, sensual writings of the likes of John Donne and the more scientifically-minded *Aristotle's Master-Piece*.

The moral backlash against this kind of literature is best articulated by a Stuart-era voice: in *A Treatise on Self-Denial* (1675), the nonconformist minister and polemicist Richard Baxter opined that, 'Another part of self-interest of sensuality to be denied is the use of wanton filthy discourse, and of wanton books, and songs and ballads, commonly called Love songs. As these are the fruits of vain minds that do invent them, so do they breed and feed the like vanity in others. Indeed they are the Devil's psalms and liturgy'.[2]

Among the words used for sexual activities were:

Fornication: sexual intercourse, usually of the premarital or adulterous variety—pretty much any kind of sex outside wedlock. This word was usually used by the more puritanical.

Fucking: sexual congress, generally used in a vulgar manner (it is not, for example, listed in Henry Cockeram's *The English Dictionarie of 1623*[3]).

Swiving: a term for having sex with, comparable with 'fucking'.

Frigging: masturbation.

Tupping: another word for 'fucking'.

The erotic literature of the time also contained a good deal of content that may reasonably be considered the stuff of the average Stuart-era man's nightmares—for example, scenarios involving impotence and inability to satiate a woman's sexual desires.[4] After all, during this period it was assumed that 'Women are more prone than Men to amorous desires'.[5] Indeed, this idea was so thoroughly entrenched that women who enjoyed sex and had strong sexual desires would often feel embarrassed or even guilty. Such was the case with young widow Mary Capel Somerset (1630–1715), who battled with her highly-sexed nature and her wish to remain virtuous.[6]

The School of Venus, or The Ladies Delight, originally published in France in 1655 as *L'Escholes des filles*, was translated into English and published in 1680. It comprises dialogues between an innocent and sheltered young woman, Katy, and her much more sexually experienced cousin, Frances. The latter explains the ins-and-outs of lovemaking and, when she discovers that a young gentleman named Roger is madly in love with Katy but has been effectively 'cock-blocked' (in modern parlance) by her mother, Frances advises Katy to give Roger her virginity, or maidenhead, and use him as her 'Fucking Friend'.[7] Given the opportunity, due to Frances's scheming, Roger and Katy proceed to have sex, and the subsequent dialogue reveals the various sexual positions and the frequency with which the lusty young couple engage in vigorous bed-sport.

On 13 January 1667/68, Samuel Pepys stated that he bought a new book in French, which he hoped his wife would translate for him, until he realised it was 'the most bawdy, lewd book that ever I saw, rather worse than *Putana errante* so that I was ashamed of reading in it'.[8] Nearly a month later in his diary entry of Sunday 9 February, Pepys wrote: 'Up, and at my chamber all the morning and the office doing business, and also reading a little of *L'escholle des filles* which is a mighty lewd book, but yet not amiss for a sober man once to read over to inform himself in the villainy of the world'.[9] After reading this book (during which time he had an erection, culminating in masturbation and ejaculation),[10] Pepys decided he had had his fill of its 'information' and proceeded to burn it rather than have it become a shameful addition to his book collection.

The other work Pepys referred to, *La Puttana Errante*,[11] was an earlier Italian publication of two parts: a poem, and a dialogue between two women, Maddalena and Giulia. The latter part lists and describes thirty-six sexual positions, which are wonderfully and amusingly named, including: 'The Frog', 'Lodging his Host', 'Running the Ring', 'Fucking, German-style', 'Ride his Donkey', 'Kiss a Doggy', and 'The Saint in Ecstasy'.[12] *La Puttana Errante* was reworked and translated into English and published as a periodical by John Garfield in London in 1660 as *The Wandering Whore*. In this version, the two women are named Magdalena and Julietta. At the end of each part there appeared a list of prostitutes currently working in London[13]—presumably for the convenience of readers who found their passions aroused. Among the bawds listed are Damaris Page and Priss Fotheringham—two of the most notorious in Stuart Britain.[14]

The Dialogues of Luisa Sigea, written by Nicolas Chorier in 1660, is a sexually explicit dialogue between two women, Ottavia and Tullia. Their conversations cover wide-ranging sexual topics, such as loss of virginity, fingering, male ejaculation, lesbian sex, vaginal odour, and more.

Scientific and anatomical reference books were also sometimes considered risqué. For example, *Aristotle's Master-Piece*, published in 1684, caused a stir among Stuart-era folks. Whilst not a particularly sexy read, especially when compared with *The School of Venus*, it nonetheless titillated readers with its frank descriptions of male and female sexual reproductive organs (it was not written by Aristotle).

In the same vein as *Aristotle's Master-Piece* was an earlier publication, *The Secret Miracle of Nature* (1658). Later, the *Complete Midwife's Practice Enlarg'd* (1680), was much more scientific with its images and information, but it still might well have titillated readers. *Bartholinus Anatomy*, published in 1665, boasted having 'one hundred and three figures'—some of these were full-frontal drawings of naked men, and some were of penises.[15] Another popular work of literature was a 1658 publication of an English translation of an Italian work by Giovanni Benedetto Sinibaldi entitled, *Rare Verities: The Cabinet of Venus Unlocked, and Her Secrets Laid Open.* Whilst this work did not contain sexual images, it nevertheless discussed topics relating to sex and procreation.

Aristotle's Master-Piece was often sold next to well-liked pornographic works such *Aretino's Postures* and *Satyrica Sotodica*.[16] The *Postures* were written by Italian Pietro Aretino (1492–1556), who created pornographic literature that was still popular with those who read that genre during the Stuart period. Other erotic works included *Erotopolis* (1684) and *The Cabinet of Love* (1714).

In the 1680s, a French work called *l'Académie des Dames* was published, and written by Nicolas Chorier (although misattributed to Aretino). At the back of this voluminous erotic work are several sexually-explicit engravings of orgies, outdoor sex, woman-on-top sex, a nun 'frigging' another woman, a man ejaculating after a 'hand-job', a woman masturbating herself with a dildo as she watches a couple having sex, and even a man penetrating a woman whilst both are riding a horse!

The year 1650 saw the (brief) publication of a book called *The English Rogue: Being a Complete History of the Most Eminent Cheats of Both Sexes*. The author, Richard Head, was an Irish-born writer whose minister father had been killed in the Irish Uprising of 1641.[17] This bawdy novel was considered so graphic that it was banned in the year of its publication, and is even now rather difficult to obtain.

Another title, *Moll Flanders*, by Daniel Defoe (1660–1731), is one of the most popular books that was published during the early eighteenth century, but Defoe himself lived most of his life during the Stuart era and Moll Flanders itself was set during the late seventeenth century and even finishes with the line, 'Written in the year 1683'. The novel is about a young woman who finds herself embroiled in prostitution, adultery, theft, and incest. Defoe's other book about a 'kept woman', *Roxana: The Fortunate Mistress* was published in 1724 yet was also set during 'the time of King Charles II'.[18] The protagonist of this story has a series of rich lovers and some misadventures, but the story has a relatively happy ending.

Sexy poetry

John Donne's *The Flea*—arguably his most famous poem—exudes a subtle, but nevertheless potent, sensuality:

> Mark but this flea, and mark in this,
> How little that which thou deniest me is;
> It sucked me first, and now sucks thee,
> And in this flea our two bloods mingled be;
> Thou know'st that this cannot be said
> A sin, nor shame, nor loss of maidenhead,
> Yet this enjoys before it woo,
> And pampered swells with one blood made of two,
> And this, alas, is more than we would do.

Sir John Suckling (1609–c.1641) was an English courtier who sided with the King during the English Civil Wars. Although he was a man of many abilities, which included developing the game of cribbage, Suckling is best known for his erotic poem about the Stuart-era femme fatale, Lucy Hay, Countess of Carlisle, *Upon My Lady Carlisle Walking in Hampton Court Garden* in which he wrote of his undressing her with his eyes. Suckling's romantic works are excellent examples of sensual, less overtly erotic poetry of the seventeenth century. His *Love's Representation* is quite an intimate view of two (presumably illicit) lovers, post-tryst:

> Leaning her head upon my breast
> There on Love's bed she lay to rest;
> My panting heart rock'd her asleep,
> My heedful eyes the watch did keep.[19]

After some inward reflections, he continues:

> Love granting unto my request,
> Began to labour in my breast;
> But with this motion he did make,
> It heav'd so high that she did wake.
> Blush'd at the favour she had done,
> Then smil'd and then away did run.[20]

In a similar vein, Robert Herrick's *The Vision to Electra*, part of his *Hesperides* (1648), is a romantic and very sensual poem about (presumably, his) erotic dreams about a woman:

> I dream'd we both were in a bed
> Of roses, almost smothered:
> The warmth and sweetness had me there
> Made lovingly familiar;
> But that I heard thy sweet breath say,
> Faults done by night will blush by day;
> I kissed thee, panting, and I call
> Night to the record! That was all.
> But, ah! If empty dreams so please,
> Love, give me more such nights as these.[21]

Shrewd Stuart-era publishers sometimes gave their publications a saucy title in the hope of luring people into buying works that actually had quite innocent and romantic content.[22] Such was the case with *The Amorous Abbess, Or, Love in a Nunnery* (1684), which sounds as though it will be a Marquis de Sade-like journey into a convent full of naughty nuns and horny abbesses, but actually turns out to be a rather sentimental epistolary novel about a young man torn between two sisters.[23]

Discomfort with nudity

The Stuart period saw an enormous number of nudes portrayed in paintings and sculptures, but not everyone was comfortable with so much flesh on display, even if it was in art. Samuel de Sorbière, a Frenchman, recorded his observations when he visited London in 1698. One incident involved him escorting a (presumably English) lady to Hyde Park Corner, whereupon they came across several naked statues. The lady expressed her offense at these nudes, which prompted a conversation. Sorbière asked, 'Why should Nature be so offensive since a very great part of the World yet defies clothes, and ever did so; and the parts they do most affect to cover, are from a certain necessity only'.[24] She didn't have much of a reply to that.

A similar discomfort regarding nudity manifested itself in the 1640s, when, according to historian E.J. Burford, some nude statues were either destroyed entirely or had their exposed genitalia covered up with decorative features such as fig leaves and clothing—this is not unlike efforts made by similarly puritanical persons during the later Victorian period.[25]

In the Late Stuart era, Ned Ward opined 'I think it a Shameful Indecency for a Woman to expose her Naked Body to the sight of Men and Boys' because it would arouse the 'beastly appetites of Lecherous Persons'.[26]

Pornographic imagery

Agostino Carracci (1557–1602) was an Italian Late Renaissance/Early Baroque artist perhaps best known for his Biblical paintings, *The Penitent Magdalene* and *The Last Communion of St. Jerome*. He also engraved sexually-explicit depictions of popular mythological couples in the heat of copulation, including Oenone and Paris of Troy, Mars and Venus, Achilles and Briseis, and Juno and Jupiter. These engravings vividly depict the penis entering the vagina, in a manner not-too-dissimilar to modern pornography.[27] At least one of Carracci's works (though they were not erotic engravings) was purchased by King Charles I, sold during the Interregnum, then reacquired during the reign of his son, King Charles II.[28]

Sensual Stuart-age erotica

Some less overtly sexual images still retained a powerful sensuality. Dutch painters are notable for their large oeuvre dedicated to depictions of everyday life—one such is a charming drawing by Gersina Ter Borch, from 1653, showing a young blond couple blushing—post-tryst, perhaps?

Rembrandt's *The Jewish Bride* also shows a couple; his hand tenderly brushing against her breast.[29] This painting was once believed to depict a father and daughter, but the body language between the two subjects is more likely to be that of two lovers. Rembrandt also etched *The French Bed* in 1646, in which he depicted himself mounted atop a smiling woman as they engaged in lovemaking. The woman, it later transpired, was his beloved wife, Saskia—a fact which caused some scandal when it was discovered, since she came from a respectable family.[30]

In the 1670s, King Charles II commissioned the Italian Baroque painter Benedetto Gennari to paint a series of erotic paintings for his private viewing pleasure.[31] Indeed, Charles's mistress of sixteen years, Nell Gwynn, posed for a few titillating portraits—one, by an anonymous artist, depicts the cheeky actress handling sausages in a suggestive manner, while another, by Peter Lely, depicts her as the goddess Venus.

Artist Marcellus Laroon II's late-seventeenth-century etching of a prostitute is memorable in that it depicts a young woman who regards the viewer with a knowing look as she sits in front of two men with her leg propped up on the table, clearly showing them her naked genitalia.[32] One man peers between her legs and adopts a fascinated expression, whilst the man behind him has a lascivious smile upon his lips. Is she perhaps a prostitute masturbating in front of two clients?

Saucy Stuart stage-plays

Sir John Vanbrugh (1664–1726) is best-known for his architectural masterpieces, Blenheim Palace in Oxfordshire and Castle Howard in Yorkshire (both of which he designed with Nicholas Hawksmoor). But Vanbrugh was, like so many gentlemen of his time, multi-talented. He was in fact primarily known as a playwright during his lifetime, and two of his plays are noted for their sauciness. *The Relapse* (1696) contained a great deal of sexual content, whilst *The Provok'd Wife* (1697) had adultery as one of its main themes.

Perhaps the most explicit play of the time, however, is *The Farce of Sodom*, which, although published anonymously in 1684, is sometimes attributed to John Wilmot. According to Suffolk Archives, *Sodom* is 'the first literary work ever to be censored in England for obscenity'.[33]

A striking aspect of Restoration-era plays (and, indeed, many Stuart-era plays in general), is how often rape or sexual violence is used as a plot device.[34] Even in the Late Elizabethan and Early Stuart periods, William Shakespeare wrote *The Rape of Lucrece*, the character Lavinia in *Titus Andronicus* is horrifically raped and mutilated, and some of his male characters are would-be rapists or actual rapists, including Cloten in *Cymbeline*, Caliban in *The Tempest*, and Proteus in *The Two Gentlemen of Verona*.[35]

The Restoration comedy, *Love for Love* (1695), by William Congreve elicited this from Jeremy Collier in 1698: '*Scandal* solicits Mrs. *Foresight*; She threatens to tell her Husband. He replies, *He will die a Martyr rather than disclaim his Passion.* Here we have Adultery dignified with the stile of Martyrdom: As if 'twas as Honourable to perish in Defence of Whoring, as to dye for the Faith of Christianity.'[36]

Furthermore, William Wycherley (1641–1715) raised more than a few eyebrows with his plays, among which were *The Country Wife* (1675) and *The Plain Dealer* (1676). *The Country Wife* shocked Stuart audiences due to its sexual content: in this story, a rake named Horner concocts a plan to spread false rumours that he is 'as bad as a eunuch'[37] so that husbands will think it safe to leave their wives alone with him—and so that he can then bed as many of them as he wishes: 'Now may I have, by the Reputation of an Eunuch, the Privileges of one, and be seen in a Lady's Chamber in a Morning as early as her Husband, kiss Virgins before their Parents, or Lovers'.[38] Things don't quite work out as the protagonist intends, however, and Wycherley's brilliant use of double entendres throughout this play just oozes Stuart sexiness!

Scandalous Stuart pamphlets

There is much similarity between the scandal-mongering pamphlets of the Stuart period and the tabloid culture of our own time. The celebrities may be different, but sexual relationships still feature highly! Also, then, just as now, those who were mentioned were usually not happy having their dirty laundry displayed before the world.

In 1709, a salacious work entitled *Secret Memoirs and Manners of Several Persons of Quality* was published in London. Although given fake names, the thinly-veiled Duke and Duchess of Marlborough are mentioned several times,[39] along with references to Churchill's past sexual relationship with Barbara Palmer (née Villiers).[40] Speaking of whom, *The Night-Walker: Or, Evening Rambles in search after Lewd Women* (1696), is dedicated to Barbara and the anonymous author poured scorn on her having 'defiled the marriage bed'[41] when she engaged in adultery with King Charles II.

Chapter 4

Prostitution: Or, Whoredom in Stuart Britain

But whatere it cost me, Ile have a fine Whore,
As Bold as Alice Pierce, as Fine as Jane Shore,[1]
And when I am weary of her, Ile have more.[2]
- 'A Prophetick Lampoon', George Villiers,
2nd Duke of Buckingham

Prostitution

Often referred to as 'the oldest profession in the world', the history of providing sexual services in exchange for monetary, or other, remuneration goes back at least to the beginning of documented history. In Stuart Britain, when a woman 'played the whore', she was said to *meretricate*,[3] and some of the words used for prostitutes included, 'harlot', and 'punk'.[4]

Prostitutes were widely looked-down-upon and it is not difficult to find derisive language about them in the literature—particularly religious works—of the time. The prevalent opinion was that a prostitute was a 'degenerate woman, unwomaned, of both modesty and chastity'.[5] The Biblical Whore of Babylon is a symbolic woman whom Stuart religious works often mentioned. In Revelation 17.16 of the Bible: 'they [the ten kings] hate the whore, who did seduce and bewitch them; They...burn her with fire'.[6]

A 'strumpet', according to Thomas Dekker in 1620, is a 'cockatrice that hatcheth...egges of evils'.[7] It's little wonder, then, that prostitutes were seen by many as almost subhuman and fully deserving of scorn, and even violence. An anonymous author of a Stuart-era song suggests that people 'brand them like Cain, let Whores wear whorish marks... whores [shall] have neither Coin, nor Food, nor Rest'.[8]

Nonetheless, prostitutes were sometimes seen as creatures worthy of one's pity and compassion, for they had fallen from innocence into sin, for 'without any exception, all lewd Women, have for some yeares bin [sic] pure Virgins'[9] or so opined Daniel Brevint in his 1672 work, *The Depth and Mystery of the Roman Mass*. Of course, some women didn't want to go into prostitution at all, but were forced into it by their father or husband who pimped them out.[10] These women were thought to be more worthy of compassion than those who had willingly become prostitutes.

Despite all these negative opinions and the cultural zeitgeist being one of moral castigation, prostitution was rife during the period. Men who comprised the clientele of prostitutes were known as 'whoremongers', 'palliards', and 'pandars'.[11]

The ballad *The Two-Penny Whore* (c. 1666–1679) includes a dialogue between a spendthrift man who is down to his last two pence and a prostitute whose services he previously used when he had more money.[12] She replies that half a crown is her pay and she will not be a 'two-penny whore'. This suggests that among those in her trade, there was a sort of hierarchy, and this particular prostitute found it beneath her dignity to be paid so little for her services. The song ends with a moralistic warning: 'The best way I know of, for you to prevent it (poverty), is to keep your goods out of the hands of a Whore'.[13] This advice goes hand-in-hand with the words of John Milton, who, in his great Stuart-era epic poem, *Paradise Lost*, wrote, '…the bought smile of Harlots, loveless, joyless, unendear'd, casual fruition…'.[14] Even the notorious Stuart-era libertine John Wilmot, 2nd Earl of Rochester, complained—after sex with his whore—that 'she bereaves me of [both] money and cunt'.[15]

The Life of Epicurus, published near the end of the Stuart period in 1712, may have been a work about the ancient Greek philosopher, but the moralising tone against prostitution was directed at a Stuart-era reading audience:

> 'Now although he [Epicurus] allow'd his Wiseman to Marry upon certain Considerations, yet he always was against the illegal use of Women. There was nothing he had more in Abomination, than those common Prostitutes, who may be properly styl'd, The Sinks of Luxury and Lasciviousness, and who may be said to be carried away with the Torrent of their Passion'.[16]

Other uses for 'whores'

The word 'whore' was not just a term used for those who made money from the selling of sexual favours—it was also frequently used as a derogatory term: 'she is a very noted whore and sells tobacco, and run at two seafaring men, first with a spit and afterwards with a drawn rapier'.[17] 'The Queen is a whore…and she left a bastard at Newark-upon-Trent!' shouted one Thomas Beres in 1647, referring to King Charles I's wife, Henrietta Maria, in the presence of many witnesses.[18] For calling her a whore, and for which he was found guilty, Beres was fined one hundred marks and sentenced to be imprisoned for some time.[19]

Even intangible concepts such as glory were made feminine and then labelled as whores—for example: 'Thus glories fortune in inconstancy; For her I care not, she's a fickle whore'.[20] In one publication from 1641, the failure of the Gunpowder Plot of 1605 was likened to 'Rome brought to England with the whores miscarrying'.[21]

In the anti-Catholic-missionary treatise, *The Missionarie's Arts Discovered* from 1688, Catholics are seen as being on the same level as prostitutes—i.e. very low down: 'What Barbarities have they [the Catholics] not committed?...In whose mouth is Whore and Bitch more frequent, than her that is a common Prostitute?'.[22]

Astrologers warned that 'if a trades man set up while Saturn is Lord thereof, he will be sure to swallow a spider, especially if he be given to whoring, drinking, and gaming, as too many of them be'.[23] Not an attractive thought, particularly for lecherous tradesmen who happened to be arachnophobic, too!

Prostitution in the arts

Prostitution was depicted in many artworks of this period. In Hendrick Goltzius's 1615 painting entitled *Unequal Lovers*, a couple is portrayed on the verge of kissing. The leering man clearly has some form of disease—his nose looks particularly unhealthy—and he's some thirty years her senior. She gives him a cold smile while accepting the bag of money he is proffering. It seems likely, therefore, that this painting illustrates a wealthy elderly man visiting a nubile young whore.

Even music—that wonderful entertainment so beloved of mankind throughout the world—was considered, by some, to be the domain of prostitutes: 'And, indeed, it [music], softens the mind; the curiosity of it, is fitter for women than men, and for courtesans than women'.[24] Note how the author, Owen Felltham, makes a clear distinction between women and courtesans.

Male brothels

Although most prostitutes were female, there were male prostitutes as well. These seem to have been more lowly regarded even than were their female counterparts, as they were associated with all things sodomitical.[25] Male brothels, or *spintries*, existed in the Early Modern period—there was a popular one in Hoxton during Elizabeth I's reign.[26] Molly houses probably began to develop late in the Stuart period, but really came into being during subsequent historical periods, being mostly associated with that of the eighteenth century.

Houses of ill repute

This excerpt from the *Middlesex Sessions Rolls*, dated 11 January 1627 clearly demonstrates that whorehouses had a very poor reputation:

> '[Brothels and] diverse other places within this county are pestered with many immodest, lascivious and shameless women generally reputed for notorious common and professed whores, who are entertained into victualing or other houses suspected for bawdry houses and other base tenements for base and filthy lucre and gain to the landlords and tenants'.[27]

From Thomas Dekker's *The infection of the* Suburbs (1620): 'He saw the doors of notorious Carted Bawdes (like Hell gates) stand night and day wide open, with a pair of Harlots in Taffata gownes'[28]—the sight of which was more conducive to entering the establishment than any old sign. Men or women who ran brothels or bawdy-houses were known as 'bawds', and in *An Act for Suppressing the Detestable Sins of Incest, Adultery, & Fornication* (1650), anyone fitting this description was regarded as guilty of a secondary offense felony. The punishment for this was for the bawd to be whipped in public and then placed in the pillory, where they would then have the letter 'B' (for 'bawd') branded into their forehead with a hot iron. There was more to come: the bawd would then be sent to prison for three years without bail. If, upon release, they re-offended, they would then be executed.[29]

One of the most successful prostitutes and brothel keepers was Damaris Page (1610–1669).[30] So well-known was she, that Page was even mentioned by Samuel Pepys in his *Diary*. In *The Life and Death of Damaris Page, That Great, Arch, Metropolitan (Old-Woman) of Ratcliff High-Way,* published by R. Burton, London, 1669:

> 'Death on her house of Clay at last did seize,
> And sack't the same worse then the 'Prenctices;
> There many a Seaman hath sat with his Doxy
> And spent his Coyn till he grew Foxy, Poxy'.[31]

One of Page's contemporaries and fellow Madams was Elizabeth Cresswell. Referred to (in the nineteenth century) as 'a celebrated English procuress, during the reign of Charles II',[32] it is likely that Cresswell began her career as a prostitute in the 1650s before working her way up to the status of bawd.

In the Bawdy House Riots of 1668, female prostitutes and their brothels were subjected to attacks from mainly young men, who proceeded to vandalise and destroy these properties.[33] *The Poor Whore's Petition*, published in March of 1668, was a petition addressed to Barbara Palmer, Lady Castlemaine on behalf of her poorer sister prostitutes[34]—and was one of the direct consequences of the Bawdy House Riots. Needless to say, this did not go down well with the king's tempestuous mistress! As Pepys observed, 'My Lady Castlemaine is horribly vexed at the late libel, the petition of the poor prostitutes about the town whose houses were pulled down the other day'.[35] Both the aforementioned Damaris Page and Elizabeth Cresswell were listed as signatories at the bottom of the *Poor Whores' Petition*.

In 1638, a James Wall provided information to authorities about the existence of an Irish brothel located in Drury Lane, London.[36] This is unsurprising; the Covent Garden area was a magnet for prostitution, coffee shops, and taverns—so much so that by the eighteenth century, it was considered notorious.[37]

Elizabeth Holland, another famous London bawd, ran an upscale brothel in the heavily Dutch-populated Paris Garden, Bankside, called 'Holland's Leaguer' or 'Hollands laager' for three decades, beginning in 1603.[38] Her establishment became very popular, and King James I himself, along with many of his courtiers, is reputed to have been among the clientele.[39]

Another infamous bawd and prostitute, Priss Fotheringham (c.1615–1668) was listed in Garfield's *The Wandering Whore* as 'Priss Fotheringham at the Chuck Office'.[40] This was a reference to Fotheringham's popular lewd trick of standing on her head, her legs spread to show off her genitals, at which point her spectators would literally chuck coins at her, which she would catch with her vulva.

Women who were indicted for keeping a brothel usually faced a large fine and had to provide sureties for good behaviour. This was the case with Elizabeth Elye in 1693, who kept a 'House of evil Repute' in Fetter Lane [41]—she received a fine of 20*l* and was imprisoned until she paid it.[42]

Some prostitutes faced a prison sentence—though not exactly for prostitution, as was the case with Sarah Pridden (born c. 1690). Pridden was a famous prostitute who began her career during the Late Stuart period, and ended it during the early Georgian period incarcerated in Newgate Prison after she non-fatally stabbed one of her lovers.

During the reign of Queen Anne (1702–1714), the Society for the Reformation of Manners, which had been founded during the reign of William and Mary in 1691, was given the clear instruction 'to have stews rooted out, and the streets cleansed from lewd and impudent women, and detestable sodomites that infest them'.[43]

Camp followers and sexual violence during wartime

The English Civil Wars, also known as the British Civil Wars or the Wars of the Three Kingdoms, were an incredibly bloody time during the Stuart period. Families and towns were divided between Parliamentarian and Royalist, and it is believed that between 180,000[44] and 800,000[45] people died as a direct and indirect result of the warfare. Non-combatants, including women, were often a target for the enemy on both sides.

Camp followers were women who followed armies as they marched from one battle to the next. These women—most of whom were either married to, or somehow related to, the soldiers they were following—would cook and wash clothes, along with performing other useful and necessary tasks. Sometimes camp followers included prostitutes.[46] Perhaps the most devastating and notorious example of foul behaviour against women camp followers was following the Battle of Naseby in June of 1645, when hundreds of women were viciously attacked by Parliamentarian troops: their faces were deliberately mutilated and disfigured, and many of the women were murdered.[47] The victims, who were probably Welsh, were mistaken for Irish—for whom there was a vehement antipathy in England. This kind of extreme violence was also perpetrated against women camp-followers in Methven in the same year.[48] Although we lack conclusive evidence, it's likely that some of these women were sexually assaulted as well.

Sexual violence in political propaganda

Propaganda was rife during the Stuart period, especially at times of heightened political upheaval—such as during the civil wars. One of the most upsetting aspects of some publications of this time was the depiction of sexual violence in order to agitate people against an enemy. For example, following the Irish Uprising of 1641, numerous pamphlets and engravings were made of the most horrific things imaginable. One shows a man, a 'Papist', knife in hand, kneeling over the corpse of a woman, her belly ripped open, viscera clearly on show. The woman had been pregnant, and she was raped by the same men who had murdered her husband, then her baby was cut out from within her. This horrific image shows the babe then being tossed into a fire in the background. Sexual violence is such a powerful propaganda tool because it is the stuff of nightmares.

Chapter 5

Stuart Players & Femmes Fatales

Some of the earliest actresses in Britain began performing during the Stuart period, and this was extremely controversial—for playacting, and indeed many other aspects of theatre, were deemed by some to be immoral. William Prynne urged his readers to follow the example of the early Christians, who 'concluding their meetings with a psalm and a prayer; and then departing, not to a Tavern, a Whorehouse, or a Playhouse, as some of us do: but to their own houses with Temperance and Sobriety'.[1]

During the Interregnum, plays were banned—but not everyone did as they were told. Up in Oxford, England, the antiquarian Anthony Wood stated, 'They would not suffer any common players to come into the University, nor scholars to act in private but what they did by stealth'.[2]

'Compleat Female Stage Beauty'

Before women were legally allowed to tread the boards, young men were often hired for female roles, such as Ned Kynaston, who 'being then very Young made a Compleat Female Stage Beauty, performing his Parts so well, especially Arthiope and Aglaura'.[3] But men playing women didn't go down well with some: 'What higher strain of invirility can any Christian name, then for a man to put on a woman's raiment, gesture, countenance, and behaviour, to act a Whore's, a Bawd's, or some other lewd, lascivious female's part? If this be not effeminacy in the superlative degree, I know not yet what effeminacy means'.[4]

Stuart masques & plays

Stuart-era masques were hugely extravagant, popular, and expensive court entertainments which involved elaborate costumes and set design, combined with dialogue, music, and dance. Although they were performed for the Late Stuart monarchs, they are most associated with the reigns of King James VI & I and his successor, King Charles I. The most famous masques of this period were written by Ben Jonson with set and costume design by Inigo Jones. William Shakespeare incorporated a masque into his play *The Tempest*, which was performed before newlyweds Elizabeth Stuart and Frederick V of the Palatinate in 1613.[5]

These entertainments were not only a feast for the senses; they were also of symbolic and political importance. Masques were written and performed in honour of major royal and aristocratic weddings, such as that of the aforementioned Elizabeth Stuart and Frederick V, and Frances Howard and Robert Carr—both of which took place in 1613.[6] Upon the subject of Frances Howard, she performed in at least two masques: Ben Jonson's *The Masque of Queens* in 1609, and in Samuel Daniel's *Tethys Festival* in 1610, the latter part of the celebrations for Henry Stuart's investiture as the Prince of Wales.[7]

Masques were such an integral feature of Jacobean court culture that the Native American, Matoaka (Pocahontas), and her fellow Powhatan advisor Uttamatomakkin attended Ben Jonson's *The Vision of Delight* at St. James's Palace in the winter of 1617.[8]

Royals, of both sexes, took part in these extravaganzas—to the displeasure of some subjects—but, while the women were allowed to dance and wear costumes, they weren't supposed to have any speaking parts, for this simply wouldn't have been acceptable for a respectable lady.[9] The attractive Lady Anne Clifford (1590–1676), an English peeress now famed for her letter-writing and her diary, took part in many Jacobean masques. Clifford is believed to have been painted in 1610 wearing one of the costumes designed by Inigo Jones for *The Masque of Queens* in 1609.[10] She had previously had a role in Ben Jonson's 1608 masque, *The Masque of Beauty*.

During the subsequent Caroline era, Queen Henrietta Maria took part in masques—including *The Shepherd's Paradise* of 1632, in which she had a substantial role. One writer in particular, William Prynne, made known his dislike of acting and of the whole scene associated with plays. In his notorious *Histrio-Mastix, Or, The Players Scourge* (1633), he railed against play-houses, and those who frequented play-houses and acted in plays. According to Prynne, such establishments were cesspits of vice and moral uncleanliness, and he entreated readers, to 'join hands, join hearts, and judgements with me in censuring, in condemning stage-plays, because they contaminate and defile both their actors, their spectators' souls and bodies; because they thus instigate, nourish, and enflame their inseparable full fleshy lusts which war against their souls, which should be mortified and subdued, not fostered, not fomented, as they are'.[11] Lucy Hutchinson was also not a fan, taking particular umbrage against the Jacobean court: 'To keep the people in their deplorable security, till vengeance overtook them, they were entertained with masks, stage plays, and various sorts of ruder sports'.[12] Another critic was James Collier, who, in his *A Short View of the Immorality, and Profaneness of the English Stage* (1698), stated 'nothing has gone farther in Debauching the Age than the Stage Poets, and Play-House'.[13]

Plays were nevertheless very popular, and many people ignored and rebelled against such criticisms. Anthony Wood, for example, listed the various plays that were performed in Oxford in 1661, and there, 'the players at Oxon at the King's Armes, acted on the stage in the yard: first, to spite the Presbyterians'.[14]

The first actresses

Although some high-born women had—scandalously—taken part in masques at the Jacobean and Caroline courts, it was in 1661—following the Restoration—that King Charles II made it legal for women to act upon the stage.[15] Such women were an incredible novelty, and the phenomenon was even titillating for some men. Anthony Wood wrote, 'these plays wherein women acted, made the scholars mad, run after them'.[16]

The most beautiful and famous actresses tended to attract very wealthy and powerful men. Margaret 'Peg' Hughes, one of the first women—if not *the* first woman—to act professionally, performed the role of Desdemona in William Shakespeare's *Othello* in 1664.[17] Hughes had several lovers, including Sir Charles Sedley and Prince Rupert of the Rhine, the latter fathering their illegitimate daughter, Ruperta, in 1673.

Elizabeth Barry, another Restoration actress, was acclaimed for her portrayals of Shakespeare's tragic heroines. She became John Wilmot, 2nd Earl of Rochester's mistress, and it is popularly said that she owed her successful stage career to him. According to Graham Greene, Rochester's 1974 biographer, this is due to his accepting a wager to see if she would become a popular actress within six months; he then took her under his wing and privately tutored her to master her voice and acting.[18]

Barry later returned the favour when she was ordered by King Charles II to tutor a very shy Princess Anne to speak well—a characteristic the princess demonstrated when she became Queen Anne (although she never really got over her shyness in public).[19] In terms of her appearance, Barry was not considered beautiful; her appeal rather came in the form of her remarkable facial expressiveness and her moving voice.[20] Her vocal quality was again commented upon by her contemporary, the actor and prompter John Downes, who said that her Monimia in *The Orphan* and Isabella in *The Fatal Marriage*, 'forced tears from the eyes of her auditory, especially those who have any sense of pity for the distressed'.[21]

The most famous of all Stuart-era actresses is undoubtedly Nell Gwynn. There is something remarkable about an impoverished orange seller who rose to become a celebrated comedic actress and a favourite mistress of a king. More about her later!

Another woman who rose from a poor background to become a successful actress was Anne Oldfield (1683–1730). For over a year she played secondary characters with few lines, but was suddenly thrust into the spotlight when the main actress of the company, Mrs Cross, up and left to go to France with her lover.[22] Among Oldfield's lovers was the English author and Whig politician, Arthur Maynwaring.[23] In *The Life and Posthumous Works of Arthur Maynwaring, Esq.* (1715), this love affair was expanded upon: 'the Famous and Excellent Actor, Mrs. Oldfield, whom Mr. Maynwaring lov'd for about eight or nine Years before his Death, and with a Passion, that could hardly have been stronger, had it been both her and his first Love'.[24]

Anne Bracegirdle (c.1663–1748) delighted audiences, particularly with her performance as Belinda in Vanbrugh's provocative 1697 play, *The Provok'd Wife*.[25] Sometimes, two major actresses were in the same production: Bracegirdle and Barry, for example, performed together in fifty-six different plays.[26]

Playwrights and political women

Some women did not remain within the expected sphere of activities for their sex. A number of female writers emerged during the Stuart period—these were outliers rather than the norm for their time. Aemelia Lanier, an English-born poetess of Venetian Jewish heritage, who published *Salve Deus Rex Judaeorum* (1611), is recognised as the first Englishwoman to have published original poems and written professionally.[27] Aphra Behn, another English writer, is generally accepted to be the first woman to have made a living by her pen, writing several plays including *Abdelazar: Or, The Moor's Revenge*, and *Oroonoko*.

Whilst Aphra Behn's works have seen a renaissance in recent years, very few people seem to know of her contemporary and fellow successful female playwright, Susanna Centlivre (aka Susanna Carroll). Two other women who were also playwrights during the late 1660s and early 1670s were Frances Boothby and Elizabeth Polwhele.[28]

Margaret Cavendish, Duchess of Newcastle, was at the time referred to derisively as 'Mad Madge' by Samuel Pepys, but she authored several works—some of which became popular once again in the 2010s: *The Blazing World*, *Covent of Pleasure*, *The Bridalls*, and *The Sociable Companions*. As Stuart-era biographer William Winstanley wrote, 'Now was his (the Duke of Cavendish) Duchess no less buried in those ravishing Delights of Poetry, leaving to Posterity in Print three ample Volumes of Her studious Endeavours; one of Orations, the second of Philosophical Notions and Discourses, and the third of Dramatick and other kinds of Poetry'.[29]

Celia Fiennes (b. 1662) was one of the first women to become a kind of travel expert, as she wrote her observations of the places she had visited around the country.[30]

Nadine Akkerman of Leiden University has done exceptional work uncovering the histories of female spies, or *she-intelligencers*, in seventeenth-century Britain. Both men and women were involved in espionage during the Stuart period. Those who were caught could be tortured for information, regardless of their sex, and men would be executed by hanging, while women, if accused of witchcraft, would be drowned—but most she-intelligencers were released after a short period.[31] Elizabeth Murray, the supremely intelligent, intellectual, and gorgeous Countess of Dysart, was another Stuart-era female spy, whose name is often associated with The Sealed Knot—a secret royalist organisation—though she worked with another such group, the Great Trust.[32] Susan Hyde, sister of the well-known author of *The History of the Rebellion* and a once-powerful advisor to King Charles II, Edward Hyde, Lord Clarendon, was yet another she-intelligencer—one whose work in espionage on behalf of the royalists was not even mentioned in her brother's *History*, despite the fact that she held the position of Postmistress in the Sealed Knot and is believed to have died in custody.[33]

Stuart femmes fatales

Frances Howard was considered to be one of the great beauties of the Jacobean court. Prince Henry was even rumoured to have been a potential suitor at one point. Aged fifteen, she was married in 1606 to Robert, 3rd Earl of Essex, who was eight months her junior. This was a prestigious match between two powerful families—but any love between the two was lamentably one-sided, coming only from Robert, who was a grandson of Lettice Knollys, Countess of Leinster.[34] The match proved unhappy, and Frances began to look elsewhere for love and, possibly, sexual satisfaction—for in 1613, annulment proceedings took place on the grounds that Robert was impotent.[35]

Lucy Hay, Countess of Carlisle, was a major—and fascinating— Stuart *intrigante*. Born in 1599, Lucy was married to James Hay, the 1st Earl of Carlisle, in a wedding ceremony that was attended by King James VI & I, Prince Charles, and the great favourite, George Villiers, the future 1st Duke of Buckingham. Marriage didn't stop her from enjoying herself with other men, though it's hard to say with certainty whether these affairs were of the sexual variety.

Beautiful and clever, the Countess of Carlisle had several high-profile, very different, intimate friends (possibly lovers)—all of whom were very powerful—including George Villiers, Duke of Buckingham,[36] Thomas Wentworth, 1st Earl of Strafford, and John Pym. She was even the muse behind Sir John Suckling's dialogue poem *Upon My Lady Carlisle's Walking in Hampton Court Garden*. She became a Lady of the Bedchamber to Henrietta Maria, and, despite the queen's initial dislike of her, the two became very close. The teenaged queen looked up to the worldly-wise, sophisticated Lucy—who was ten years her elder and who, in due course, taught the young queen how to apply makeup.

When King Charles I attempted to arrest the 'Five Members' of Parliament (John Pym, John Hampden, Denzil Holles, Arthur Haselrig and William Strod), in early January 1642, he was taken aback that they were not present, and remarked, 'The birds have flown'. It was a lovely little bird who tweeted them the news: Lucy had both the opportunity to hear private conversations between the royal couple and the inclination to help her friend (and possible lover) Pym. Henrietta Maria blamed herself for having blurted out that 'Pym and his confederates are arrested before now', in Lucy's presence, but Lucy probably eavesdropped on Henrietta Maria's earlier conversation with Charles I in which it was decided he would arrest the MPs. Being the only one with the opportunity to hear private conversations and the inclination to help Pym was enough to make Lucy the culpable party. Why? Lucy was attracted to powerful men. She had been close to Thomas Wentworth, 1st Earl of Strafford, until his downfall, and then gravitated towards Pym.[37] Henrietta Maria could not deny that Lucy was the only one who could have informed Pym of the plan; and Royalists, in general, looked upon Lucy as a betrayer. That said, Lucy was a shrewd player of the political game and she was eventually in communication with King Charles during his imprisonment at Carisbrooke Castle. Her legacy comes through to us in the form of Milady de Winter in *The Three Musketeers*, for Lucy is reputed to have been the muse for Alexandre Dumas's memorable villainess.

Another Stuart-era lady reputed as a 'femme fatale' was the beautiful Elizabeth Seymour, Duchess of Somerset, who was married thrice. Elizabeth (neé Percy) married her first husband, seventeen-year-old Henry Cavendish, Earl of Ogle, at the tender age of twelve—a marriage which was probably never consummated due to her age and his death only a year later.[38] In 1681, she was forced into a second arranged marriage, despite believing herself to be in love with Count Karl von Königsmarck, this time with the extremely wealthy yet dissolute Thomas Thynne of Longleat.[39] In a dramatic course of events, she escaped to Holland to be with her lover, Count Königsmarck, who had Thynne murdered by hiring assassins (Colonel Vrats and others) who shot him five times in the abdomen.[40] This episode proved scandalous and was the talk of the court. John Evelyn remarked, in his entry of 10 March 1682 (the day Thynn's assassin Colonel Vrats and some of his accomplices were executed for murder): 'He went to execution like an undaunted hero, as one that had done a friendly office for that base coward, Count Königsmarck, who had hopes to marry his widow, the rich Lady Ogle, and was acquitted by a corrupt jury, and so got away'.[41] Elizabeth's dalliance with the dashing Königsmarck was at an end, but she went on to marry Charles Seymour, 6th Duke of Somerset in 1682, and the couple had no fewer than thirteen children together.[42] Nonetheless, Seymour never fully lost her reputation of being a femme fatale.

Chapter 6

Virginity & Pre-Marital Sex: Or, Fornication!

'O the daily filthiness that lodgeth in the thoughts and imaginations of some men! They can scarce look on a woman of any comeliness, but they have presently some filthy thought.'[1]

—Richard Baxter. A Treatise of Self-Denial, 1675

Importance of virginity and chastity

'Virginity untouch'd and taintless, is the boast and pride of the fair sex'[2]

- Aristotle's Complete Master-Piece.

Elizabeth I fully appreciated the propaganda potential of her own virginity. Accordingly, she had it symbolised in her portraits—particularly in those that were painted following her cousin Mary Queen of Scots' fall from power in the late 1560s. Mary's reputation, by contrast, was that of a wanton woman. Mary, mother of Jesus, is revered by Christians as the *Virgin* Mary—something that has been a profoundly powerful aspect of her character: for she is clean, unspoiled, holy. Dr John Wallis confronted any doubts about Mary's virginity thusly: 'And when they question the being born of a Virgin, may they not as well question how the first Woman was made of the Rib of Man?'[3]—in other words, he thought it absurd to question anything that had come into being through divine power.

A woman's sexuality—and sexual chastity—was of paramount importance, and violating the person of a high-ranking woman could be considered treason. According to the old Statute of Treasons, 'Violating or Carnally knowing the Queen, King's eldest unmarried daughter, or Prince's wife' was considered treasonous.[4]

If a couple had not engaged in sexual intercourse prior to their wedding night, it was assumed that the woman would bleed when her husband's penis ruptured her hymen membrane, and in doing so, took her virginity and 'deflowered' her. A woman's bleeding during her first sexual experience has been interpreted by many cultures as a sign of her innocence—which was both expected and desired in a wife. Indeed, according to *The Ladies Dictionary* (1694), a woman's virginity was 'the fairest and richest Gage of [a woman's] Love'.[5]

But, of course, every human body is different; and whilst many (if not most) virgins experience some pain and blood loss in their first sexual coupling, not all do. Men whose new wives fell into this latter category were comforted by the advice found in works like *Aristotle's Masterpiece*, which defended such women:[6] 'he has no reason to think her devirginated, if he finds her otherwise sober and modest; seeing the Hymen, or *Claustrum Virginale*, may be broken so many other ways, and yet the woman both chaste and virtuous'.[7] Nevertheless, the author goes on to warn virgins to 'take all imaginable care to keep their Virgin Zones entire'[8]—virginity was, in some respects, akin to a woman's treasure.

The character of Laurentia in *A Woman will have her Will* (1616), states, 'Why was I made a Mayde, but for a Man?'.[9]

Greensickness

'…their Desire of Veneral Embraces becomes very great, and at some critical Junctures almost insuperable'.
—Aristotle's Master-Piece (1684)

Paradoxically, however, some Stuart literature reveals the opposite attitude: that virginity was a waste, and even harmful to a woman's health. In *A Magnificent Entertainment*, published in 1604: 'This jewell of the Land; England's right Eye: Altar of Love; and sphere of Majestie: Greene Neptunes Minion, bou't whose Virgin-waste, Iris is like a Cristall girdle cast'.[10] In William Shakespeare's beloved tragic play Romeo and Juliet (c.1590s), Romeo's famous monologue is full of references to virginity—and how it's not good:

'But soft! What light through yonder window breaks?
It is the East, and Juliet is the sun!
Arise, fair sun, and kill the envious moon,

Who is already sick and pale with grief
That thou her maid art far more fair than she.
Be not her maid, since she is envious.
Her vestal livery is but sick and green,
And none but fools do wear it. Cast it off.'[11]

There was also a prevailing belief that remaining a virgin for too long would lead to 'greensickness' (hence Romeo's line 'sick and green') and the line 'and none but fools do wear it' clearly urges against letting one's sexuality go to waste. We find more in this vein from *Aristotle's Master-Piece*:

> '...the Use of these so much desir'd Enjoyments being deny'd to Virgins (sex), is often followed by very dangerous, and sometimes dismal consequences...or else it brings them to the Green Sicknesses, or other diseases...But when they are married, and those desires satisfied by their husbands, those distempers vanish, and their Beauty returns more gay and lively than before'.[12]

In other words, marriage (and the womb's subsequent intake of sperm) was the recommended cure for greensickness. Another work, *The English Housewife* (1631), prescribed 'white wine and a handful of rosemary, a handful of worm-wood, an ounce of *cardus Benedictus* seed, and a dram of clove'[13]—all of which would then be put in a jug for about twenty-four hours and then given to the young woman suffering from greensickness.

Bundling

A traditional practice during courtship, which dated to medieval times, was known as bundling. This involved a (usually) young man and young woman sleeping in the same bed overnight. The idea was to allow a young couple to enjoy some intimacy before marriage allowed them full rein with each other's bodies. Sometimes other family members would also be sleeping in the same room and sometimes a board would be placed between the couple to thwart actual penetrative sex that might result in pregnancy. However, it's reasonable to assume that the couple might have waited until everyone else was asleep and then managed to quietly indulge in some sexual activity nonetheless! After all—according to historian Maureen Waller—by 1700, one in ten English brides was already with child by the time they got married.[14]

Pre-marital sex

Premarital sex has been very much frowned upon throughout most of history, with penalties ranging from fines to much more severe punishments. A woman's maidenhead—a popular term for virginity— was an important aspect of her reputation and sexual identity. At the beginning of one of the bawdiest books of the Stuart period, *The English Rogue*, the narrator's mother has had premarital sex (though she thought otherwise), become pregnant, and her parents 'were much troubled…to hear how their daughter had shipwrecked her fortune (as they judged it) in the unfortunate losing of her maidenhead'.[15]

In the colony of Pennsylvania, one James Lowns and his wife Shusanah were brought before the court 'for committing fornication' out of wedlock; they were fined ten shillings and the case was then dismissed.[16] In a similar case, on 6 April 1688, Thomas Eveson and Elizabeth Woodward were brought before a court for 'ye sin of fornication': 'The said Thomas Eveson acknowledging ye fact and not willing to plead thereunto puts himself upon ye mercy of ye King and Governor'. The couple were fined £40 and forced to marry each other 'at or before ye 6th day of ye 5th month next'.[17] One wonders whether they regretted succumbing to the desires of the flesh.

In a memorandum from the colonies dated 4 February 1638, there is a paragraph which states that a maidservant, Dorothy Temple, in the employ of Mr Stephen Hopkins, was pregnant with an illegitimate child fathered by Arthur Peach, a highwayman and murderer recently executed for his crimes. As Temple owed over two years to Hopkins due to the terms of her indenture, there was some question as to whether she should continue under Hopkins' roof for the remainder of the contract. Four days later, another entry states that her indenture with Hopkins was bought out by one Mr John Holmes of Plymouth for £3, and that Dorothy and her child would 'serve all the residue of her time with the said Mr Holmes'.[18] What became of this mother and child is not known.

A similar situation arose in the Colony of Pennsylvania, and was brought to inquest in June 1689. Mary Turberfield, who was a maidservant under contract with Nathaniel Evans, 'committed fornication with John Eldridge in a boate upon ye river and confesseth her self by ye said act with child'—Eldridge also confessed.[19] Turberfield's employer, Evans, demanded remuneration as apparently Mary was often running off—presumably to meet her lover—and consequently, her work was neglected. The court records mention Mary again, this time around October 1689: 'Mary Turberfield was called to ye Barr and Judgment awarded to receive 10 strips upon her bare back well laid on at ye Common Whipping Post at Chester'.[20] But that wasn't the end of Mary's troubles, for she was mentioned yet again in January of 1689/90, in relation to an argument about the fees associated with her case.[21]

Chapter 7

Stuart-era Gender Roles

In Stuart Britain gender roles were generally binary, and there was widespread inequality—however, people of the time typically regarded this as a natural and normal state of affairs. A Stuart person's sex could determine a great deal about their lives. For example, although this only pertained to a tiny part of the population, 'none of the honours bestowed by the king on a family, can be lost, *but by want of Issue Male*, except where the Patent extends to Issue Female'.[1] Men were regarded as being naturally superior to women (this belief was, with the exception of some radical ideologies, universally held).[2]

Stuart-era women, meanwhile, were multi-skilled homemakers with knowledge of cookery, sewing, distillery, some medicine, and the raising of children.[3] Women, in general, were seen as temptresses, as per the tradition of their being descended from Eve. In the *Anatomy of Melancholy,* author Robert Burton stated: 'She sets you all afire with her voice, her hand, her walk, her breast, her face, her eyes…though they say nothing with their mouths, they speak in their gait, they speak with their eyes, they speak in the carriage of their bodies. And what shall we say otherwise of that baring of their necks, shoulders, naked breasts, arms and wrists, to what end are they but only to tempt men to lust?'[4]

Stuart Britain saw the publication of a great deal of 'conduct' literature—or literary works which encouraged men and women to behave in a godly and respectable manner. Slightly before this period, in 1598, the English Protestant ministers John Dod and Robert Cleaver published *A Godly Forme of Household Management*, in which they urged women to be humble and helpful wives, and for men to love their wives as if they were their own flesh, and be dominant over them. The emphasis on traditional gender roles and a chaste and dutiful Christian way of life was a standard theme for this genre of literature throughout the rest of the subsequent Stuart period.

In general, men dominated women, whether in the form of a father, an uncle, a brother, a husband, or a son.

This said, men thought women had lesser—but still considerable—powers of their own. In his *Advice to a Daughter* (1688), George Savile, 1st Marquess of Halifax wrote, '...there is inequality in the sexes, and that for the better economy of the world, the men, who were to be the lawgivers, and the larger share of reason bestow'd upon them...you have more strength in your looks, than we have in our laws, and more power by your tears than we have by our arguments'.[5] Although men ruled the world, a woman, via her feminine charms, could often persuade a man to do things her way.

The belief that men and women are very different creatures prevailed; this can be gleaned from casual lines in letters from the time. Take, for example, the Duke of Shrewsbury's letter to King William III & II from June 1695: 'But on this subject I write so like a woman, that I ought not to expect to be regarded'.[6] A woman was not to be taken seriously, since she was not a man's equal.

Certain characteristics were gendered. Boldness, for example, was a manly characteristic, and was considered grotesque if found in a woman. 'If boldness be read in her face, it blots all the lines of beauty, [and] is like a cloud over the sun'.[7]

There were, however, radical groups that emerged during the Stuart period, including the Quakers. The most prominent Quaker, William Penn, held that, 'sexes make no difference; since in souls there is none: and they are the subjects of friendship' and that 'between a man and his wife, nothing ought to rule but love. Authority is for children and servants; yet not without sweetness'.[8] On this latter point, William Haughton noted that parents who dealt with their children in an overly heavy-handed, authoritarian manner could see their efforts backfire: 'the Girles are wilfil, and severitie May make them carelesse, mad, or desperate'.[9]

Again in his *Advice to a Son* (1673), Francis Osborne offered the following thoughts about the differences between the sexes in the state of marriage: 'However the patient submission to the Institution of Marriage is the more to be wondered at, since Man and Woman not being allowed of equal strength, are so far prevailed upon by Policy, as quietly to submit themselves to one Yoke'.[10] In *The Lady's New-Year's Gift, Or, Advice to a Daughter* (1688), George Savile, Marquis of Halifax, wrote:

'Your Behaviour is therefore to incline strongly towards the Reserved part...A close behaviour is the fittest to receive Virtue for its constant guest, because there, and there only, it can be secure'.

Women who nagged and berated their husbands (the opposite of the meek and 'reserved' ideal) could find themselves wearing a 'scold's bridle' as punishment.[11] This torturous contraption comprised of an iron muzzle that would be placed around her head, with another piece of metal which inserted into her mouth. It would have been both physically painful and embarrassing to wear in public.

According to English scholar Robert Burton's *The Anatomy of Melancholy* (1638), 'Passion...is more outrageous in women than men... by reason of the weakness of their sex'.[12] Burton continues, quoting Dutch philologist and historian Joseph Justus Scaliger (1540–1609), that women have 'inconstancy, treachery, suspicion, dissimulation, superstition, pride (for all women are by nature proud), desire of sovereignty...bitterness and jealousy'.[13] In a 1705 publication, Thomas Brown warned of women who had too much self-love: 'When once a Woman is so far infatuated with Self-Love, as to shake hands with her Modesty, she becomes the most dangerous and ungovernable Monster that is'.[14]

Men, however, were also under moral pressure to properly fulfil their roles as husbands. The English Puritan Isaac Ambrose stated that although a husband should maintain his authority over his wife, he must also nevertheless 'tenderly respect'[15] her, 'carefully provide for her', and according to Colossians 3.19 of the Bible, must 'never be bitter against her'. And, wrote Ambrose, when arguments and unpleasantness arise, the husband can reprove his wife, but with words of 'meekness and love'. While admonishment was acceptable, a husband must 'never to lay violent hands on her'.[16]

Domestic abuse

Physical violence within some relationships is sadly nothing new, and examples of this can be found in both Stuart fact and fiction. Our first history is that of Elizabeth and Holcroft Blood (a son of Thomas Blood, he who attempted to steal the Crown Jewels in 1671). Theirs is a tale which combined years of probable verbal and emotional abuse with physical violence. Although Holcroft Blood eventually came to have a successful and distinguished military career, his behaviour in his private life left much to be desired. Elizabeth's personality wasn't so endearing either, but there was probably good reason for her to be irritable. Married in 1686, Elizabeth had put up with her husband's extramarital affairs, in which he openly indulged. What's worse, he would invite one of his mistresses, a Mary Andrews, to their house and spend several hours of the night in her chamber—or he would have sex with his mistress *in the same bed* where Elizabeth slept. In 1699/1700, he tried to rape another female visitor, Dorothy Green, who again slept beside his wife.[17] Following a brutal marital rape in 1700, Elizabeth had finally had enough.[18] She packed up and left her husband.

From Maryland, in 1656, comes a disturbing account of a pregnant wife being beaten so violently by her husband that she miscarried a three-month-old male foetus shortly thereafter. 'When the child was born it was all bruises and the blood black in it'.[19] Prior to this horrid incident there had been more beatings, including one when 'he did beat her with a cane' so viciously, it broke into little pieces.[20]

Anne Younge's physically violent relationship with her husband, James, came to light in 1608 when she went to court to sue for a separation.[21] The court heard that she had, on one occasion, been beaten so badly with his fist that her face was black and blue.[22]

Evidence of men being beaten by their wives is scant, but this may, at least in part, be because such a circumstance would have been even more embarrassing for men in Stuart Britain than some feel it to be today. Wife-on-husband physical abuse did, however, appear in the literature of the time. For example, in William Wager's play, *Tom Tyler and his Wife* (reprinted in 1661), a hardworking man laments how his shrewish wife spends all the little money he makes, and when he complains, she responds by physically attacking him:

> 'Besides this unkindness whereof my grief grows,
> I think few Tylers are matched to such shrows,
> Before she leaves brawling, she falls to deal blows...
> The more I forbear her, the more she doth strike me'[23].

Undoubtedly both women and men could be physically abusive. The penalty for a wife killing her husband, however, was much more severe than if the husband killed his wife—the crime was regarded as

'Petit-Treason' and as tantamount to a servant killing their master: 'The punishment for a woman convicted of High Treason, or Petit-Treason, is all one; and that is, to be drawn and burnt alive'.[24]

This is precisely the sentence that was meted out to Elizabeth Ridgeway, who murdered her husband William in 1684 by poisoning his soup with white mercury.[25] Female serial killers often use poison to murder their victims, and William Ridgeway was not her first victim.[26] A popular belief during the Stuart period was that the corpse of a murder victim would bleed in the presence of the killer. In accordance with this superstition, *A True Relation of Four Most Barbarous and Cruel Murders Committed in Leicester-Shire by Elizabeth Ridgway* (1684), states that Elizabeth's father-in-law, John Ridgway, asked to her touch her husband's corpse, and in doing so, blood oozed out of the deceased's nose and mouth.[27] In killing her husband, she had not only committed murder but Petit-Treason (or petty treason). She was found guilty and, after confessing to the further murders of her mother, a servant, and a suitor, was garrotted and burned to death on 24 March 1684.[28]

A woman's role

Not all women matched the obedient, mild-mannered, and loyal ideal widely desired during this time. A rather amusing piece of advice from *The Ladies Dictionary* (1694) warns: 'And let this Notice be given to all Husbands...the more a Woman is forbidden or denied anything, the more she desires and covets it'.[29] This, of course, is a two-way street.

In the political realm, women were often the instigators of very significant events. It was a woman, for example, who reputedly threw a stool in a Scottish church, starting the outcry against the Book of Common Prayer in Scotland, which led to the Bishop's War—a forerunner of the English Civil Wars, or British Civil Wars. In January 1686, women were part of a group hurling insults at Catholics as they emerged from a priest's house.[30] In May 1649, hundreds of Leveller women marched into the House of Commons bearing a petition in which they argued for the right to suffrage, or to vote.[31] They were met with amused ridicule and told to go home and look after their homes and families.

Other women assumed the traditionally male role of defending their homes during times of siege, such as Brilliana Harley and Lettice Digby. In 1643, Harley successfully defended her home of Brampton

Bryan Castle, Herefordshire, from Royalist troops during the English/ British Civil War. Lettice Digby, 1st Baroness Offaly, was in her early sixties when she also successfully held her family home, Geashill Castle, during the Irish Uprising of 1641.

Elizabeth Lilburne, the wife of the radical Leveller writer galloped on horseback from London to Oxford—despite being pregnant—in order to save her husband's life. This would have been against the received wisdom of the time, for such a decision could have easily imperilled her unborn child's life (even walking up a hill was considered unwise),[32] but such was her devotion to her husband that it became a secondary consideration.

Mary Frith (c. 1584 – 1659), who notoriously became known as 'Moll Cutpurse', was a pickpocket and highwaywoman.[33] She cross-dressed, smoked, and became even more well-known when Thomas Middleton and Thomas Dekker based a play on her—*The Roaring Girl* (published 1611).[34] The fictional character in the play is both heroic and unusual, since she differs from other women in her behaviour and appearance, both of which strayed out of the bounds of social norms.[35]

Unwanted advances

Then, just as now, not all attractions were mutual—but if a man found himself rejected by a woman in Stuart times this could lead to unpleasant repercussions for the woman's family. Take, for example, the *Report of the Conference about an Impeachment against Lord Mordant*: 'Here is an illegal Dispossession and arbitrary Imprisonment of William Tayleur Esquire, by the Lord accused, because Mr. *Tayleur's* Daughter would not prostitute herself to his Lust'.[36] The general wisdom of the time found the woman responsible in such cases: 'Mankind, from the double temptation of Vanity and Desire, is apt to turn every thing a Woman doth to the hopeful side; and there are few who dare make an impudent Application, till they discern something which they are willing to take for an Encouragement. It is safer therefore to prevent such forwardness, than to go about to cure it'.[37]

Famed Stuart-era diarist Samuel Pepys certainly made unwanted sexual overtures towards women, but not all of his targets should be seen as helpless victims—some of them fought back. In August of 1668, one woman, annoyed by his constant touching of her hands and body during a church service, threatened to stab him with pins she had removed from her pocket. He quickly relented, and turned his attentions to another young woman nearby.[38]

Sometimes, a young woman simply wasn't interested in the man who was attempting to woo her. Take, for example, Jane, Duchess of Norfolk—whose beauty so enraptured the Duke of Ormonde that he sent her gifts and appropriated a portrait of her from the Duchess of Richmond.[39] Norfolk eventually found Ormonde's romantic attentions exasperating and wrote to her ardent suitor: 'If you are prepared to establish a genuine and agreeable friendship with me my lord, such as is accompanied with recreation, but which has no other motive, I consent. But my lord if you intend anything further you must withdraw your troops and lay siege to a heart easier to conquer than mine'.[40] It is doubtful whether many finding themselves in such a position today would reply in so elegant a manner.

Other unwanted advances took a decidedly sinister—and sometimes downright-murderous turn. The aforementioned female serial killer, Elizabeth Ridgeway, at one point had two suitors vying for her hand in marriage—Thomas Ridgeway, a tailor, and John King, a servant. She chose the former, but King appears to have become something of a nuisance to her. She 'continued to keep the said John King company until she had the opportunity to season him some draught which sent him into the other world'.[41] In other words, she poisoned him.

In 1665, Frances Jennings (later the Duchess of Tyrconnell) and her friend Goditha Price decided to have a wild night out by pretending to be orange-selling wenches—but they weren't planning on actually being treated like them! One Thomas Killigrew, a notorious libertine and theatre manager, immediately took advantage of the situation and fondled Frances's breasts—something about which she was none too happy.[42]

Depictions in art

Throughout history, different European civilisations have gravitated towards certain myths from the ancient world which resonated with their own culture and time. In the Stuart period, one of these popular myths was that of Apollo and Daphne, a powerful tale of an unrequited love. Following his row with Eros, the god of love, Apollo, the god of the Sun, was shot with an arrow of love, whilst the nymph Daphne was shot with an arrow of hatred (a truly bad combination!) and the latter was lustily pursued by the impassioned god. The 1616 publication *The Workes of the Most High and Mightie Prince James*, includes a scene from this tale. The letter 'I' is within a beautifully illustrated box which depicts the moment when Daphne transforms into the laurel tree—thus escaping her unwanted lover. This myth also served as a subject for the great Italian sculptor Gian Lorenzo Bernini in the early-to-mid 1620s.

Another ancient tale, the Biblical story of Susanna and the Elders from the Book of Daniel, was very popular during the Stuart period. Believing herself to be in the privacy of her own garden, the beautiful and virtuous Susanna disrobes and bathes herself. Unbeknownst to her, two lecherous and powerful elders are watching her and make themselves known, threatening to tarnish her reputation with accusations of adultery unless she has sex with them. This moment, when Susanna is naked and exposed before the men's leering faces, was the inspiration for many a work of art, notably Artemisia Gentileschi's 1610 painting (Gentileschi's reputation and talent were such that she was eventually invited to England by King Charles I, an avid art collector). The same story inspired many other great artists of the period, including Rembrandt, Guido Reni, Guercino, Annibale, and Carracci.

Misogyny and misandry

Some would have us believe that Stuart Britain was rife with misogyny— outright hatred of women. There is little evidence to support this claim, but it is fair to say there was a widespread *distrust* of women. After all, were not women (as Daughters of Eve) to blame for man's fall and expulsion from the Garden of Eden? In an entry from 1666, Pepys comes across as being rather frightened by some angry women: 'To the office; the yard being very full of women, (I believe above three hundred) coming to get money for their husbands and friends that are prisoners in Holland; and they lay clamouring and swearing and cursing us, that my wife and I were afraid to send a venison-pasty that we have for supper to-night, to the cook's to be baked, for fear of their offering violence to it: but it went, and no hurt done'.[43]

Some men certainly were openly hostile to women. Anthony Wood stated that one P. Sthael, was 'a great hater of women'.[44] Sir Isaac Newton, the genius mathematician no doubt better known for his contributions to mathematics and science than for his volatile temperament, had an intense dislike of his mother,[45] and appears to have had little regard for women in general. Newton never married, and would probably best now be described as a misogynist. Further, the author of the broadside *The Character of a Bad Woman* (1679) closes his four-page rant with the line: 'All this of a Bad Woman's understood, But prithee (Reader) shew me One that's Good'.[46] Presumably, the male author of this work had had negative personal experiences with the opposite sex.

In Francis Beaumont and John Fletcher's Jacobean play, *The Woman-Hater*, published in 1607, the main character, Gondarino, is very much a woman-hater and comically gets his comeuppance at the hands of women by the play's end.[47]

From the English writer Owen Felltham (1602–1668), however, we find a more balanced view: 'Some are so uncharitable, as to think all women bad; and others are so credulous, as they believe, they all are good'.[48]

Witchcraft

'Thou shalt not suffer a witch to live'
- Exodus 22:18, KJV Bible

Accusations, interrogations, and executions of 'witches' tarnish the Stuart period with much blood. With the witch trials in Lancashire in the 1610s, the so-called Witchfinder-General Matthew Hopkins terrorising East Anglia during the 1640s, and the infamous Salem Witch Trials of 1692, among many others, it's little wonder that witchcraft and the Stuart period are considered closely connected.

Things that couldn't be explained were usually attributed to the supernatural. Women were far more likely to be accused of witchcraft than were men. Indeed, according to historian Owen Davies, eighty percent of the people who were tried for witchcraft in Britain were women.[49] Why was this the case? According to John Bell's 1697 work, *Witch-Craft Proven, Arreign'd, and Condemn'd in its Professors, Profession and Marks* the reason is to be found in Original Sin, when Eve—a woman—fell for the Devil's lies and ate of the apple: 'the woman was by Satan first deceived, or that that Sex is more readily circumvented, or else for that more of them than of men be thus deceived'.[50] Quite often, old, widowed, and/or eccentric women would be targeted. Widowed women in particular were believed to be exceptionally easy prey for the Devil, who could take advantage of their loneliness and attempt to seduce them.[51] In 1653, Barbara Bartle—a widow—of Stepney, was suspected of being a 'common witch and inchantrix' who used her dark powers against a spinster named Elizabeth Gyan.[52] Petty grievances, long-held grudges or perceived slights, could lead to an accusation of witchcraft.

There is a strong element of sexuality in Stuart-era notions of witchcraft: 'the *Incubusses* also serve to satisfie the lust of the Witches, and the *Succubusses* the lust of the Wizzards'.[53] Succubi (or succubæ) were female demons who would target sleeping men in order to have sex with them. Incubi, on the other hand, were male demons who would do the same, but with women.

Strangely enough, one of the most active witch-hunters of the Stuart period was the king himself.[54] King James was profoundly interested in a variety of supernatural topics, especially witchcraft, and his interest intensified shortly before becoming King of England.[55] He is credited with writing the book, *Dæmonologie* (1597), which covered topics such as necromancy, witchcraft, and spectres. In this, he stated that an entire nunnery was believed to have been used for the purpose of sexual abuse by incubi and was burned down for this reason.[56] Furthermore, he stated that these supernatural entities steal 'the sperme of a dead bodie',[57] and that this sperm, being used on a living victim, 'seemes intollerably cold'.[58] This idea of cold ejaculate and body would be mentioned later by some accused of witchcraft, notably in the trial of Susanna Edwards in 1682:

> 'Susanna Edwards to confess, that she was suckt in her Breast several times by the Devil in the shape of a Boy lying by her in her Bed; and that it was **very cold unto her**. And further saith, that after she was suckt by him, the said Boy or Devil had the carnal knowledge of her Body Four several times'.[59]

Even three decades after the publication of *Dæmonologie*, in 1637, there was a great debate in France about the existence of *succubi* and *incubi*—which suggests that many people still believed in them.[60]

The emphasis on witches' teats and other parts of their anatomy that were 'sucked' by the Devil or by his imps were another sexualised aspect of Stuart-age thinking about witchcraft. In 1619, the trial of the 'Witches of Belvoir' centred on Joan Flower and her two daughters, Margaret and Philippa, for the deaths of Henry and Frances Manners—heirs to the 6th Earl of Rutland. Margaret confessed (quite possibly under torture)[61] that she had been sucked by two spirits—one of whom performed a kind of cunnilingus on her:

> 'She confesseth, that she hath two familiar Spirits sucking on her, the one white, the other black spotted; the white sucked under her left brest and the black spotted within the inward parts of her secrets'.[62]

According to Hopkins' *A Discovery of Witches* (1647), the inspection of a woman's naked body and any abnormalities found therein could lead to her doom: 'Witch, who was thereupon apprehended, and searched, by women who had for many yeares knowne the Devills marks, and found to have three teats about her, which honest women have not'.[63] In 1645, Hopkins and his assistant, John Stearne, travelled to Bury St Edmonds, where one of the accused women—Jane Linstead—'confessed' to having refused the Devil consent to have sex with her when he arrived before her in the form of a man.[64]

In Devon, 1682, another witch trial took place which again had strong sexual connections: Mary Trembles of Biddiford confessed that after she had made a bargain with the aforementioned Susanna Edwards (also accused of witchcraft), the Devil had come to her and had sex with her:

> 'And that after the Devil had had knowledge of her Body, that he did suck her in her Secret parts, and that his sucking was so hard, which caused her to cry out for the pain thereof'.[65]

This idea of woman as witch was also an integral part of the imagery of the period. The frontispiece of 1643's *A Most Certain, Strange, and true Discovery of a Witch*, for example, shows an old, unattractive woman with unkempt hair and bare feet, balancing herself with a cane on a narrow board as she floats down a river, with two black birds hovering about her.[66] The story therein of the 'Witch of Newbury' was that soldiers saw her unnaturally and effortlessly sailing down the river, they set upon her and shot her, but she—cackling—caught the bullets and chewed them. This type of horror tale was quite common during the intensely stressful chaos of the English, or British, Civil Wars, and stories of witches were often included in pamphlets of the time.

Matthew Hopkins rose to prominence during the chaos of the 1640s, when England—and indeed the rest of Britain—was plunged into civil war. Approximately three hundred innocent women were hanged following his interrogations,[67] yet, due to the political chaos of the years in which he operated (again, he was self-appointed, and was not working for the government), he was never brought to justice. Hopkins remains a figure of dread and horror in British history despite him 'witchfinding' for a period of only three years.[68]

His notoriety notwithstanding, Hopkins was not the only person who claimed to be able to discover witches. Around the year 1649/1650, two sergeants named Thomas Shevel and Cuthbert Nicholson went to Scotland to hire the witch-finding services of a Scotsman, and doing so, they brought him to Newcastle. There, 'thirty women were brought into the town-hall, and stript, and then openly had pins thrust into their bodies, and most of them was found guilty, near twenty-seven of them by him, and set aside'.[69] Other historians have mentioned this, but it bears repeating: seeing these women stripped naked and humiliated—in public—must have been an erotic sight, especially for the more sexually-repressed of the community.

Although there were these accusations of witchcraft, some contemporary writers expressed clear scepticism on the topic. One of these was Thomas Ady, in his 1656 publication *A Candle in the Dark: Or, A Treatise Concerning the Nature of Witches & Witchcraft*. In the section entitled 'The Reason of the Book', Ady writes: 'The Grand Errour of these latter Ages is ascribing power to Witches, and by foolish imagination of men's brains, without grounds in the Scriptures, wrongfull killing of the innocent under the name of Witches.'[70]

Chapter 8

Stuart Marriage: Or, Legal Sex!

Marriage more inclines the mind to serious, and necessary
business, then the wandring lusts of Stews and Concubines[1]
– An Account of Marriage (1672)

Whilst some people engaged in premarital sex, the prevailing attitude of
the time was that sex was best left until after marriage; for it was only
through wedlock that a couple could have sex without the stigmas and
legal troubles associated with fornication and bastardy. Marriage 'in all
Civilized Nations was made the Foundation of Posterity',[2] so great was
its importance.

Marriage was considered a sacred gift from God, a union of 'two
sexes'—man and woman, for God ordained that because 'it was not good
that the Man should be alone, gave him a Help-meet, and commanded
them both to Increase and Multiply, and imprinted in them an eager
desire to unite themselves together for the Propagation of their Species'.[3]
It was through marriage that a man could obtain *levament*—a comfort
which only a wife can provide.[4]

According to Daniel Defoe, Matrimony 'is God's holy Ordinance'
and 'the married Life has a Sanction too, and ought to be preserved
sacred, not to be debauched with criminal excesses of any kind'.[5]
He continued: 'The great Duty between the Man and his Wife, I take
to consist in that of Love, in the Government of Affection, and the
Obedience of a complaisant, kind, obliging Temper; the obligation is
reciprocal, 'tis drawing in an equal Yoke; Love knows no superior or
inferior, no imperious Command on one hand, no reluctant Subjection
on the other'.[6]

For most men and women of Stuart Britain, the most important
decision of their lives was that of making a good choice of spouse, since
this would affect nearly everything else in their life. It's therefore no

wonder that some people turned to astrology to determine what time would be best to look for a spouse. In *His Perpetual Almanack* (1663), Jack Adams stated that 'the eighth House give judgement of Fathers and Children...and when a man ought to look out for a Husband for his Daughter, what portion he should give her'.[7]

Marriage was also meant to satiate the lust of the body and 'thereby more securely enjoy his [mankind's] impure pleasures',[8] and it was recommended that 'new or young married folks ought not licentiously to go together, before they have first upon their knees, secretly in their chamber, commended themselves unto God by prayer'.[9]

The spiritual reasons for marriage aside, there were practical elements involved in the selection of a spouse. This was an age in which women came to a marriage with a 'portion' or dowry (money, property, or other assets). The more bountiful a dowry, the likelier a woman would be to secure an advantageous match. This said, marrying solely for money was discouraged.[10] A 'jointure' would be whatever a bride brought to her marriage that could be used to sustain her should she survive her husband.[11]

Wedding practices

The Marriage Act of 1653 made it mandatory for all wedding ceremonies to be conducted before a local Justice of the Peace.[12] As with births and burials, the registry of marriages was maintained by local parishes. Marriage registration required at least twenty-one days' notice, and the intention of the couple to marry would be announced either in the church or in the marketplace by the church on three occasions over the course of three weeks.[13] The age of consent was for the most part sixteen for a man and fourteen for a woman, but by the end of the century Henri Misson wrote that 'in England, a boy may marry at fourteen years old, and a girl at twelve, in spite of parents and guardians, without any possibility of dissolving their marriage'.[14]

What would the bride and bridegroom have worn for their special day? Traditionally, a wedding meant new outfits, but as clothes were costly and generally tailor-made, some people would have simply worn the best clothes they had. The wealthiest, however, would indulge in sumptuous wedding garments. The outfit that James, Duke of York, wore to his 1673 wedding ceremony with Mary of Modena (his second marriage), survives to this day, and is a wool suit, lined with vibrant red silk and beautifully and intricately decorated with silver and silver gilt thread. Princess Elizabeth Stuart, James's aunt, who wed Frederick V of the Palatinate in 1613, wore a gown made from an elaborately embroidered Florence cloth of silver and with sleeves that were encrusted with diamonds.[15]

The man's wedding vow—again according to the 1653 Marriage Act—was to be said as follows:

> 'I, [man's name], do here in the presence of God the searcher of all hearts, take thee, [woman's name], for my wedded Wife; and do also in the presence of God, and before these witnesses, promise to be unto thee a loving and faithful Husband'.

The woman, in turn, was to reply:

> 'I do here in the presence of God the searcher of all hearts, take thee, [man's name], for my wedded Husband; and do also in the presence of God. And before these witnesses, promise to be unto thee a loving, faithful and obedient Wife'.[16]

According to Monsieur Misson in 1698, the vows were the same for both husband and wife until the end, when the husband would give the wife her wedding ring and say, 'with this ring I thee wed, with my body I thee worship, and with all my worldly goods, I thee endow' and the wife would reply that she will love, cherish, and obey him.[17] The wife was the only one of the two whose vows included the promise to obey.

Monsieur Misson mentioned the bestowing of the wedding ring, above, and this brings us to the subject of rings. There was a popular trend during the seventeenth century whereby women took to wearing their wedding ring on their thumb, rather than on their ring finger.[18] However, those of a more puritanical persuasion looked unfavourably upon the ritual of wedding rings altogether, thinking it to be too Popish.[19] Gimmel, or Jimmal, rings were popular during the sixteenth and seventeenth centuries and served as betrothal rings or wedding rings.

Julia, I bring
To thee this Ring,
Made for thy finger fit;
To shew by this,
That our love is,
(Or sho'd be) like to it.[20]

– Robert Herrick

As evidenced by Herrick's poem above, rings were symbols of love and a promise to 'let our love as endless prove, And pure as Gold for ever'.[21]

The diarist John Evelyn described his wedding to Mary Browne, the daughter of the English ambassador in Paris: 'On Thursday, 27th of June, 1647, he married us in Sir Richard Browne's chapel, between the hours of eleven and twelve, some few select friends being present'.[22]

Some wedding ceremonies were not performed in a church, but instead took place in the parental home of either the bride or the groom. Alice Thornton described her wedding to William Thornton in 1651 as having taken place in her mother's house in Hipswell, and mentioned that the couple were married by a Mr Siddall.[23]

There were some rather entertaining wedding practices. After the wedding feast and other celebratory festivities, the newly-married couple would be escorted into the bedchamber by the wedding guests, then the bridesmaids would undress the bride and settle her into the bed, whilst the groomsmen would take the groom into another room to undress him. Both the bride and groom would be relieved of their stockings, which would then be flung. After this, the couple would be given a caudle to drink (this was a creamy and delicious concoction made of egg yolks, milk and wine, and flavoured with sugar, nutmeg, and cinnamon) to help stoke the fires of their desire.[24] The groom was then supposed to shoo everyone away so he could be alone with his bride. Sexual consummation of the marriage was expected to occur after this. The following morning, the couple would be awakened by family and friends with merriment and some sack-posset to refresh them.

Politics & marriage

The English historian and diarist Narcissus Luttrell often included news of marriages of the nobility in his *Brief Historical Relation of*

State Affairs, as evidenced by his entry from 1694: 'The Lord Spencer, son to the Earl of Sunderland, is married to the youngest daughter of the late Duke of Newcastle; and the Lord Feversham's niece is to be married to the old Earl of Strafford'.[25] Such marriages were worth noting because they could, and often did, have political repercussions.

Colonel Thomas Rainsborough, the Parliamentarian officer and prominent Leveller who famously declared 'I think that the poorest he that is in England hath a life to live as the greatest he', had two sisters—one of whom married Governor Winthrop of Massachusetts,[26] while the other married Winthrop's son, Stephen. This proved useful—for Stephen fought in Rainsborough's regiment, and quite a number of men in this regiment had also come from Governor Winthrop's New England colony.[27] Marriages—and the connections they brought—could be used by military leaders like Rainsborough to their own advantage.

Again from Luttrell, we learn about a foreign match: 'the Elector of Bavaria met his Electoress at Wesel, and the ceremony of his marriage was consummated'.[28] It may strike us as odd that anyone in Britain would care about the sex life of people who lived so far away, but Maximilian II Emanuel's marriage to the Polish Princess Teresa Kunegunda Sobieska in 1695 had political and dynastic ramifications throughout Europe.

Marital advice

Much Stuart-age marital advice makes sense, no matter the time period. For example: 'make not a celebrated beauty the object of your choice; unless you are ambitious of rendering your house as populous as a Confectioner's shop; to which the gaudy Wasps, no less than the liquorish Flies, make it their business to resort, in hope of obtaining a lick at your Honey pot'.[29] In other words, if she's especially attractive, good luck in warding off other men who will try to obtain sexual favours from her, making one a cuckold in the process!

Hannah Woolley (1622–c.1675), a successful English writer of works on household management, gave very sensible advice about love in *The Gentlewoman's Companion* from 1675: 'Look well before you like; love conceived at first sight seldom lasts long, therefore deliberate with your love, lest your love be misguided; for to love at first look makes an house of misrule'.[30]

Also, marrying too young or too old was frowned upon, as Daniel Defoe explained: 'It is the opinion of some, that after there is no more room to expect children, it is not lawful to marry'.[31] Defoe then asks us to consider a hypothetical scenario in which a fifty-five-year-old woman has recently married, knowing she is past childbearing years. She cannot say she wants to marry to have children, nor to have someone look after her affairs, so that only leaves her desire to have sex with the man she intends to have as her husband. 'She ought to say that she married merely to lie with a man. And is not this Matrimonial Whoredom? If not, what then must it be called, and by what words, that will not be criminal in themselves, can we express it?'[32]

Marrying for love was the romantic ideal, but marrying for love whilst being impoverished was—realistically—asking for trouble. After all, 'poverty in wedlock, is a great decayer of love and contention'.[33] Thomas Bentley, in his *The Sixt Lampe of Virginitie*, warned men against marrying 'an idolatrous and superstitious woman', because such a woman was 'dangerous both to bodie and soule'.[34] This said, unlike the aristocracy, the majority of Stuart people had more freedom to choose their spouse based on genuine affection rather than political advantage.[35]

Some unions were prohibited. During the Cromwellian conquest of Ireland, Cromwell's soldiers were strictly forbidden from marrying Irish women, the penalty for disobedience being a severe flogging.[36]

Age differences

Throughout the Stuart period, there are examples of men marrying much-younger women. There was good reason for this, since by this time a man would typically be financially, and materially, stable enough to provide for a wife, especially in the case of the aristocracy. Lucy Hutchinson (1621–1680) wrote that her father was 'then forty-eight years of age' and her mother, 'not above sixteen' when they married.[37]

The fifty-year-old Sir John Denham shocked everyone when he married Margaret Denham—a great court beauty who was twenty-seven years his junior. Sadly for him, his young wife soon got into bed with the young and very handsome James, Duke of York. Their affair was so passionate and indiscreet that everyone, even her husband, knew about it. Denham was so incensed and hurt by being thus cuckolded that some feared for his sanity.[38] In the midst of this affair, Lady Denham suddenly became ill and died—leading many to believe she had been poisoned.[39]

As discussed later, in Chapter 16, one of the problems with having a much-older husband was the potential for his being impotent. 'In old men there is not so much vigor and heat as to prick them on to lust',[40] wrote Sinibaldi. He also warned that an old man's seed, or sperm, is less likely to be healthy, and that people should be wary of having too great an age gap between man and wife.[41] Indeed, impotent men were considered unfit for marriage because they would not be able to sire offspring.[42]

An older spouse could spell problems in the bedchamber, as well. In John Wilmot, 2nd Earl of Rochester's 'A Song Of a Young Lady to her Ancient Lover', the young lady has to give her much-older lover a 'hand-job' in order to help him have an erection: 'And, south'd by my reviving Hand, In former Warmth and Vigour stand'.[43]

Sir Edward Coke (1552–1634) made an unwise choice when, following the death of his first wife Bridget, he married the stunningly beautiful Lady Elizabeth Hatton, who was twenty-six years his junior. The couple had almost nothing in common and ended up arguing and, finally, living in separate households.[44] A similar situation was found in Hortense Mancini's marriage to the much-older Marquis de la Meilleraye. Things became so bad between the two, that Hortense took her jewellery and left her husband.[45]

The Ladies Dictionary (1694), warns that in a marriage between a young woman and a much-older man, there is a strong probability that the man will be inordinately jealous 'if she chances to cast her Eye on any one more comely than himself', at which point he may 'conclude that an Assignation is being made by the Language of her Eyes'.[46]

Differences in rank

Another potential problem with Stuart love and marriage was when spouses came from very different social classes. When a couple from different backgrounds married, this was noteworthy enough for the gossipmongers. Anthony Wood wrote about, 'Wright Croke', who 'lives at Merston and in the latter end of August 1684, he being then about twenty-six years of age, married his maid'.[47]

Although this next union was not a difference in rank, John Evelyn's wry observation about the match proves rather comical, for he found the bridegroom simply…strange: 'I went to congratulate the marriage of Mrs Gardner, maid of honour, lately married to that odd person, Sir Henry Wood; but riches do many things'.[48] Evelyn was of the opinion that Mrs Gardner could turn a blind eye to Wood's oddities because he was wealthy.

On 29 March, 1686, John Evelyn had something to say about George Fitzroy, Duke of Northumberland's recent marriage: 'The Duke of Northumberland (a natural son of the late King by the Duchess of Cleveland) marrying very meanly, with the help of his brother Grafton, attempted in vain to spirit away his wife'.[49] The woman to whom Evelyn referred in this entry was Catherine Wheatley, daughter of a Berkshire poulterer and therefore very much a commoner.[50] However, despite the derision with which some, like Evelyn, looked upon the marriage, George and Catherine stayed married until her death in 1714. George later remarried a Mary Dutton, but that marriage was short-lived, since he himself died in 1716.

King James II & VII was none-too-pleased when his illegitimate son, James FitzJames, the Duke of Berwick, married Honora de Burgh, Countess of Lucan—for she was the penniless nineteen-year-old widow of the Irish Jacobite soldier and former MP of Ireland, Patrick Sarsfield.[51]

Chapter 9

Contraception & Fertility: Or, How to Sheathe Your Sword

'For all physicians agree they must both spend together to get a child'[1]

– The School of Venus, 1680.

During the Stuart era, fertility was considered an important matter, and despite a lack of sure-fire methods of contraception, infertility was a common problem.[2] Motherhood was an extremely significant aspect of the Stuart woman's life and of her identity as a woman. Sexual union in wedlock and the subsequent offspring who arose from this coupling were an essential factor in the glue that held society together. In Genesis 9:7, God commands us: 'And you, be ye fruitful, and multiply; bring forth abundantly in the earth, and multiply therein'.[3]

Men had their seed (sperm), but women, as mentioned in Chapter One, were also believed to have their own, internal, seed. These seeds would come together to form a new human being.

The prevailing belief during the Stuart era (as in the previous Tudor era) was that mutual sexual pleasure was required for a woman to become impregnated.[4] Indeed, Stuart-era people believed it was essential for both the man and the woman to reach orgasm in order for the woman to conceive.[5] This belief presented a problem when it came to pregnancy which resulted from rape: if the victim conceived, then she was considered to have enjoyed the copulation, and so couldn't have been raped.[6]

An advertisement on the back page of *The Post Boy* newspaper from October 19, 1708 (during the reign of Queen Anne) recommends that the quintessence of Bohee-Tea and cocoa-nuts into a dish of tea or chocolate 'prevent miscarriages, cause procreation and conception'.[7]

Scientific discoveries

A great many scientific and medical advances were made during the seventeenth century. The use of microscopes greatly increased, and figures such as Antonie van Leeuwenhoek, Regnier de Graaf, and Robert Hooke made crucial discoveries which not only clarified aspects of human reproduction but impacted our understanding of biology itself.

It was van Leeuwenhoek (1632–1723), however, who examined his own semen under a microscope.[8] What he saw was ground-breaking, for he was the first person to see sperm cells.[9] He recorded his findings and submitted them to The Royal Society in London as a work entitled, *De Natus E Semine Genital Animalculis* (1677/78). Leeuwenhoek included in his observations his theory of the Humunculus, or the idea of a miniature human *in utero*. This was the idea that a human male's sperm contained a tiny complete human which was transferred to the woman in the man's ejaculate, and which the woman would nurture and grow within her womb. This theory is, of course, completely incorrect. We now know that a man's sperm races towards an egg, and usually one sperm 'wins' and is able to penetrate the thick outer membrane, thus beginning conception. The woman's womb then creates the placenta, which was sometimes referred to as the *secundine* during this period.[10]

Furthermore, Regnier de Graaf, a Dutch anatomist and physician, who lived from 1641 to 1673, is credited with the discovery of the ovum (the egg cell) in the year before his death.[11]

Barrenness and infertility

Although we assume Stuart-era women were pregnant almost all the time, infertility was, in fact, a problem for quite a number of people, including some well-known figures such as Samuel and Elisabeth Pepys. Despite having access to the best physicians of the day, not even royals escaped the emotional pain of infertility and the loss of a child. In fact, post-Restoration, the House of Stuart endured significant gynaecological problems that had repercussions for the entire dynastic line.

Those couples who had trouble conceiving could find a plethora of advice—written and oral—regarding what might make a woman more likely to become pregnant. *The English Housewife* (1631) recommended:

'let her drink mugwort steeped in her wine, or else the powder thereof mixed with her wine'; for this was thought to help fertility. Another book, this time published in 1702, recommended the use of *Herba Jacobi*, Rag-wort, to get rid of so-called 'barrenness'.[12]

In *The Cabinet of Venus Unlocked* (1658), the author maintained that barren women were sexually unsatisfied because their bodies had too much blood and heat, and this created a toxic environment for a man's sperm, or seed.[13] According to Isaac Ambrose (1604–1664), an English vicar from Preston, Lancashire, married couples should rid themselves of all the 'exorbitant pollutions of the Marriage-bed', for if they did not, 'God should punish such a couple with no children, or with misshapen children, or with Idiots, or with prodigious wicked children'.[14] In other words, if people did not lead lives as free of sin as possible, then they could expect to be punished with barrenness or with physically or mentally disabled children. This is very much in keeping with Stuart-era beliefs: misfortunes were generally considered punishments from God for transgressions. William Gouge, in *Of Domesticall Duties* (1622), implied that some people thought barrenness was tantamount to impotence. He argued that although procreation is the main purpose of marriage, even a union which does not produce children is inviolable and 'cannot be broken for want of children'.[15]

Quack doctors

Infertility during the Stuart period was just as emotionally painful for couples as it is in our age, but the treatments for it were quite interesting—and sometimes downright bizarre. John Wilmot, 2nd Earl of Rochester (yes, he's back!) adopted the role of a quack physician named 'Dr Bendo'. Supposedly infertile women would seek the services of Dr Bendo, who promptly impregnated them himself—or so Gilbert Burnet implied.[16]

One advertisement for a quack doctor, in 1650, marketed their supposed ability to guess the number, time, and place that a marriage would take place, how many children—and of what sex—the couple would have, and whether a man would marry the woman he fancied.[17] The mysterious future would be foretold in much the same manner as one would expect from fortune tellers and the like.

Contraception

But what did Stuart-era people do when they wanted to have sex without this leading to a pregnancy? There was always the 'pull-out' method, or *coitus interruptus*, in which the man withdraws his penis from the woman's vagina just before ejaculation occurs. The semen, or ejaculate, would be squirted onto the man's sexual partner or into some receptacle. Although this method is probably the oldest kind of birth control in history, it was not a sure-fire method of preventing fertilisation, for even if the man had the self-control to withdraw his penis in time, pre-ejaculatory fluids can contain spermatozoa which can cause pregnancy.

Coitus interruptus not being the most dependable form of contraceptive, Stuart-era people looked elsewhere. The prostitute, Julietta, in *The Wandering Whore* mentions that she urinates following sex,[18] but whilst this would have been helpful in preventing urinary tract infections for women, it was unlikely to have contraceptive effects (some women even today believe this myth).[19] Again, from *The School of Venus*, 'some will tie a Pig's Bladder to the Top of their Pricks, which receives all without hazard'.[20]

Let's examine Stuart-era condoms more closely. In accordance with the description provided by *The School of Venus*, they were indeed made from preserved and treated animal organs shaped into a sheath, which would then be tied onto a penis with a ribbon. These sheaths were mainly used by the nobility (even the Earl of Rochester wrote *A Panegyrick Upon Cundom*), and were less likely to be used in whorehouses, for they were expensive.[21]

In 1985, a team of archaeologists excavating Dudley Castle's latrines came across the remains of ten condoms.[22, 23] They had been thrown into the latrine sometime before or during the two sieges of Dudley Castle at the time of the British Civil Wars.[24] It is unclear whether they were primarily used for contraception or as a defence against venereal diseases, but nonetheless these seventeenth-century sheaths remain some of the oldest-surviving condoms in the world.[25]

Chapter 10

Bigamy, Widowhood, & Remarriage

Clandestine weddings

William Gouge's *Of Domesticall Duties* (1622), stated that clandestine weddings were performed in secret, often in the dark and without adequate witnesses or even a reputable clergyman present. As such, he maintained, they were doomed to be unsuccessful.[1] Twenty-nine-year-old poet John Donne wed his sixteen-year-old wife during Advent of 1601 in a secret ceremony, without banns having been read and without the consent of the bride's father (since she was underage).[2] When this was discovered, Donne lost his job, was arrested, and was sent to the Fleet prison.[3] Due to a lack of records, it is possible that the English Baroque composer, Henry Purcell, and his wife, Frances, had a clandestine marriage as well, following Purcell's twenty-first birthday.[4]

Clandestine marriages became a problem that was ultimately deemed to require legislation. This arrived in the form of the Marriage Duty Act, which was passed in 1696 during the reign of William III, and which meant that everyone who intended to marry needed to purchase a license or certificate and have their banns read out.[5] Any clergyman who did not obey this law could face a fine of £100.[6]

Stuart bigamy

Bigamy is the state of being married to more than one person at a time in a country that views monogamy as the only legal marital state. The average Stuart's views on bigamy are probably best captured by Thomas Bentley: 'A man ought to be the husband but of one wife. For to have more than one at once is a signe of incontinencie'.[7] Monsieur Misson was of the opinion that 'polygamies, easily conceal'd', were 'too much practis'd'.[8]

77

Charles II's arguably most notorious mistress, Barbara Palmer, Lady Castlemaine, later inadvertently married a bigamist. She had fallen for the much younger rakish hunk Robert Fielding, who was seducing several wealthy women simultaneously.

Bigamy was by no means the preserve of the aristocracy—commoners committed the crime too, although sometimes they were not even aware it *was* a crime, or they had to go to court to prove they had not committed it. Take for example, Thomas Middleton, a tooth-drawer from Ludgate Hill during the reign of Charles II. Middleton was indicted for bigamy, for he was believed to be married to two women at the same time. At his trial, he produced evidence that he had been granted a divorce from his first wife on the grounds of her adultery.[9] Thomas Hearne (1678–1735) recounted a story he'd heard 'of one who got by that means a pretty woman to be his wife, who had been at ye same time married to another, and her husband still living'.[10]

Delarivier Manley, a popular writer known for her scandalous 1709 work *Secret Memoirs and Manners of Several Persons of Quality, of Both Sexes, from the new Atalantis* is believed to have been in a bigamous union to the already-married Tory MP John Manley.

The loss of a spouse

> 'These divorces by death'
>
> —John Donne

The death of a spouse was just as emotionally difficult as it remains to this day, though the practicalities of living could be exponentially more difficult (due to the loss of the spouse's income and there being no welfare state, for example). By the late sixteenth century, some literary works suggested that widowhood was seen as 'a plague of God upon the ungodly'.[11] After all, in Exodus 22.22: 'If my wrath be kindled, saith the Lord, against you for your oppression, then will I kill you with the sword, and your wives shall be widows, and your children fatherless'.

Stuart-era peoples reached out to those who had been bereaved. John Donne, for example, wrote a moving consolatory letter in 1624 to a lady following the death of her husband: 'We are not bound to think, that souls departed, have divested all affections towards them, whom they left here; but we are bound to think, that for all their love to us, they would not be here again'.[12]

Although the majority of his life was lived during the Tudor period, the influence of Guy Fawkes and the other Gunpowder Plotters on the Stuart period cannot be underplayed. According to his most recent biographer, Nick Holland, Fawkes may have had a secret Catholic wedding to Maria Pulleyn.[13] A son was born, but the mother and child died. His heart utterly broken, Fawkes eventually turned more towards Catholicism and the extremist strains that led him to take part in one of the most infamous plots in British history.

Melford Hall, a stately home in Suffolk, came into the possession of Lady Savage following the death of her husband, Thomas, Viscount Savage in 1635. Staying true to her family's religious and political views (she was a Catholic and a Royalist) caused the widow much trouble during the English Civil Wars that followed, and in 1642, a mob ransacked her homes at St. Osyth and Melford Hall. This, along with fines and other troubles, rendered her penniless, and she died within a few weeks of being incarcerated in a debtor's prison in 1651.[14]

Widows sometimes appear in legislative documents from this period. In 1698, for example, Rebecca Lassels, a widow, sought, and was enabled via an Act of Parliament to 'sell copyhold lands and houses in Ealing, in the County of Middlesex'.[15] Lassels' actions are understandable, especially given the context of what widowhood meant. According to *Angliæ Notitia: Or, The Present State of England* (c.1679), 'all the chattels personal the wife had at the marriage, is so much her husband's that after his death, they shall not return to the wife, but go to the executor or administrator of the husband, as his other goods and chattels, except only her paraphernal, which are her necessary apparel'.[16] In other words, a wife wouldn't automatically receive everything upon the death of her husband; nor did she have the right to keep belongings that were hers before the marriage.

Remarriage

Death being so common as a result of the various diseases prevalent during the Stuart period and, of course, death from childbirth, remarriage occurred more often than we might think. This commonly produced step-mothers, step-children, step-siblings, and half brothers and sisters. It's therefore no surprise that some fairy tales from this time period included stories of wicked stepmothers. The seventeenth-century French writer, Charles Perrault, is famed for his version of *Cinderella*, in which the evil stepmother and stepsisters mistreat Cinderella—the only child of a recently-deceased man. One of the moral lessons imparted by this story was that a person ought to be sure of the character of their intended spouse, for the sake of previous children, as well as any future offspring.

Restoration rake Charles, 6th Earl of Dorset (1643–1706), married twice. His first wife was Frances Bagot (1645–1679). Her first husband, Charles Berkeley 1st Earl of Falmouth, having died in the Battle of Lowestoft of 1665, Frances was left a young, beautiful, and admired widow. Following her death, Dorset remarried, and his second wife was Mary Compton—his junior by some thirty years. Clearly attracted to the most gorgeous women of the Late Stuart courts, Dorset has the distinction of being the only man to have married both a Windsor Beauty (Frances Bagot) and a Hampton Court Beauty (Mary Compton).[17] He and Mary had two children. Sadly, though, his second marriage ended quickly when Mary died from smallpox aged only twenty-two.[18]

Anne Scott, 1st Duchess of Buccleuch, was married to the dashing, but doomed James, Duke of Monmouth, when she was just twelve. The couple had six children. Anne had to contend with Monmouth's licentious lifestyle, his adulteries, the ramifications of his failed rebellion in 1685, his subsequent execution, and the death of their daughter Anne in that same year. Three years after Monmouth's beheading, she remarried Charles Cornwallis, 3rd Baron Cornwallis—also a widower—in 1688.[19]

Chapter 11

Deviant Sexual Practices, Part I: Same-Sex Relations

During the Stuart period, same-sex physical relationships were considered deviant, with male same-sex liaisons running the risk of public humiliation and even execution.

Sodomy

The terms used for homosexual acts in Stuart Britain were usually 'sodomy', 'buggerie', and 'pedicate'—which means 'to bugger'.[1] 'One who useth buggerie' was a Pygist [2] and a boy who was used for buggery was a 'catamite'.[3] Sex between men was generally considered unnatural and worthy of disgust and derision, as is evident from Ned Ward's *The London Spy Compleat* (1703): 'We...jostled in amongst a parcel of Swarthy Buggerantoes, Preternatural Fornicators...who would Ogle a Handsome Young Man with as much Lust, as a True-bred English Whoremaster would gaze upon a Beautiful Virgin'.[4]

This opinion was so prevalent during the period that legislation was created to make male-male sexual activity a criminal offence. It is important to remember that Stuart Britain was very religious. In the King James Bible, published in 1611, we find: 'If a man also lie with mankind, as he lieth with a woman, both of them have committed an abomination: they shall surely be put to death; their blood shall be upon them' (Leviticus 20:13). Whilst this attitude would be controversial today, during the Stuart period men were indeed executed for engaging in 'sodomitical' acts, as we shall soon discover.

Platonic same-sex love was, on the other hand, commendable. It was good to love your friend devotedly, but to have sex with them was another matter entirely. It has become fashionable today to take a well-known figure from history and posthumously label their perceived sexuality using a modern term. William Shakespeare, for example, is a particular favourite for this kind of speculation because of his Sonnets and the connection between them and his patron, Henry Wriothesley, 3rd Earl of Southampton. Some writers suggest Shakespeare was bisexual, others that he was homosexual, but there is insufficient evidence to support either claim.[5] Some also speculate about the sexuality of the poet John Donne as well, citing his letters to a male friend—but again we ought to bear in mind that a loving, effusive, and flowery style of writing, by today's standards, was not unusual in heterosexual platonic relationships during the Stuart era.[6]

From a letter from Mr. William Prideaux, Special Ambassador to Russia, to secretary Thurloe: ''Tis said, the men are much addicted and doe exercise the abominable sinne of sodomy with boyes, and use beasts; and in those vices not inferiour to Turkes and Italians'.[7] This comparison with Turks and Italians was often found in writings of the time. Indeed, Scottish explorer William Lithgow's account is in a similar vein: 'Padua is the most melancholy City of Europe... for beastly Sodomy, it is as rife here as in Rome, Naples, Florence, Bologna, Venice, Ferrara, Genoa...a monstrous filthiness, and yet to them a pleasant pastime, making songs, and singing sonnets of the beauty and pleasure of their *Bardassi*, or buggered boyes'.[8] He also wrote of Turks: 'They are extremely inclined to all sorts of lascivious luxury; and generally addicted, besides all their sensual and incestuous lusts, unto Sodomy, which they account as a dainty to digest all their other libidinous pleasures'.[9]

One of the most notorious legal cases of sodomy was in 1631 against Mervin Touchet, Lord Audley, 2nd Earl of Castlehaven.[10] John Evelyn commented that, 'the Lord of Castlehaven's arraignment for many shameful exorbitances was now all the talk'.[11] Although he pleaded 'not guilty' to the charges laid before him, he was nonetheless found guilty and beheaded on Tower Hill in 1631. This case is notable, not only from a same-sex perspective, but also because Castlehaven was accused of forcing his servant to rape his wife, Anne Stanley, Countess of Castlehaven.[12]

In late May 1694, Mustapha Pochowachett, a Turkish man living in Stuart Britain, was accused of violently raping a fourteen-year-old

Dutch boy named Anthony Bassa—and infecting him with a venereal disease.[13] Despite Pochowachett's protestations of innocence, a physician examined his body and found him in an advanced state of the same disease. Pochowachett was found guilty and sentenced to death.[14]

Sodomy at sea

As on land, so on sea. 'If any person or persons in or belonging to the Fleet shall commit the unnaturall and detestable sin of Buggery or Sodomy with Man or Beast he shall be punished with death without mercy'.[15] So read the 32nd article of *An Act for the Establishing Articles and Orders for the regulating and better Government of His Majesties Navies Ships of War & Forces by Sea* under King Charles II in 1661.

On 9 November 1692, as *The Neptune* floated along the River Medway, a court martial was taking place on-board. Charles Cristian, a sailor on the *Windsor Castle*, stood accused of 'the unnaturall and detestable crime of Buggery' upon Richard Smith, his servant—who was sixteen years old.[16] Smith's testimony against his former employer was believed and Cristian was found guilty and sentenced to 'be hang'd from the neck 'till he be dead'.[17] Since Smith had also been involved in the act of buggery, he too could have been punished; but the court found that he had been 'under feare and constraint'[18] given the circumstances and that he was 'not consenting'—the crime was rather inflicted upon him. It therefore unanimously agreed to acquit him.

Sir Patrick Cockurn, a Scottish captain in service to Denmark from 1627, was well-respected at the British court. He had command of some 160 Danish soldiers in his company, and by 1628 was appointed Lieutenant Colonel. It was around this time, however, that he found himself in some serious trouble: by the spring of 1628, he'd been found guilty of sodomy and was incarcerated and later decommissioned for his crime(s).[19]

Throughout legal documents of this period one finds mention of men executed for sodomy. In September of 1684, for example, there is record that an unnamed 'young man found guilty of sodomy was hanged' in Portsmouth.[20] What kind of life he had led up until his execution, we will probably never know. In 1625, in the colony of Virginia, an inebriated young seaman named William Cornish went to another man's bed and raped him—and was later found guilty of sodomy and executed.[21] Governor Lord Carlisle to Secretary Coventry: 'The master's chief mate and four other men of the *Jersey* are in prison at Port Royal accused of sodomy, and will be tried for their lives on Tuesday next'.[22]

Not all who were found guilty of sodomy were killed, however; some were granted a reprieve. Such was the case with mariners Robert Stone and Richard Seawell in September of 1639, who, having been sentenced to death by Sir Henry Marten, were granted a reprieve by King Charles I.[23] The aforementioned Lord Carlisle again wrote to Secretary Coventry, on 18 February, 1679: 'A fortnight since five men of His Majesty's Ship *Jersey* were tried for sodomy, and four found guilty and sentenced to die, whereof I suffered but one to be executed, viz., Francis Dilly, who appeared to be the chief ringleader. The other three I have pardoned, white men being scarce with us'.[24] Evidently, if the men had not been white, they would have been executed.

One Captain Rigby was sentenced on 12 of December 1698, 'for blasphemy and an attempt of sodomy, that he should pay £1,000 fine, stand three times in the pillory, remain a year in prison after his fine is paid, and to find sureties for the peace for seven years after he is at liberty'.[25]

Antony Padova of *The Royal Sovereign* was court martialled in a hearing on the *Britannia* after being accused of committing buggery against Isaac Betty, but the court—Sir Cloudesley Shovell and Henry Killigrew among them—found the evidence against him inconclusive and acquitted him of the charge.[26]

Some of those who sought a living on the high seas may have found the all-male onboard camaraderie and close proximity to other men most welcome. The Stuart period coincided with the Golden Age of Piracy (c.1650–1720)—a time in which some of the most infamous pirates operated. Evidence of same-sex sexual and romantic relationships during this time is scant, but human nature being what it is means such affairs doubtless occurred at sea—and whereas the punishment for any such relations discovered in the Fleet was severe, those who became pirates had far more freedom.

Among the customs by which the latter lived was that of *matelotage*, which was a union between two pirates, usually a master and *matelot* (who was generally a subordinate), such that in the event of one of them dying, the other would have rights to all of his worldly possessions.[27] This was, in some respects, similar to marriage, and was even sometimes considered more binding than the rare cases in which one of the pirates married a woman.[28]

False accusations

In May 1613, Alban Coke, a yeoman of Hoxton, was found not guilty of sodomising twenty-year-old John Townesend.[29] This is noteworthy because it means there was either insufficient evidence (i.e. witness testimony) for a conviction, or Coke was falsely accused. Such false accusations were a convenient way of potentially getting back at someone for a perceived wrong—but, although same-sex relations were regarded negatively, falsely accusing a man of sodomy was not looked upon kindly, either. Thomas Knox, for example, was indicted for 'Subornation and Conspiracy against the Testimony and Life of Dr Oates, for sodomy, and fined 200 marks, a year's imprisonment, and made to find sureties for good behaviour for three years'.[30] Similarly, a false allegation of sodomy was directed at Sir John Bowyer of Ashton, Northamptonshire. In a lawsuit, *Bowyer v Merrell*, from 1612, Bowyer—the plaintiff— stated that Thomas Merrell and his wife, Ellen Merrell, conspired to accuse Bowyer of sodomy because they were hoping that this would lead to their gaining the forfeiture of his goods.[31]

Carnal clergymen

Clergymen of the Roman Catholic Church are not supposed to marry, while those from the Anglican Church can. Stuart-era clergymen would sometimes indulge in sexual passion with the same sex—and this could have deadly consequences.

In the autumn of 1640, the Church of Ireland's Bishop of Waterford & Lismore, John Atherton, was found guilty of the crime of sodomy along with his proctor, John Childe. Atherton, born in England in 1598, had married Joan Leakey in 1622—a union which led to five daughters.[32] Atherton was rumoured to have fathered an illegitimate child with his niece (and therefore committed incest as well) and later confessed to having engaged in 'fornication'. He was found guilty in November 1640 and executed by hanging a month later. However, John Childe's accusation that Atherton had been engaging in sodomy with him led not only to Atherton's death, but also to his own:[33] he was hanged in the following year, 1641, having been found guilty of 'Incest, Buggery, and many other enormous crimes'.[34] *The Life and Death of John Atherton*, published the year of his execution, included crude drawings of his hanging corpse.[35]

According to an intelligence letter dated 7 March 1654 in Paris, France, among three prisoners who had been tortured, one was 'an Italian priest accused of sodomy', who, 'having confessed all by the rigorosity [sic] of his pains, was condemned to be first hanged, and afterwards burnt—a sentence which was carried out the next day'.[36] William Laud (b.1573), Archbishop of Canterbury, never married and, if his erotic dreams about George Villiers, Duke of Buckingham, can be used as evidence—was sexually attracted to men.[37] Although he was executed in 1645, it was not for his sexual preferences, but for High Treason.

The theme of sodomy and carnal clergymen made its way into plays as well. In *The Devil's Charter* (1607) by Barnabe Barnes, the main character is the rather infamous Borgia Pope Alexander VI. He is sexually besotted by the young nobleman, Astor Manfredi, who isn't at all comfortable with the situation: '…Then to subject my body to the shame Of such wild, brutish and unkindly lust'.[38] Sex, murder, pacts with the Devil and more follow, with the pope finally being hauled off to Hell itself.

Tribadism (lesbianism)

Though same-sex sexual relationships between men were strictly prohibited by law (and punishable by death) in Stuart Britain, same-sex relationships between women were not. Indeed, there are some rather notable examples of 'tribades' during the Stuart period. This permissiveness on the part of Britain was extraordinarily rare in early modern Europe, where *Sapphism* was generally regarded as being just as criminal as sodomy.[39] Although there was a 1533–34 statute against all forms of anal intercourse, this affected same-sex relations between men far more than it did those between women:[40] lacking a penis, women were not believed to be able to penetrate other women sexually and were therefore regarded as exempt.

The love life of King Charles II is one of the most colourful topics of the seventeenth century, but it is perhaps not very widely known that one of his many mistresses had a passionate affair... with one of his daughters. The beautiful and exotic Hortense Mancini, Duchesa di Colonna, had developed quite a saucy reputation by the time she arrived in England in 1675. Not only had she left her husband back in Italy, but she had embarked on a series of affairs (at least one historian has labelled her a 'nymphomaniac').[41] Such a label, however, would probably not be as acceptable now as it once was—and Mancini's more open amours and penchant for dressing as a man suggest she simply was not one to conform to the strictly binary gender roles of her time. Mancini had once been regarded as a potential bride for Charles, back when he was an impoverished king-in-exile; but while she was never actually became his wife, she certainly became his mistress. King Charles II's eldest illegitimate daughter with Barbara Palmer was Anne, Countess of Essex. Her passionate attachment to Mancini proved embarrassing for her husband, who had his adulterous teenaged wife removed to the countryside. There, she pined away for Hortense, weeping over and kissing a portrait of the Italian beauty.[42]

Queen Christina of Sweden (1626–1689), who never married, had a very close relationship with her lady-in-waiting, Ebba Sparre. She frequently rejected female dress and behaviour. Christina ultimately converted to Roman Catholicism, and abdicated from the throne.

The Frenchwoman Julie D'Aubigny (c.1670–1707) was not only a talented opera singer, but she was very good with a sword, too. She was known for cross-dressing and for love affairs with both men and women.[43]

The most well-known female pirates of the Golden Age of Pirates are undoubtedly Anne Bonny and Mary Read—women who fell in love with each other on board a pirate ship. Both of these women were born illegitimately, and were encouraged by their guardians during childhood to wear boy's clothing. [44]

In *The Female Captain, Or The Counterfeit Bridegroom* (whose author remains anonymous) an eighteen-year-old woman cross-dresses and pretends to be male in order to wed a wealthy heiress. On their wedding night:

'The bridegroom had prudently got a sheep's gut,
blow'd up very stiff, as a bladder;
But what he did with it, or whether 'twas put,

I'll leave you good folks to consider:
The innocent bride no difference knew,
and seemed to be greatly delighted;
But lasses I warrant there's none among you,
that would be so easily cheated'.[45]

That a woman could be ignorant of her husband's sex and not know the difference between a blown-up pig's bladder and a man's penis was considered rather unbelievable and even comical. But there is one notable instance from the Stuart period in which two women *were* married, one (presumably) believing the groom she was marrying to be a man: Arabella Hunt (b. 1662) was famed not only for her exceptionally melodious voice but for her great physical beauty. In 1680, she began a relationship with James Howard and the couple was married in the autumn of that same year. Around six months later, Hunt sought an annulment of the marriage on the grounds that her husband was not a man…but a woman named Amy Poulter.[46] Two years later, the annulment was granted and both were free to marry again. Hunt never remarried. Was she a lesbian, or had she truly been deceived by Poulter into believing she was wedding a man?

Sexual seduction between women features as an indirect theme in a variety of Stuart-era plays. John Crowne's 1675 masque, *Calisto: Or, The Chaste Nymph*, is about the male god Jupiter, or Zeus, who is enamoured with Calisto, a favourite—and chaste—nymph of Diana. All the main roles in this play were performed by the leading ladies of the Stuart aristocracy, including Lady Mary of York (later Queen Mary II), Lady Henrietta Wentworth as Jupiter, Sarah Jennings (later the 1st Duchess of Marlborough), Lady Anne of York (later Queen Anne) as the nymph Nyphe, and Margaret Blagge as the goddess Diana.[47] In classical Greek and Roman mythologies, the king of the gods, Zeus (or Jupiter), was a sexually ravenous individual who used a wide array of ingenious disguises to seduce those he fancied. When he falls for Calisto, a devoted servant of Diana, he adopts the form of this goddess to seduce the chaste nymph—and the result is a seemingly female-female romantic pursuit.

Artwork of the time also depicted sensual and sometimes explicit scenes of physical love between women—for example, a 1690 engraving by Joannes Meursius the Younger shows two naked women rubbing their vulvas and clitorises together.[48] In Stuart Britain, or more precisely from the 1660s onwards, this sexual act was known as 'Flats'.[49]

Cross-dressing

Cross-dressing was illegal in Stuart Britain, and the penalties could be severe. That said, there were some notable exceptions due to fashion trends, which we covered earlier on. According to William Prynne (writing of men acting like women in plays): 'For since men are prohibited in the Law to put on a woman's garment, and such who do it are adjudged accursed. How much more greater a sin is it, not only to put on woman's apparel, but likewise to express obscene, effeminate womanish gestures, by the skill or tutorship of an unchaste art?'.[50] And as for women: 'Now as women's clipping of their hair like men is thus execrable in itself, because [it is] unnatural; so is their putting on of man's apparel, or men of theirs, especially for merriment'.[51]

Charles II's own first cousin, Philippe, duc d'Orléans, younger brother of Louis XIV of France, was known not only for his male lovers, but also for flamboyantly cross-dressing. Louis turned a blind eye to this behaviour due to fraternal love, despite being repulsed by it.[52]

There is some speculation that a portrait known as 'Portrait of an Unidentified Woman' is possibly that of Queen Anne's cousin, Edward Hyde, Lord Cornbury, Governor of the Province of New York and New Jersey in 1702—who gained a reputation (whether true or not) for cross-dressing.[53] Whilst the sitter in question *could* be a woman, the face appears to have a masculine 'five o'clock shadow'.

Occasionally, cross-dressing could serve as a useful and life-saving disguise. When King James II & VII was a fourteen-year-old Duke of York under house arrest in St. James's Palace, in order to escape his captivity he wore 'a woman's habit' and successfully fled England for Holland.[54] Similarly, James's youngest sister Henrietta Anna was smuggled out of England dressed as a boy—but she didn't like this scheme and her indignant protestations that she was actually a princess nearly gave her away![55]

William Maxwell, 5th Earl of Nithsdale (1676–1744), who was incarcerated in the Tower of London following his involvement in the Jacobite rising of 1715, also found cross-dressing helpful. The uprising was in support of King James II & VII's son, James Francis Edward Stuart (commonly known as the 'Old Pretender') against King George I, who had ascended the throne because he was the closest Protestant Stuart descendant via Elizabeth Stuart. In 1716, on the eve of his execution, his wife visited him, applied heavy makeup to his face, dressed him in woman's clothing, and gave him a woman's hairstyle with fake curls. The disguise worked so well that he was able to simply walk out of his cell, without drawing any attention from the guards.[56]

Similarly, Samuel Pepys recounted a conversation he had had with Sir J. Minnes about Sir Lewes Dives, an English Member of Parliament who had escaped from prison several times—once 'in woman's apparel' he leapt across a canal, much to the amusement of a soldier, who exclaimed, 'This is a strange jade!'[57]

Chapter 12

Deviant Sexual Practices, Part II: Incest, Bestiality, & Flagellation

There have always been people whose sexual appetites stray into the realm of deviant behaviour, such as paedophilia, necrophilia, and zoophilia.

Incest

An Act for Suppressing the Detestable Sins of Incest, Adultery, & Fornication (1650) defines incest as follows: 'if any person or persons whatsoever…Marry, or have the carnal knowledge of the Body of his or her Grandfather or Grandmother, Father or Mother, Brother or Sister, Son or Daughter, or Grandchilde, Father's Brother or Sister, Mother's Brother or Sister, Father's Wife, Mother's Husband, Son's Wife, Daughter's Husband, Wife's Mother or Daughter, Husband's Father or Son; all and every such Offences are hereby adjudged and declared Incest'.[1]

Throughout history—from Ancient Egyptian unions between brother and sister, through to political marriages between first cousins— incest has actually been deliberately used by some lineages in order to maintain what they thought to be a 'pure' bloodline. We now know, however, that these unions lead to a higher propensity for offspring to have severe defects. Marriage between first cousins is—in many countries—prohibited due to the close degree of consanguinity, but there were numerous examples of first-cousin marriages throughout the royal houses of Europe. The Habsburg lineage, for example, shows a consistent pattern of marriage between first cousins, which resulted in the horribly debilitating mental and physical deformities suffered by King Carlos II of Spain.[2] His death in 1700 triggered the War of the Spanish Succession, in which the British military leader, John Churchill, Duke of Marlborough, was victorious.

In the Stuart family itself, there was the union of Henrietta Anne (Minette) and King Louis XIV of France's younger brother, Philippe, duc d'Orléans in 1661—this required a Papal dispensation because of their being first cousins.[3] In Stuart Britain, two sovereigns, the married couple William III and Mary II, were also first cousins—Mary's father, James, was William's uncle (specifically, James was William's mother's brother).

During the winter of 1634, William Tilley of Babray, Somerset, was fined £100 for contempt of court for not appearing to answer charges of incest.[4] Documents in the Shropshire Archives state that on June 1616, a Griffith Howell was found guilty of committing incest and was sentenced to the pillory.[5] In Scotland, Thomas Weir (born c. 1600), who had been a major in the Earl of Lanark's regiment in the 1650s, was found guilty of both 'sorcery' and of having committed incest with his sister, Jean Weir. Both siblings freely confessed to having had sexual relations with each other. Thomas was burned at the stake, and his sister was hanged the following day.[6]

Sarah Swarton, a servant in the household of Lord Roos (son of the powerful Elizabethan statesman William Cecil, Lord Burghley), claimed she had seen her master engaging in sex with a woman who wasn't Lady Roos, his wife. There was much more to this accusation of adultery than first meets the eye, for the woman was in question was the Countess of Exeter—his step-grandmother. This, in Stuart Britain, also met the definition of incest.

The context of this event, which was part of the salacious 'Lake-Roos Affair' (1617–1620), is quite complex. Subsequent to their wedding in 1616, the relationship between Anne Lake and William Cecil, Lord and Lady Roos, had become toxic.[7] Not only did they have an unpleasant time of it with each other, but there were also family rows over finances and squabbles between the mother-in-law and son-in-law. During the first major phase of open hostilities, the mother-in-law, Lady Lake, threatened to tell everyone that Roos was impotent and to have the marriage nullified.[8] After this tactic failed, Lady Lake and her daughter tried another avenue. According to the *Cecil Papers*, in May of 1618, Sarah Swarton was found, with her 'confederates, did audaciously and without all colour of truth or good proof affirm, report and give out that your subject the said Countess had committed the said most horrible sine of incest with the said Lord Roos'.[9] This is one of many examples throughout the period of people attempting to use the laws of the day to bring about another person's downfall.

The relationship of major Stuart-era scientist Robert Hooke with his young niece, Grace Hooke, has been the subject of much speculation. She lodged with Hooke as his ward, but when she became a teenager, the two appear to have begun an incestuous sexual relationship, which continued on and off for some years.[10] Some people, however, would not have found this uncle-niece relationship so strange: the author of *The Marriages of Cousin-Germans*[11] (1673) said as much and argued that it is inadvisable for an aunt to marry her nephew not because of the inherent issue of close consanguinity, but because she goes from a position of superiority as his aunt, to one of inferiority as his wife.[12] Using references to the Bible throughout, this whole work is a defense of incestuous unions between first cousins. Unsurprisingly, perhaps, the author married his own first cousin.

There are some recorded instances of incestuous sexual molestation. According to the information given by the victim to the justices investigating these incidents, one seventeenth-century Glastonbury cobbler attempted incest with his fourteen-year-old daughter on a number of occasions, beginning by rubbing his penis against her body and then increasing the violation by inserting his finger with the intention of eventually penetrating her with his penis.[13]

Some incidents lay in a grey area between incest and adultery. Brothers-and-sisters-in-law were sometimes viewed as siblings under law, so if a sexual relationship occurred between two, this could be seen as a case of both incest and adultery. Forde, Lord Grey, was most famous for his involvement in the Monmouth Rebellion of 1685, but he also had a scandalous affair with his wife's sister, Henrietta. Seducing his wife's teenage sister, and then running off with her and deflowering her, might be considered the daytime/reality television-style antics of the day. This pairing was seen by some as the destruction of Henrietta's character, as is clearly demonstrated by the line 'to the ruin and destruction of the said Lady Henrietta Berkeley'.[14] The scandal was furthermore the inspiration for Aphra Behn's epistolary novel *Love Letters Between a Nobleman and His Sister* (1684), with a thinly-veiled Lord Grey as Philander and Lady Henrietta as Sylvia.[15, 16]

In February, 1633, a John Williams of Parke, Brecon (Wales), was fined £500—a huge sum—for having engaged in incest with 'his brother's son's wife'. Again, this couple were considered incestuous even though they were related only by law, not by blood. Indeed, some people became confused and accused couples of committing incest when they really weren't, as was the 1615 case of John Lambe v. John and Frances Wiseman of Strixton, Northamptonshire. Lambe accused them of incest, but—after an investigation—the court found that the couple was 'not within the prohibited degrees' of consanguinity.[17]

Bestiality

'Sodomy' and 'buggery' were both words used to refer to acts of sexual deviancy, with sodomy generally referring to male-male sexuality and buggery to bestiality, but they were sometimes used the other way around.[18]

With regard to bestiality, Leviticus 20:15 of the KJV Bible states: 'And if a man shall lie with a beast, he shall surely be put to death: and ye shall slay the beast'.[19] Accordingly, a person found guilty of the crime of buggery (raping/having carnal knowledge of) animals during the Stuart era would typically be hanged. Thomas Granger, a teenager in Duxbury, Massachusetts, confessed to having raped several different animals: from a cow and a horse, to goats, sheep, and even a turkey.[20] The Plymouth Colony Records show the costs for feeding Granger during his weeks of imprisonment and the fee associated with his execution and those of the 'eight beasts' he had violated.[21] Across the Atlantic ocean, in France, Charlotte-Elisabeth, Duchesse d'Orléans, better known as 'Liselotte', was disgusted by one man at court, whose sexual 'excesses extended onto animals'.[22, 23]

Back in Stuart Britain, in the summer of 1677, the sensational case was brought to trial of a middle-aged married woman who had been observed (by three witnesses through a hole in the wall) having sex with a dog.[24] She was found guilty and sentenced to death. The dog was more than likely also killed.

In Sir John Denham's poem, 'A Relation of the Quaker that to the Shame of his Profession Attempted to Bugger a Mare near Colchester', the titular Quaker not only attempts to 'bugger' the mare, but does so 'by force'.[25]

The Cabinet of Venus Unlocked, and Her Secrets Laid Open (1658) states:

> 'It is very unusual and seldom seen or heard of, that beasts have desired copulation with mankind, whereas, O wickedness! Many men have been convicted and condemned for buggery. Histories make mention of those that have had congression with a goat, and the birth proved as monstrous as the act was unnatural and abominable'.[26]

This last sentence is quite enlightening regarding what Stuart people thought could happen as a result of interspecies sex: the creation of monstrous beings, half-man, half-animal. Indeed, *Aristotle's Masterpiece* (1684), went so far as to include a drawing of a 'Monster half Man and half Dogg' – a creature which the author states was born in 1493 and 'generated of a Woman and a Dogg'.[27] Half-human/half-animal hybrids are a common feature of world mythology and folklore throughout history, but our ancestors believing that copulation between species could create such a creature shows how little they understood about reproductive biology. The idea of producing a monster would have been extremely frightening, and may well have deterred some people away from engaging in a sexual act with an animal had they been that way inclined.

Paedophilia

One of the most unpleasant topics related to sexuality is undoubtedly that of paedophilia in Stuart Britain. According to an account from 1599, there were brothels in London which supplied children aged from *seven to fourteen years old* [28]—and there is no reason to believe that this sort of trade ceased in the age of the Stuarts. Indeed, not much was done to thwart the rise of prostitution during the Jacobean period,[29] and it is reasonable to assume that many of the children born into the world of brothels, became prostitutes themselves from early ages. Even if they were not living in the dark sexual underworld, it was not unheard of for children to be targeted by sexual predators.[30]

This said, the sexual abuse of any female child under ten was considered a felony in Stuart Britain, even if the abuser stated the child had consented before a sexual act.[31]

In May 1677, a seven-year-old girl was believed to have been raped by a schoolmaster, but during the arraignment, the schoolmaster was found guilty of a lesser charge—that of assault.[32] This circumstance seems odd. How could so serious an accusation like the rape of a child become one of simple assault? Was this man's status in the community so high as to allow him get away with a mere slap on the wrist? Or, perhaps, he truly was innocent?

The ambiguity surrounding the previous case is not at all present in the next. In July 1678, an eighteen-year-old apprentice was found guilty of raping a nine-year-old girl and thereby infecting her with a sexually-transmitted disease. For his crime, the man was sentenced to death.[33]

Some literature of the time also features paedophiliac elements. In *The Farce of Sodom, or The Quintessence of Debauchery*, for example, King Bolloximian espies a handsome boy and says, 'Lust with thy beauty cannot brook delay. Between thy pretty haunches I will play'.[34] This notorious play contains a variety of appalling lines and actions, but the dialogue about having sexual relations with, presumably, a child is most unsettling.

François Rabelais' bizarre late sixteenth-century work, *Gargantua*, about a giant's life, was translated from the original French into English by Thomas Urquhart in 1693. In this, there is a brief, yet disturbing, mention of sexual assault against a child when Gargantua (who is younger than five years old) has three governesses who take his penis in their hands and work it up into an erection, then laugh.[35]

Flagellation

Another sexual activity which was frowned upon during the Stuart era was *corporal mortification* (such as whipping or flagellation). Corporal punishment of criminals or misbehaving children was considered normal, but those who practiced this before, or in lieu of, sexual activity were considered deviant. A Late Stuart-era etching entitled 'The Cully Flaug'd' depicts a man bent forward with his buttocks exposed, receiving a birching from a woman who appears to be holding a birch rod in her left hand (a 'rod' was comprised of a bundle of sticks from various trees, such as birch and willow).

In Thomas Shadwell's 1676 play *The Virtuoso*, things get so hot and heavy between the characters Snarl and Mrs. Figgup, that they discover Snarl enjoys being beaten with a rod during sex, because he was so 'used to at Westminster School [he] could never leave it off since', and he 'loved castigation mightily'.[36] Although Mrs Figgup is not keen, they are about to embark on a session of flagellation with rods from nearby curtains but are interrupted by Figgup's incensed brother.

Samuel Butler included a flagellant in his poem, *Hudibras*: 'I felt the blows still ply'd as fast, As if they 'ad been by lovers plac'd'.[37]

Fellatio and cunnilingus

Oral sex strayed from what was considered an acceptable form of sexual activity, but people did it nonetheless—of course, lovers have been doing it throughout history and all over the world. Given the scant documentation, however, there is no way we can know exactly how prevalent this kind of sexual behavior was in Stuart Britain. But the Stuarts—as we've already discovered—had a healthy respect not only for a man's penis, but also for a woman's clitoris, so it is reasonable to assume that lovers pleasured each other in this way.

Most text-based erotic literature of the time did not explicitly mention oral sex acts; but, as stated in the chapter on pornography, there certainly were engravings depicting couples engaged in oral sex. One such engraving was printed in 1690 and depicted man and woman on a luxurious bed in front of an opulent mirror and fireplace in a clearly wealthy bedroom.[38] The woman lies on her back engaging in fellatio on the man, who is above her reciprocating the favour by performing cunnilingus on her—a position now popularly known as '69'.

Sometimes, describing someone as engaging in this type of sexual activity was intended as an insult—as it is today—in those days one term being a 'suck prick'.[39]

John Wilmot, 2nd Earl of Rochester's bawdy satirical poem, *Signior Dildo*, makes a clear point of referring to Charles II's mistress Barbara Palmer's voracious sexual appetite—which, apparently, included a fair amount of fellatio:

'That pattern of virtue Her Grace of Cleveland
Has swallowed more pricks than the ocean has sand'.[40]

In *The Farce of Sodom, or The Quintessence of Debauchery*, the male character and dildo-maker Virtuoso enters a room where he has some unsatisfied female customers. They claim he modelled his substandard dildos on his own penis, but when he reveals his large member to them, they can't control themselves. The character Fuckadilla cries out, 'Oh, let me kiss it—I'll have it in my hand'.[41] The word 'kiss' in this context is likely to mean that she wishes to put it in her mouth and perform fellatio. The stage notes for *Sodom* also indicate that twelve members of the cast are to engage in sexual behaviour with each other, 'the men doing obeisance to women's cunts, kissing and touching them often'.[42]

Next, Nell Gwynn's sexual relationships with lovers was the subject of one lampoon, and the last sentence of this excerpt—'had a lick'—may refer to cunnilingus:

> Distributing her [Nell's] favours very thick,
> And sometimes witty Wilmot had a lick'.[43]

Of course, this could be interpreted in a variety of ways, but sex—in some form or another—is clearly what the author suggests.

Other sexually-deviant proclivities

According to Charles Johnson's 1724 book, *A General History of the Pyrates,* the pirate Blackbeard, whose real name was Edward Teach (c.1680–1718), married a sixteen-year-old girl, consummated the union, and then invited 'five or six of his brutal Companions to come ashore',[44] at which point, 'he would force her to prostitute herself to them all, one after another, before his Face'.[45] If we can take Johnson's word for this, was Blackbeard engaging in what we'd now call voyeurism, in masochism, or was he simply a sadist enjoying watching the degradation of another human being?

Chapter 13

Reproduction, Or, Ye Natural Consequences of Sexual Congress

Childbirth was a key part of Stuart sexuality and, of course, the Stuart lifecycle. The majority of people at this time believed that childbirth was *supposed* to be very painful, because it was woman's eternal punishment for Eve's Original Sin. Nevertheless, no one wants their loved ones to suffer, and herbal remedies—and even certain 'stones' and flowers— were used to try to counteract the pain.

Miscarriage

The experience of having a life inside one's womb, growing to love it as it develops, and then suddenly facing the physical and emotional agony of miscarriage—the death of a foetus during gestation—remains a painful (and surprisingly common[1]) issue for many women; and so it was for our Stuart ancestors. After all, as Mary Astell (1666–1731) wrote: 'our sex are by Nature tender of their own offspring'.[2] During the English Civil Wars, Parliamentarian wife Lucy Hutchinson wrote of a situation which ended in tragedy for one pregnant woman: 'This occasioning some dispute, Cooke the quarter master had utter'd some words, for which they sent for him and cast out greate threates, how they would punish him, which frighted his wife, big with child, in that manner that her child died within her, and her owne life was in great hazard'.[3]

The Englishwoman Alice Thornton (1627–1707) is now best known for her autobiography. In this, she described how, in 1652, she had to walk along a rather difficult path whilst she was almost full term and that this caused her baby so much distress that she suffered a miscarriage: 'this was the first occasion which brought me a great deal of misery, and killed my sweete infant in my wombe'.[4] Following this tragedy, her health deteriorated considerably and she 'fell into a most terrible shaking ague, lasting one quarter of a year, by fits each day twice, in much violency, so that the sweate was great with faintings'.[5]

Pepys explained how, on 7 February 1662–63, 'Ferrers telling me, among other Court passages, how about a month ago, at a ball at Court, a child was dropped by one of the ladies in dancing, but nobody knew who, it being taken up by somebody in their handkercher. The next morning all the Ladies of Honour appeared early at Court for their vindication, so that nobody could tell whose this mischance should be. But it seems Mrs. Wells fell sick that afternoon, and hath disappeared ever since, so that it is concluded it was her'. Mrs Wells, according to the Count of Grammont, was Charles II's mistress at this time, so the child might have been sired by him. Pepys wrote of Wells again later in the month, 'Mrs. Wells do appear at Court again, and looks well; so that, it may be, the late report of laying the dropped child to her was not true'. This observation does not prove she wasn't the mother of the child, since some women can recover quickly following a miscarriage, and even following childbirth.

Labour

A woman in labour would be helped not only by a midwife, but also by 'gossips'. These were other women who would provide encouragement and practical assistance during the painful (and sometimes lengthy) process of giving birth.[6] A Stuart-era woman might use a birthing-chair (a wooden chair with a semi-circular gap between the legs), some may have squatted or knelt upon the floor, whilst others would have lain on their beds. Some birthing chair arms came with handles for the labouring woman to grip during those painful contractions and when pushing.

As for the pain and duration of childbirth, there were recommended herbs and remedies in many of the how-to manuals of the time. Some things certainly didn't work, such as Artalinæ and Clysamiris, which according to Culpeper's *Pharmacopœia Londinensis:* 'being hung about Women, in labor, it causeth speedy deliverance'.[7] It's possible that hanging herbs near a woman might have had a placebo effect, but in all probability it did absolutely nothing to speed up labour. The same can be said of bezoar stones (calculus found in the stomachs of animals), which some Stuart-era people believed were powerful, healing tools to aid labouring women.[8] Gervase Markham recommended that women in difficult labour should drink 'foure spoonfull of another woman's milke' which he thought would cause the child to be 'delivered presently'.[9]

Midwifery

Midwives were an integral part of the Stuart child-birthing scene. Midwifery licenses were issued, not by any medical establishment or institution, but by the Church of England. Evidence suggests that most, if not all, licensed midwives during this period were married or widowed.[10] One of the most well-known books on seventeenth-century midwifery was *The Midwives Book: Or, the Whole Art of Midwifry Discovered* by Jane Sharp, published in 1671. Sharp was the first British woman to write and publish on this subject.

In 1680, *The Complete Midwife's Practice Enlarg'd* was published, which contained a guide for expectant mothers and covered topics including 'By what means parents may get wise children', 'how women with child ought to govern themselves', and 'how to put the womb again into its place'.[11] Of course, many pregnant women today enjoy reading guides for expectant mothers—although the topics may be a little different, we still seek such knowledge from other women!

Midwives were sometimes treated with derision by some male writers of the time. Take for example, Nicholas Culpeper's suggestion that post-partum women can drink birthwort in wine, which 'brings away both Birth and after-birth, and whatsoever a careless Midwife hath left behind'.[12]

Whilst assisting during labour was largely a woman's role during the Stuart period, Jane Sharp and Elizabeth Cellier (also known as the 'Popish Midwife') lamented the fact that women were not able to go to university like men—Cellier even petitioned King James II & VII in 1687 to remedy this situation.[13]

Male midwives often had more scientific training due to their being able to receive formal education in medicine. This resulted in a trend such that by the end of the Stuart period obstetrics became more associated with male doctors than female midwives.[14] Percival Willughby (1596–1685),[15] one of these male midwives, obtained his Doctorate and became a physician as well, but his observations on midwifery—published in 1863—are of particular note here.[16]

In one of his many accounts of childbirth, Willughby recounted the tale of Mary Baker, a penniless vagrant who likely suffered from some type of mental illness.[17] Baker gave birth—on her own—to a baby girl in Derby, England, in the winter of 1667. She appears to not have known what to do with the babe, who lay on the cold floor wailing for milk, warmth, and comfort. The child's cries attracted other people, who promptly helped both mother and child—saving their lives. According to Willughby, a difficult birth 'continueth long, and hath greater pain than ordinary' and 'will afflict four or five days, or longer, and, usually, the child dieth in that time, and sometimes the mother with it'.[18]

In another case, Mr. James Yonge, a physician, wrote to Dr. Hans Sloane in November of 1705 and described a recent—horrific—labour he had attended: a thirty-year-old woman had been in labour for four days with her first child, whose head was too big to pass through the birth canal. Those in attendance were left with the grisly and unenviable task of deciding whether to save the mother's life or let both die. And so, Yonge 'directed my son to open the child's head, and take out the brains, with so much of the skull as he could; and then by a cord fastened round the neck with a noose, to pull it out, which was soon and easily done'.[19] The deceased infant's body was then found to be 'corrupted' and 'stunk much'.[20]

Finally, there is a rather touching letter from a servant in the early seventeenth century to a great lord about the latter's wife, who at the time was in the midst of a difficult labour: 'If there be not health enough in the world for us all, I pray God give them both a liberal portion thereof, and that He let it be abated out of mine'.[21]

Death in Childbirth

Death during childbirth, or due to subsequent infections, was far more common during the Stuart period than it is today. Taking only two examples: Alice Thornton, who survived multiple births, recorded in 1645 the death of her sister during the birth of her sixteenth child, a son named Francis, who survived the trauma of birth.[22] And in mid-December 1599, Joan Apsley died in childbirth, leaving her husband, Richard Boyle (later Earl of Cork), a widower.[23]

If a woman died during childbirth, but the child within her womb still lived, a caesarean section would be performed—but Robert Barret,

Brother of Surgeons Hall, warned: 'a Surgeon must never practice this cruel Operation whilst the mother is alive; but when she is dead, he ought not to neglect it, and what he does, he must do it quickly, because delay will certainly be the Death of the Child'.[24]

Stuart-era breastfeeding

Some Stuart-era midwives recommended that, immediately after birth, babies should be bathed and swaddled and then, just before having their first drink of milk, they should be placed close to the mother's heart. This was believed to draw all the potential evils from the baby through the mother and out with the rest of the discharge and material from her womb.[25] The belief that a baby should lie on his or her mother's chest following birth endures today in the practice of 'skin-to-skin', which is advocated by midwives in the United Kingdom due to the many health benefits associated with this simple act.[26]

Medical texts of the time sometimes cautioned against breastfeeding—especially what we now consider to be the most nutritious milk: colostrum. Why was this? If you recall, we learned that menstruation was considered a filthy part of a woman's being. Breastmilk, by the same token, was sometimes considered to be menstrual blood that had transformed into milk.[27] Colostrum, the thickest and most beneficial breastmilk that comes shortly after giving birth, was thought to have dangerous properties, and another woman's milk was recommended for the first two days.[28]

Most Stuart-era women breastfed their babies themselves. Sometimes, however, a woman's breasts have trouble creating milk, or a sufficient amount thereof, and lactating women wishing to increase their milk supply would seek herbal remedies, including drinking coleworts[29] boiled in strong posset ale.[30] A common problem associated with breastfeeding—even to this day—is chapped and very sore nipples. A remedy for this, recommended in *The English Housewife*, involved using chopped violet leaves boiled in milk or water mixed with wheat bran or wheat breadcrumbs.[31] This mixture would then be applied to the sore breasts.

Wet-nurses were often employed by more aristocratic families even when the mother had no difficulty producing milk. This is rather lamentable, given that modern-day research has concluded that a mother produces milk specifically attuned to her child's needs—this milk helps provide the child with a variety of health benefits, including a strong intestinal microbiome.[32] Even back in the seventeenth century, however, there were those—for example midwife Jane Sharp (1641–1671)—who suspected as much, and did not agree with the practice of women unnecessarily giving their babies away to other women to nurse.[33]

Elizabeth Clinton, dowager Countess of Lincoln, who had given birth to eighteen children,[34] also expressed her opposition to this trend, stating in her 1622 work, *The Countesse of Lincolnes Nurserie*: 'Oh impious, and impudent unthankfullnesse; yea monstrous unnaturalnesse, both to their own natural fruit borne so neare their breasts, and fed in their owne wombs, and yet may not be suffered to sucke their owne milke'.[35] Clinton felt that women had both a religious and a moral duty to breastfeed their babies, and she was not alone in this belief. Others, including many Puritans agreed that the feeding of a baby was the mother's responsibility.[36]

In a similar vein, the English nonconformist minister Henry Newcome's pamphlet *The Compleat Mother* (1695) urged women to reconsider using a wet-nurse and to feed their babies themselves: 'Look on your own Breasts, which soon after the Birth spring full of Milk. Did Nature intend no more in this, but to put you to the trouble of drying them?'[37] Newcome, like Clinton before him, argued that to refrain from feeding one's own child was an affront not only to nature but also to one's religious duty.

These considerations aside, the more aristocratic a lady was, the more likely she would be to employ a wet-nurse.[38] 'Thou hast sucked wisdom from thy teat',[39] says the Nurse in Shakespeare's *Romeo and Juliet*. The fictional Juliet has a closer bond to her nurse than to her own mother, with whom Juliet has a much more formal and distant relationship. This makes sense, for in such a noble household, Juliet would often have been in the company of her nurse—who would have nurtured and loved her as if she were her own daughter.

How did a woman become a wet-nurse? Fairly typically, in an age of high child mortality, Juliet's nurse had lost her own daughter, Susan. A bereaved mother still produces milk, and when the wealthy Capulet family sought a wet-nurse, she found employment. Choosing a suitable wet-nurse was a big decision—and even the prospective hire's physical attributes were taken into consideration. Sinibaldi, for example, stated that blonde women were more wanton than brown-haired women.

'Physicians advise to choose a nurse that's brown (haired), for by her temperate natural heat, she breeds good milk'.[40]

Whilst the babe was nursed by a wet-nurse, the still-lactating new mother would take measures to dry up her own supply of milk.[41] To help achieve this, *The English House-wife* (1631) recommended warming a mixture of red sage and wine vinegar in a flat dish over hot coals, soaking brown paper in this, and then applying this paper across the breasts.[42] In normal cases, however, Stuart women would seek to stop their lactation as their baby was weaned onto solid foods,[43] or following the death of a nursing child. And, of course, after a while without having been sucked, milk production gradually comes to a halt naturally.

Child mortality

Throughout the history of mankind, the great joys inherent in parenthood have often been cut short by tragedy with the death of offspring. There is a terrible myth that suggests that parents somehow managed to love their children less in the past because they didn't wish to become attached to them, knowing how likely they were to die. This cannot be further from the truth. Life wasn't cheap, and people felt the death of a loved one just as acutely as we do today—there are countless examples of bereaved Stuart-era parents who were horribly devastated by the death of a child.

After 'six fits of a quartan ague...died my dear son, Richard' wrote John Evelyn on the 27 January, 1657/8. His son had been five years old and a source of great pride and happiness for his father. The pages Evelyn devoted to remembering Richard make for an extremely moving read. He concluded with the heartrending sentence, 'Here ends the joy of my life, and for which I go even mourning to the grave'.[44] Even worse, only a few days later, on 15 of February, 1658, another of Evelyn's sons, George, also died. And in an entry dated 26 March, 1664, sorrows once again came to the Evelyn household. A clearly heartbroken John Evelyn states that his healthy one-month-old son, another Richard, died suddenly. He and his wife suspected that the child's nurse had accidentally smothered, or 'overlain him; to our extreme sorrow, being now again reduced to one: but God's will be done'.[45] It's important to note how Evelyn took this tragedy as being the will of God; this belief no doubt helped to comfort the bereaved.

A moving Stuart-era letter of condolence was sent from one anonymous gentleman to his friend after the loss of the latter's only son: 'It is in no power of mine, to give you any solid comfort in this great loss of yours, but the good God of Heaven, both can, and will completely do it'.[46] Again, we see the power of Christianity as a source of comfort.

Thomas Browne, a respected English writer and physician, married Dorothy Mileham in 1641, and the couple had eleven children—only five of whom survived into adulthood.[47] Staunch royalists during the English/British Civil Wars Richard and Ann Fanshawe, had a staggering twenty-three children together—only three of whom survived.[48] It is difficult to even imagine how these people must have felt, losing so many of their children.

The renowned Early Stuart-era dramatist, Ben Jonson, and his wife, Anne, also suffered from the loss of their children, and the grief inspired two poems. A daughter named Mary was the sad theme of 'On My First Daughter': 'at six months she parted hence With safety of her innocence'.[49] Next, a son, who died aged seven, was the impetus behind 'On My First Sonne':

> 'Farewell, thou child of my right hand, and joy,
> My sin was too much hope of thee, lov'd boy:
> Seven years thou wert lent to me, and I thee pay...'[50]

The reference to Jonson's 'sin' again shows how Stuart-people believed that hardships and bereavements were punishment from God for personal moral failures and sins.

Frances and Henry Purcell, the greatest English Baroque composer of the seventeenth century, lost their first-born child in 1681, which would have undoubtedly been a blow to the young couple.[51]

Major Stuart-era political intrigante, Lucy Hay, Countess of Carlisle, had one child, a son, who was born in 1618—a year after her wedding to James Hay. This child died approximately one month after his birth—and Lucy is not known to have become pregnant again.[52] The poetess Aemelia Lanier (1569–1645) had a daughter named Odillya who lived less than a year after her birth in 1598.[53]

The Great Plague of London in 1665 also affected a huge number of people, and few who were born at this time survived.[54] Smallpox was yet another disease which took the lives of many children, as well as adults, and John and Elizabeth Lilburne lost both of their sons to it—a tragedy which John (who had been incarcerated in the Tower of London) regarded as worse than his imprisonment.[55]

Illegitimate children

Illegitimate children, also known as bastards, were often more delicately referred to during this period as 'natural' children. Illegitimacy was very much looked down upon, however, and the rate of children being born out of wedlock was very low[56] compared with Europe in the twenty-first century in which it is now common for unwed persons to have children.[57]

Gossip could be a problem, and even a married pregnant woman wasn't necessarily immune from malicious speculation. In a letter dated 27 March 1648, Robert Baillie informed his cousin, Reverend Spang, about his concerns over the moral character of a woman of his acquaintance: 'Try, with all the diligence you can, who that Jean Dalyell, spouse to James Reid, can be, who got a testimonial from the ministers of Gorcome of the birth of her son. I deadly suspect she is a whore who is retired to bear her child to some man of quality near us: it were good to find out'.[58] One is apt to wonder what about her behaviour (or perhaps appearance) caused Baillie to think her a 'whore'.

In Autumn of 1638, Thomas Boardman and his wife, Luce, were accused of having begotten their child out of wedlock—a charge to which they confessed. Thomas was 'severely whipt' and the heavily pregnant Luce's punishment was, 'to be censured when she is delivered, as the Bench shall think fit'.[59] In Chester County, Pennsylvania, Elinor Arme of Springfield was presented before the court in November 1692 for 'being with child and having no husband'.[60] In a harsher sentence for a similar crime (though these two were not married, apparently), Thomas Poe and Sarah Buller went before the court in January 1693, 'and the court gave Judgement that the said Thomas and Sarah do stand at the Common whipping post and for the officer to declare their offence to the People'.[61] Classic public humiliation, which perhaps worked to persuade would-be fornicators from following the same path.

Other men, however, refused to accept the fact that a child was on the way. In 1637, a curate got his mother's maidservant pregnant (who knows if their sexual relationship was consensual or not?). Considering the social and legal consequences of premarital sex and having an illegitimate child, the maidservant was naturally frightened, and she informed the curate of her condition. He told her not to tell anyone and to meet him the next day, which she did. But instead of meeting him by herself, she brought along her sister, in whom she had also confided. Angered by this, the curate refused to talk to her and told her to meet him alone that evening instead. The next morning, the pregnant woman was found dead, having been strangled with her own apron strings—and 'someone had had the use of her before or after her strangling'.[62] In other words, the corpse showed signs that someone had copulated with her before—or after—her murder.

Sometimes, however, illegitimate children could overcome the state into which they were born, and flourish. Take, for example, Frederick Nassau-Zuylenstein, an illegitimate son of Frederick Henry and Margaretha Catharina Bruyns, a mayor's daughter. Frederick was given the post of governor for the young William III, Prince of Orange (who later became King William III of England).[63]

Sir William Davenant, a popular playwright and poet, claimed to have been William Shakespeare's 'natural'—*viz.* illegitimate—son.[64] His biographer, William Winstanley, omitted any mention of Shakespeare in his entry on Davenant,[65] and this connection to the Bard was probably just wishful thinking on Davenant's part.

Born in 1682, Henrietta Crofts was the illegitimate daughter of the equally illegitimate James Scott, Duke of Monmouth, and his mistress, Eleanor Needham. Despite being the bastard daughter of a bastard son of King Charles II, she nevertheless married well and became the Duchess of Bolton.

George Howard (1622–1677) was the illegitimate child of Lady Howard and probably her servant, George Cuttford. His mother had been separated from her husband for eighteen months before his birth, so his illegitimacy seems likely. Despite this, Howard went on to become MP for Tavistock.[66]

Chapter 14

Rape, Abortion, and Infanticide

Rape, or a sexual act performed as a result of force or coercion, is the unsavoury topic of this section. During the Stuart era the word 'rape' also had other, non-sexual meanings: throughout documents of the period there are references to the Lewes 'rape', Hastings 'rape', Pevensey 'rape', Chichester 'rape', Arundel 'rape', and the Bramber 'rape'—these were actually ancient divisions of land in the county of Sussex. Pity the poor people who had Rape as their surname, too—a Balthazar Rape was listed as the plaintiff in a lawsuit against John Chambers in 1660.[1]

The terms 'rape' and 'ravish' could be used interchangeably, both meaning to forcibly abduct someone.[2] For example, in Alice Thornton's autobiography, she stated: 'the great deliverance I had from a *rape* by Captain Innis, a Scot, who did swear to *ravish* me from my dear mother's ground; but his own servant that I cured a wound did discover it to me, and I was saved'.[3] Thornton previously wrote that she was delivered from 'the violence of a rape by Jeremy Smithson'.[4]

What constituted a rape in Stuart Britain? Straight from Michael Dalton, an English barrister who lived from 1564–1644:

> 'If a Man take away a Maid by Force and ravish her, and after she giveth her consent and marrieth him, yet it is a Rape. Ravishment here taken in one and the same signification with Rape, which is the Violent Deflowering of a Woman, or carnal Knowledge had of the body of a Woman against her Will'.[5]

Following a rape, Dalton continues, a woman had to seek help from 'credible persons' and make a legal complaint within forty days of the attack.[6] If she took longer, she had no case. Furthermore, if a rape victim became pregnant, this would be taken as her having given her consent and she could no longer claim to have been raped.[7]

During the reign of William III (1694–1702), a John Tayler was convicted for the rape of Sophia Page, who was the daughter of Sir Gregory Page.[8] Sophia's privileged social status no doubt worked in her favour—had she been a scullery maid, her assailant might never have been convicted.

Rape, along with other horrors, was common during the English Civil Wars.[9] We will never be able to determine how many people were raped during this tumultuous period, but the accounts that exist make for disturbing reading.

Abortion

Among all the possible consequences of copulation, the greatest and most life-changing is surely that of conceiving a child. Whilst raising children is arguably one of the supreme joys a human can experience, throughout history there have been women, who, for one reason or another, did not want to have the child they conceived. This is still a very controversial issue, bound up with rights and morality of the mother, the father, and the child. During the Stuart period, women sometimes sought to abort their child due to the intense stigma surrounding conception outside wedlock, especially if the child was conceived as a result of adultery, incest, or rape, due to economic concerns—or, in some cases, because of a psychological fear of childbirth.

It is known that women (and sometimes the men who fathered the baby) would seek assistance from apothecaries or cunning women who claimed to have a good knowledge of herbs in order to cause miscarriage and expel the unwanted child from the womb.[10] Although frowned upon by Stuart culture in general, herbal remedies which may have had abortifacient effects were described in some of the popular household literature of the day. According to Gervase Markham, Water of Rew, 'drunk at morning and at night, at each time an ounce, it provoketh the termes in women'.[11] If a herb could cause menstruation in a woman who was late, surely it could also potentially have abortifacient properties? In *The New London Dispensatory* (1702), Turbith or Turpethi—a drug made from the root *Operculina turpethum*—was considered dangerous for pregnant women to consume,[12] so may have been used in an attempt to induce abortion. But such measures could harm not only the child, but the mother as well.

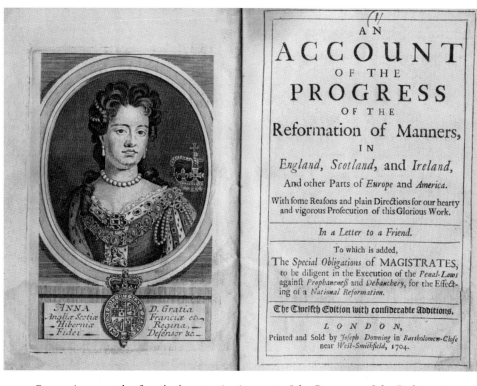

Queen Anne on the frontispiece to *An Account of the Progress of the Reformation of Manners*, (Joseph Downing, London, 1704). The Seventeenth Century Lady Archives.

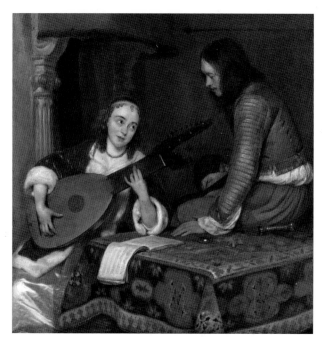

A Woman Playing the Theorbo-Lute and a Cavalier, c.1658, Gerard ter Borch the Younger. Bequest of Benjamin Altman, 1913. (Courtesy of Metropolitan Museum of Art, NYC, under Creative Commons CC0 1.0, www.metmuseum.org).

Right: *Portrait of Arnold Joost van Keppel*, 1712-1713. (Courtesy of the Rijksmuseum, Amsterdam, under CC0 1.0 Universal (CC0 1.0), http://hdl. handle.net).

Below left: *Queen Anne*, 1702, John Smith, after Sir Godfrey Kneller. (Yale Center for British Art, Gift of John Hay Whitney, Yale BA 1926, Yale MA (HON.) 1956, transfer from the Yale University Library and the Yale University Art Gallery, http:// collections.britishart.yale.edu).

Below right: *Sarah Churchill, 1ˢᵗ Duchess of Marlborough,* 1746. The Seventeenth Century Lady Archives.

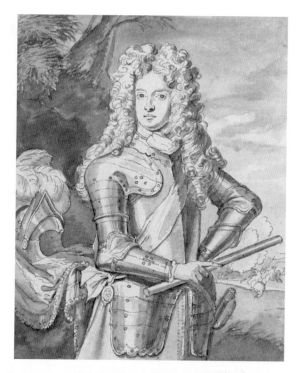

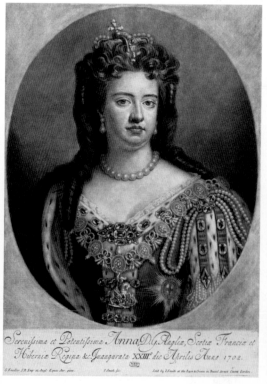

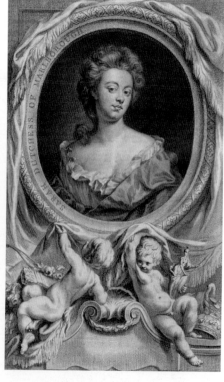

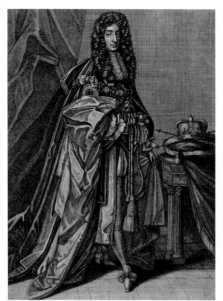 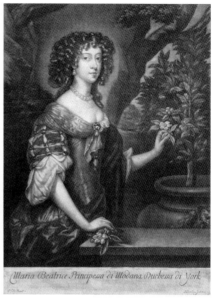

Above left: *King James II; table with a crown in the background*, engraving by P. Landry, 1693. (Wellcome Collection, CC BY 4.0, https://wellcomecollection.org).

Above right: *Portrait of Maria Beatrice of Modena*, engraved by Abraham Bloteling, after Peter Lely (Sir), 1673-1690. (Courtesy of the Rijksmuseum, Amsterdam, under CC0 1.0 Universal (CC0 1.0), http://hdl.handle.net).

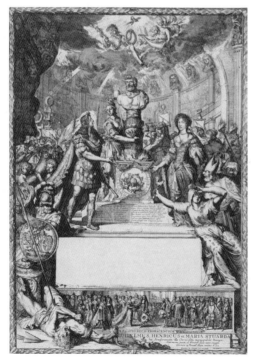

Allegory on the marriage of Willem III and Mary Stuart, engraving, 1677. (Courtesy of the Rijksmuseum, Amsterdam, under CC0 1.0 Universal (CC0 1.0), http://hdl.handle.net).

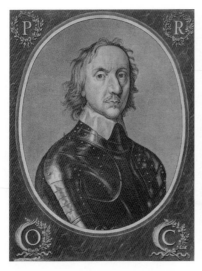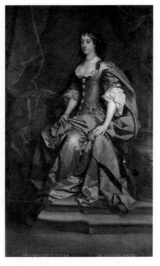

Above left: *Oliver Cromwell,* after 1653, Jan van de Velde IV. (Courtesy of Metropolitan Museum of Art, NYC, under Creative Commons CC0 1.0, www. metmuseum.org).

Above right: *Barbara Palmer, Duchess of Cleveland.* (Courtesy of Metropolitan Museum of Art, NYC, under Creative Commons CC0 1.0).

Below left: *Charles II (1630-1685), King of England*, style of Samuel Cooper (British, probably after 1672). Bequest of Millie Bruhl Fredrick, 1962. (Courtesy of Metropolitan Museum of Art, NYC, under Creative Commons CC0 1.0, www.metmuseum.org).

Below right: Queen Catherine, Charles II's long-suffering wife.
  Title: *Catherine of Braganza, 1661*, etching, by Wenceslaus Hollar, Bohemian. Courtesy of Metropolitan Museum of Art, NYC, under Creative Commons CC0 1.0. https://www.metmuseum.org/art/collection/search/412446

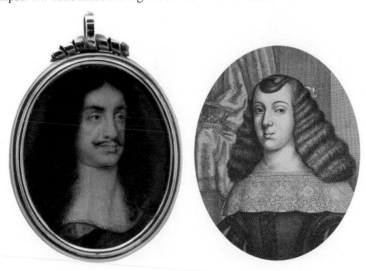

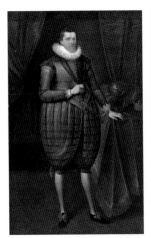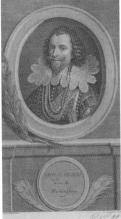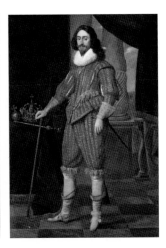

Above left: James I of England (James VI of Scotland), 1618, attributed to Paul can Somer, c.1576-1621. (Yale Center for British Art, Paul Mellon Fund, http://collections.britishart.yale.edu).

Above Middle: George Villiers, 1st Duke of Buckingham, undated. Ch. Imonneau. (Yale Center for British Art, Paul Mellon Collection, http://collections.britishart.yale.edu).

Above right: King Charles I was a man who enjoyed sex, but unlike many other members of his family, he was almost impeccably faithful.
 Charles I, King of England,1629, Daniël Mijtens. (Courtesy of Metropolitan Museum of Art, NYC, under Creative Commons CC0 1.0, www.metmuseum.org).

Below: King Charles I of England with his wife Henrietta Maria of Bourbon, Robert van Voerst, after Anthony van Dyck, 1634. (Courtesy of the Rijksmuseum, Amsterdam, under CC0 1.0 Universal (CC0 1.0), http://hdl.handle.net).

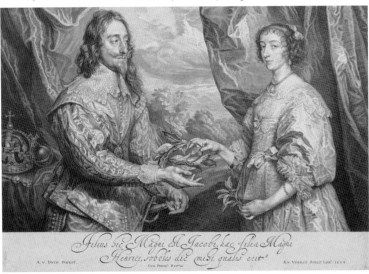

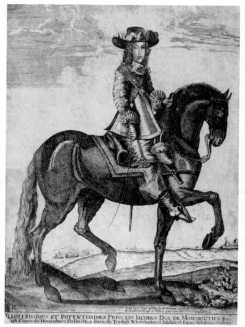
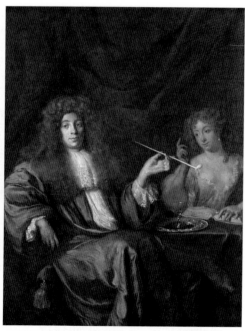

Above left: *Duke of Monmouth as a Boy*, between 1673 and 1685. Print made by Francis Barlow, c.1626-1704. (Yale Center for British Art, Gift of John Hay Whitney, Yale BA 1926, Yale MA (HON.) 1956, transfer from the Yale University Library and the Yale University Art Gallery, http://collections.britishart.yale.edu).

Above right: *Portrait of Adriaan van Beverland, Writer of Theological Works and Satirist, with a Prostitute*, Ary de Vois, c.1675. (F.G. Waller Bequest, Amsterdam).

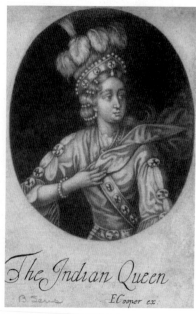

Print made by Bernard Lens, 1659–1725, The Indian Queen, 1680-1690s. (Yale Center for British Art, Paul Mellon Fund, http://collections. britishart.yale.edu).

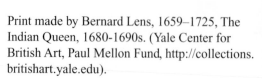

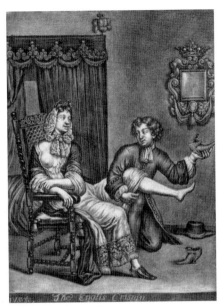
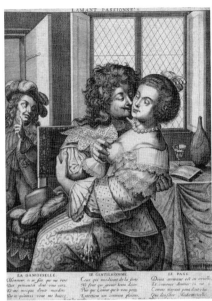

Above left: *The Englis Crispin*, Jan van Somer, 1655-1700. (Courtesy of the Rijksmuseum, Amsterdam, under CC0 1.0 Universal (CC0 1.0), http://hdl.handle.net).

Above right: *Minnekozende jongeman en vrouw in interieur (een herberg of bordeel?)*, purchased with the support of the F.G. Waller-Fonds. (Courtesy of the Rijksmuseum, Amsterdam, under CC0 1.0 Universal (CC0 1.0), http://hdl.handle.net).

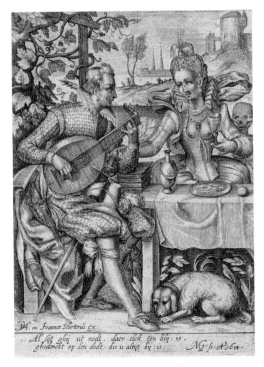

Paartje aan een tafel (Pair at a table). Nicolaes van Geelkercken, after Pieter Feddes van Harlingen, 1614. (Courtesy of the Rijksmuseum, Amsterdam, under CC0 1.0 Universal (CC0 1.0), http://hdl.handle.net).

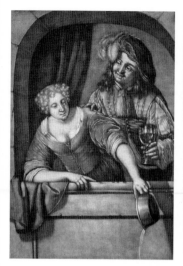

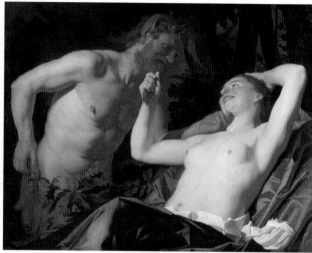

Above left: *Young Man and Woman Leaning out of Window*, print made by Pieter Schenck, 1660-1719, after Jacob Ochtervelt. (Yale Center for British Art, Paul Mellon Fund, http://collections.britishart.yale.edu).

Above right: *Satyr and Nymph*, Gerard van Honthorst, 1623. (Courtesy of the Rijksmuseum, Amsterdam, under CC0 1.0 Universal (CC0 1.0), http://hdl.handle.net).

Right: *Amor en Psyche*, Jacob Matham, after Abraham Bloemaert, 1607. (Courtesy of the Rijksmuseum, Amsterdam, under CC0 1.0 Universal (CC0 1.0), http://hdl.handle.net).

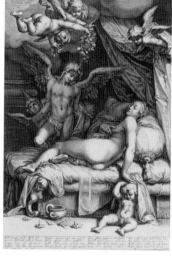

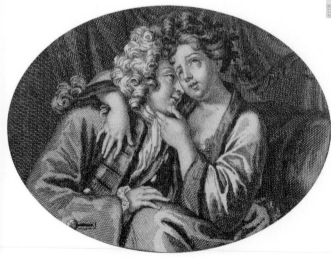

Paar dat elkaar omhelst (Couple hugging each other), Bernard Picart, 1683-1733. (Courtesy of the Rijksmuseum, Amsterdam, under CC0 1.0 Universal (CC0 1.0), http://hdl.handle.net).

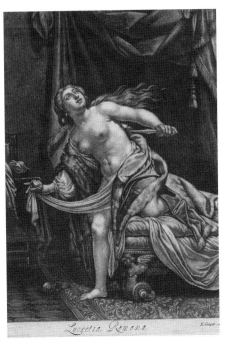

The rape of the noblewoman, Lucretia, in Ancient Rome was a subject which again was popular in literature (Shakespeare's Rape of Lucrece) and in art. Lucretia, the victim of rape, was seen as heroic when she commits suicide.

Lucretia Romana, between 1678 and 1717. Print made by William Faithorne, 1656-c. 1701. (Yale Center for British Art, Paul Mellon Fund, http://collections. britishart.yale.edu).

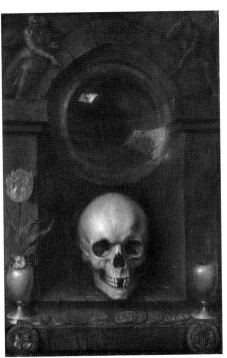

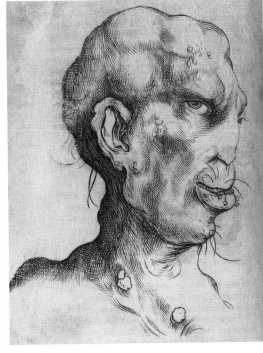

Above left: *Vanitas Still Life*, 1603, by Jacques de Gheyn II. (www.metmuseum.org).

Above right: *Head illustrating symptoms of syphilis*. Engraving, 1632. (Wellcome Collection, CC BY 4.0, https://wellcomecollection.org).

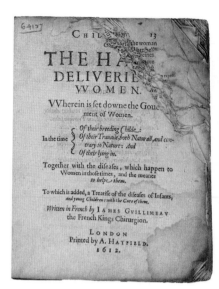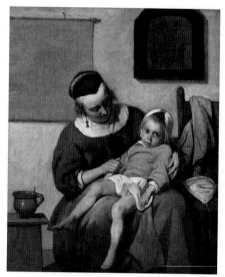

Above left: Titlepage: *Childbirth, or the happie deliverie of women*. (Wellcome Collection, CC BY 4.0, https://wellcomecollection.org).

Above right: *The Sick Child*, Gabriël Metsu, c.1664-c.1666. (Courtesy of the Rijksmuseum, Amsterdam, under CC0 1.0 Universal (CC0 1.0), http://hdl.handle.net).

Below left: *A Gypsy Mother with Three Children*, 1650s. Cornelis Visscher. Purchase, Director's Fund and Clement C. Moore Gift, 2016. (Courtesy of Metropolitan Museum of Art, NYC, under Creative Commons CC0 1.0, www.metmuseum.org).

Below right: The subject of rape or abduction was a popular subject, both in Stuart-era artwork and as a plot device for plays.
Roof van een Sabijnse vrouw, vooraanzicht (Rape of a Sabine woman, front view), Jan Harmensz. Muller, after Adriaen de Vries, 1596-1600. (http://hdl.handle.net).

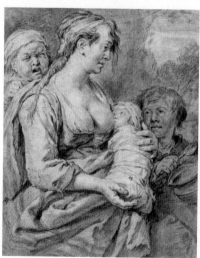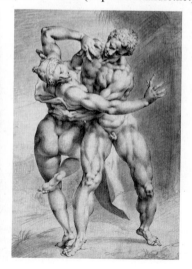

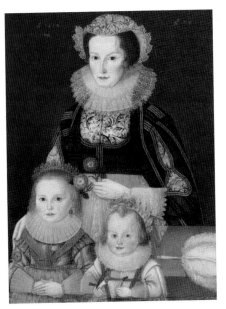 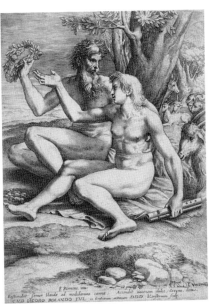

Above left: *A Lady and Her Two Children*, 1624, unknown artist. (Yale Center for British Art, Paul Mellon Collection, http://collections.britishart.yale.edu).

Above right: *Two Nude Shepherds*, 17th century, Lucas Vorsterman I., Joseph Pulitzer Bequest, 1917. (Courtesy of Metropolitan Museum of Art, NYC, under Creative Commons CC0 1.0, www.metmuseum.org).

Below: Sheep and goats under a tree, Charles II Errard (attributed to), 1616 - 1689 http://hdl.handle.net/10934/RM0001.COLLECT.108488

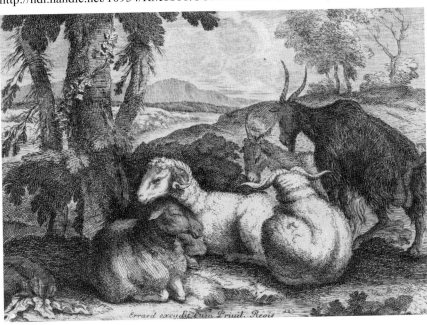

Unwanted advances go back to the dawn of civilisation. The Biblical tale of Susannah and the Elders is an example of this, and the story resonated with Early Modern people and was often recreated in art during the period.

Susannah and the Elders by Johann Carl Loth, 1632-1698. (Digital image courtesy of the Getty's Open Content Program, www.getty.edu).

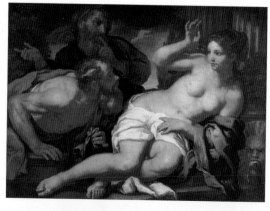

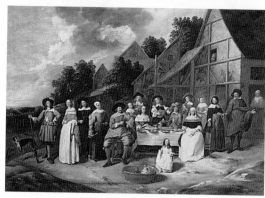

Stuart-era marriage provided the only legal and socially/morally permissible route for a couple to have sex and children. *Group Portrait: A Wedding Celebration*, Gillis van Tilborgh. (Courtesy of Metropolitan Museum of Art, NYC, under Creative Commons CC0 1.0, www.metmuseum.org).

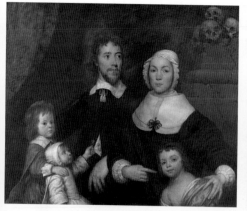

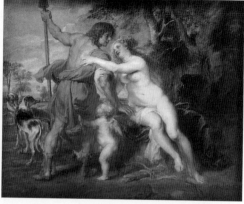

Above left: Portrait of a Family, Probably that of Richard Streatfeild, c.1645, William Dobson, 1611-1646. (Yale Center for British Art, Paul Mellon Collection http://collections.britishart.yale.edu).

Above right: Venus and Adonis, probably mid-1630s, Peter Paul Rubens. (Courtesy of Metropolitan Museum of Art, NYC, under Creative Commons CC0 1.0, www.metmuseum.org).

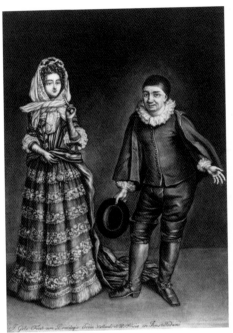
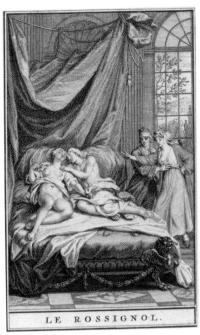

LE ROSSIGNOL.

Above left: Raymond Poisson was one of the leading French actors of his day, and also one of the founders of the Comédie-Française in 1680. Here he is with an unknown actress.

Title: Raymond Poisson en een actrice (Raymond Poisson and an actress), Jacob Gole, 1670-1724.(Courtesy of the Rijksmuseum, Amsterdam, under CC0 1.0 Universal (CC0 1.0), http://hdl.handle.net).

Above right: Young couple caught by parents, Bernard Picart, 1683-1733 (http://hdl.handle.net).

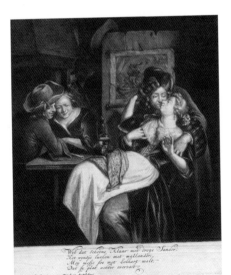

Love Scene. Print made by Jacob Gole, 1660-1737, after unknown artist. (Courtesy Yale Center for British Art, Paul Mellon Fund, http://collections. britishart.yale.edu).

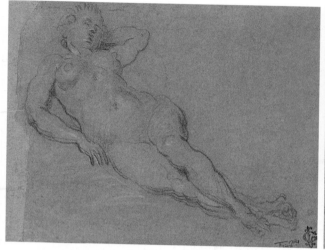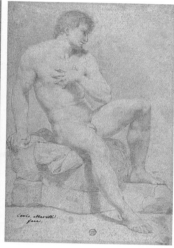

Above left: *Reclining Female Nude*, early 17th century, Domenico Tintoretto, Robert Lehman Collection, 1975. (Courtesy of Metropolitan Museum of Art, NYC, under Creative Commons CC0 1.0. www.metmuseum.org.

Above right: *Nude Male Figure,*1625-1713, ascribed to Carlo Maratti, gift of Cephas G. Thompson, 1887. (Courtesy of Metropolitan Museum of Art, NYC, under Creative Commons CC0 1.0. www.metmuseum.org).

Below: *Brothel Scene*, Wallerant Vaillant, after Gerard Pietersz. van Zijl, 1658-1677. (Courtesy of the Rijksmuseum, Amsterdam, under CC0 1.0, Universal (CC0 1.0), http://hdl.handle.net).

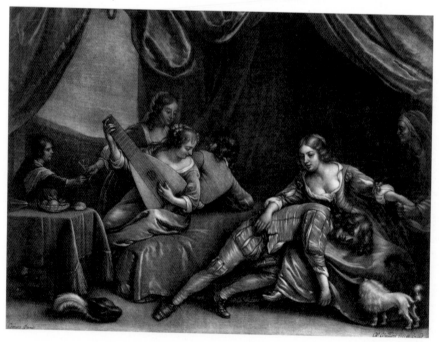

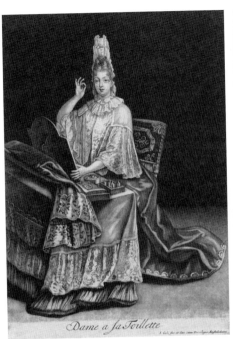

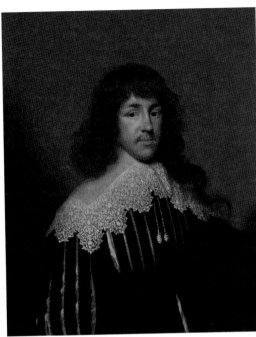

Above left: This elegant woman is wearing a towering fontange headdress, and is applying face patches, also known as 'mouches'. *Lady at her Dressing Table,* Jacob Gole, c.1690-early 18th century. (Courtesy of the Rijksmuseum, Amsterdam, under CC0 1.0 Universal (CC0 1.0), http://hdl.handle.net).

Above right: The man in this portrait is sporting a lovelock; very much in style among the fashionable and lambasted by the likes of William Prynne. *Portrait of a Man, probably Sir Francis Godolphin,* 1633, Cornelius Johnson, 1593-1661. (Yale Center for British Art, Paul Mellon Collection, http://collections.britishart.yale.edu).

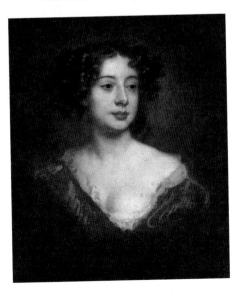

Study for a Portrait of a Woman, 1670s, Sir Peter Lely (Pieter van der Faes), Rogers Fund, 1906. (Courtesy of Metropolitan Museum of Art, NYC, under Creative Commons CC0 1.0, www.metmuseum.org).

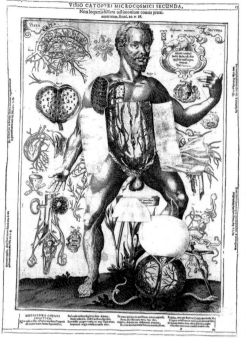

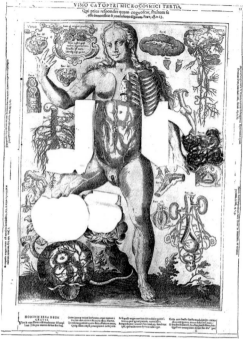

Above left: J. Remmelin, 1660: Male anatomy. (Wellcome Collection, CC BY 4.0, https://wellcomecollection.org).

Above right: J. Remmelin, 1660: Female anatomy. (Wellcome Collection, CC BY4.0, https://wellcomecollection.org).

Below: *Hermaphrodite*,1639. Giovanni Francesco Susini. (Gift of Mr and Mrs Claus von Bülow, 1977, courtesy of Metropolitan Museum of Art, NYC, under Creative Commons CC0 1.0, www.metmuseum.org).

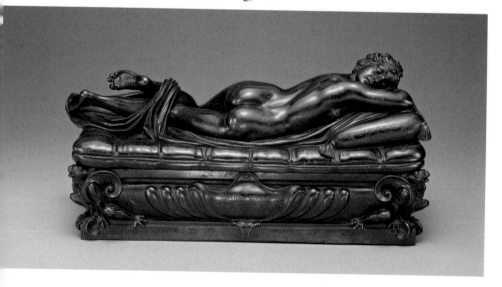

Infanticide

'We detest the Wickedness and Cruelty of a poor Wretch,
who to hide her Shame strangles her Bastard'[13]
— The Compleat Mother (1695)

There are, sadly, many examples of infanticide, or the murdering of
children, throughout the Stuart period, and some disturbing examples
are forthcoming in this section.

Although sexual activity outside of marriage was statistically rare,[14]
infanticide nevertheless became problematic, even in the early part of
this period, and new legislation—the Infanticide Act of 1624—was
passed in order to 'prevent the Destroying and Murdering of Bastard
Children'.[15] Indeed, it appears to have been common for those women
who had babies out of wedlock to murder the baby, hide the body, and, if
found, claim the baby had been born dead.[16] According to *The Countrey
Justice*, an influential Stuart-era legal manual, if a woman was discovered
to have drowned or otherwise killed her bastard child, she would be as
guilty as any other murderer.[17] If she claimed that her child had been
stillborn, she would need witnesses to vouch for the veracity of her
claim—but she would be unlikely to be able to do this, given that unwed
pregnancy was seen as a legal and moral crime.

*The Bloudy Mother, Or, The Most Inhumane Murthers, Committed
by Jane Hattersley*, published in 1610, describes the history of a serving
maid named Jane Hattersley who was seduced and impregnated by
her employer, Adam Adamson. Jane was sent away and gave birth to a
healthy child who she then killed, probably by smothering. She returned
to Adamson, and the two continued their illicit liaison, resulting in
more pregnancies, births, and Jane's murder of these infants, too. The
orchard where she had interred the bodies of three of her child-victims
was searched, the remains discovered, and Hattersley was found guilty
and hanged in 1609.[18] This story, though shocking, was by no means an
isolated case. Maidservants were considered fair game by dishonourable
male employers and there are numerous accounts of servants having
been impregnated by their masters.[19]

Abigall Hill, of St. Olaves, Southwark, was entrusted with caring for
and nursing poor parish children—a duty for which she was paid. Four of
these infants were found to have been murdered by her—the very person

who was supposed to be looking out for their well-being. Hill managed to avoid suspicion for some time, but eventually her crimes were discovered and she was executed in Cheapside on 22 December 1658.[20]

In July of 1648, an enquiry was held into the brutal murder of a four-year-old girl, Martha Clark, in the colony of New Plymouth. Her throat had been cut so deeply it had severed her windpipe. The confessed murderer was none other than the little girl's mother, Allis Bishop.[21] In a time when motherhood was so integral to a woman's role in society and personal identity, what could have compelled this mother to commit such a bloody deed against her own child? After questioning by authorities, Bishop confessed and showed some remorse. She was eventually executed by hanging for her crime.

Premarital sex, along with adultery and infanticide, are the combined themes of our next example. Mary Martin was an unmarried English twenty-one-year-old maidservant who embarked upon an affair with a married man. It's not clear who the man was, but by 1646 Martin arrived in Boston, pregnant. She kept her pregnancy a secret and eventually gave birth to a healthy child... whom she proceeded to smother. When this was not fatal, she—even more horrendously—battered the child to death.[22]

In the summer of 1679, a Katherine Tumince was found guilty and sentenced to death for the murder of her baby boy—whom she had left under a pile of rubbish in an attic.[23] Later, in 1683, Elizabeth Neal was found guilty and sentenced to death for murdering her infant son by strangulation.[24] A further two years later, in 1685, Katherine Brown was found guilty of killing her new-born child by drowning it in a brook.[25] Also, a number of women gave birth to their children and then disposed of them in a 'House of Office' or a privy or toilet, causing—horrifically—the newborns to die choking on the filth of human effluence. This was the manner in which Frances Boddyman disposed of her newborn son in 1695.[26]

What did these women have in common? They all had given birth to illegitimate children. While their deeds are abhorrent, most of the woman were probably not inhuman monsters, but were rather in a state of utter despair and desperation, fearing the shame and punishment which was sure to follow, and the bleak prospects of ever being able to provide for their children.

Chapter 15

Sexually Transmitted Diseases: Or, Ye Curse Upon Fornicators!

We might wonder whether the average sexually-active Stuart-era person worried at all about sexually transmitted diseases. Well, they did—especially if they frequented brothels or engaged in casual sex with more than one sexual partner.[1] So whilst people would have a merry old time rolling in the hay, they sometimes shared more than bodily fluids and sexual pleasure, and ended up getting much more than they bargained for.

Venereal diseases are infections that are passed from one sexual partner to another. They have been a nasty consequence of sex for many centuries and are one of the reasons why promiscuity was looked down upon. Venereal disease, wrote Stuart-era chirurgeon Richard Wiseman, is 'a venomous contagious Disease gotten either Immediately or Mediately from an impure Coition'.[2]

Common sexually transmitted infections of the Stuart era included gonorrhoea, syphilis (French or Spanish 'pox'), herpes, genital warts, and pubic lice. Then, just as now, promiscuous people were more likely to contract a sexually transmitted disease. However, though the stigma of venereal diseases was combined with the stigma associated with promiscuity, a person could have sex with only one partner and still be unfortunate enough to contract an STD—as eighteenth-century author Phil-Porney wrote in *A Modest Defence of Publick Stews*:

'Men give it to their Wives, Women to their Husbands, or perhaps their Children; they to their Nurses, and the Nurses again to other Children; so that no Age, Sex, or Condition can be entirely free from the Infection'.[3]

Gonorrhoea

Gonorrhoea, popularly known as 'the clap', is very easily transmitted from one person to another via unprotected vaginal, oral, or anal sex.[4] Again, according to Richard Wiseman:

> 'when a man hath had to do with an impure woman, either he hath some heat of inflammation on the Penis with excoriation, which ariseth soon after coition, and is caused by the affliction of a virulent humour, or else he finds a heat in his Urine, and in a day, two or three, a Gonorrhoea or issuing of virulent matter out of the seminal vessels through the urethra'.[5]

Gonorrhoea, akin to many other STDs, includes symptoms which affect both men and women, such as a 'burning' pain while urinating and discharge from the penis or vagina[6]—which may have led people to assume that they had a urinary tract infection (which could nevertheless be fatal during the Stuart period if the infection spread to the kidneys). Gonorrhoea was very dangerous for pregnant women since it could cause miscarriage and, even if that didn't happen, the bacteria could cause permanent damage to the child's vision.[7]

Of course, the Stuarts didn't have antibiotics at their disposal, but suggestions for the treatment of Gonorrhoea were available in many herbal remedy books of the time. William Salmon's *Pharmacopœia Londinensis: Or, The New London Dispensatory* (1702) suggested that Gonorrhoea could be treated with a drink made from *Iris Florentina* mixed with vinegar.[8]

John Wilmot, 2nd Earl of Rochester—one of the most infamous seventeenth-century hedonists—had a solution for when he wanted the services of a prostitute but worried about contracting a venereal disease: 'I send for my whore, when for fear of a clap, I spend in her hand, and I spew in her lap'.[9] In other words, he opted for a 'hand-job' and ejaculated on her lap. Later in the same poem, however, he has no such qualms when he has sex with (or anally rapes?) his page.[10]

Syphilis

Syphilis is believed to have been brought to Europe from the New World by conquering Europeans[11] (who also took smallpox to the Americas, devastating the indigenous populations).[12] It is one of the most notorious sexually transmitted diseases because the ulcers that are associated with it are intensely painful and, if the disease is left untreated, it can lead to blindness[13] and even insanity.[14]

There are four stages to syphilis, which increase in severity: *primary* (in which generally painless chancres appear), *secondary* (a large rash appears and fever occurs), *latent* (symptoms go away), and *tertiary* (in which any number of internal organs can be severely affected, potentially leading to death). Regarding genital sores, men who suffered from syphilis could have extremely painful ulcers appear on their penis and perineum, and women on their vulva. Pregnant women who had syphilis passed the disease on to their children. The effect of congenital syphilis on children is particularly heart-rending, due to the disfigurement and painful ulcers the disease causes.

The aforementioned John Wilmot, 2nd Earl of Rochester, is believed to have suffered from several sexually-transmitted illnesses, including syphilis. According to John Aubrey—whose short biographies in his *Brief Lives* should be taken with a pinch of salt—Elizabeth Broughton was 'a most exquisite beauty, as finely shaped as nature could frame'.[15] This beauty, Aubrey went on to write, moved to London, where she became a courtesan. She was eventually spotted by Richard Sackville, 3rd Earl of Dorset (1589–1624), who made her one of his (many) mistresses. Unfortunately, Elizabeth contracted 'the pox'—and died from it.

Prosthetic noses were popular with those whose nose had become deformed following a collapse of the bridge due to syphilis. These fake noses would be applied to the face using some kind of adhesive or with a string or ribbon.[16] Some good examples of these prosthetics can be seen in the Science Museum, London, today. William Davenant, the Restoration playwright and theatre impresario, contracted syphilis in 1631, and subsequent portraits show that his nose had collapsed due to the ravages of the disease.[17] He was ridiculed for this disfigurement and may have worn one of these prosthetics, though there is no direct evidence that he did.

Genital herpes

Although syphilis and gonorrhoea are usually the venereal diseases that are mentioned when it comes to Stuart Britain, these were by no means the only sexually-transmitted infections with which our Stuart ancestors had to contend. *Herpes genitalis* (genital herpes) was present as well. This disease has plagued mankind since at least Mesopotamia—the cradle of civilisation. It can spread to the mouth via oral sex, and thereafter also be contracted (for example, by children) from saliva via non-sexual means.[18]

Pubic lice

Pubic lice, or 'crabs', are not so much a disease but an infestation of *Pthirus pubis*—parasites. These parasitical infestations—which find new hosts via sexual contact—are as old as head lice and were documented as being in existence in Roman and Medieval England.[19] As with head lice, pubic lice could be eliminated, at least temporarily, by removing the hair—usually by shaving.

Cures

'One night with Venus, a lifetime with Mercury'. This phrase refers to the way that just one night in the arms of a lover could lead to a sexually transmitted infection that would often be treated with a dangerous 'cure': the highly toxic chemical element, mercury (also known as *quicksilver*, or by its periodic table Hg).[20]

Gervase Markham's *The English Housewife* tackled the pox with three entries: 'For the French or Spanish pox', 'To put out the French pox', and 'To make the scabs of the French pox to fall away'.[21]

Richard Wiseman, one of King Charles II's physicians, wrote about the treatment 'of the Lues Venerea' in his book, *Eight Chirurgical Treatises*. He recommends that, along with other commonly prescribed remedies such as bleeding, purging, vomiting, salivating, sweating, and the administration of cordials and opiates, various 'preparations of mercury' be added.[22] Bathing, taking exercise, and sleep were also recommended as part of the cure, 'but Venery ought to be avoided during their course of Physick'.[23]

Urethral syringes manufactured during the early 1700s and later discovered in the shipwreck of the pirate Blackbeard's ship *The Queen Anne's Revenge* still contain traces of the mercury that had once been administered via these medical instruments to pirates suffering from syphilis.[24]

Chapter 16

Libido & Masturbation: Or, Ye Art of Self-Pleasuring

The libido, or sex drive, is an inherent part of human sexuality, and various factors, including hair colour, diet, even the time of year all were believed to affect a person's libido during the Stuart period.

According to Sinibaldi's *The Cabinet of Venus Unlock'd* (1658), red-haired people were considered prone to sexual self-control (*incontinency*) and vice, blondes were thought to be 'for the most part wanton', brunettes more 'temperate', and those possessing 'leadish' coloured hair were 'insatiable in venery'![1]

Sinibaldi also stated that women, being 'cold and moist', are more given to lust during the heat of summer, while men, being hot, find their sexual drives hindered by that season and their lust more comfortably suited to winter.[2]

Diet

Stuart-era people believed that their libido could be influenced by what they ate and drank. Some viewed coffee (along with tea, spices, and tobacco) as being 'unnatural for English Bodies; for a Cold Regimen is proper to Cold Countries, as the Hot Regimen for Hot Regions'.[3] They didn't think it was suited to the bodies of Englishmen, Welshmen, Scotsmen, or Irishmen—this belief can be seen in a variety of texts from the period, including Nicholas Culpeper's *Pharmacopœia Londinenseis,* the advertisement for which states that his complete method of physick can help a man preserve his health using 'things only that grow in England, they being most fit for English bodies'.[4]

The Women's Petition Against Coffee (1674) stated that the increasingly popular consumption of coffee was making the husbands who imbibed

117

it impotent. It was far better, they said, to drink cock ale, because that would give a man strength and vigour in the sack!

But, despite the alleged consequences of drinking coffee, Stuart men couldn't stay away from it—and coffee houses grew in popularity. *The Men's Answer to the Women's Petition* (1674) even asserted that, on the contrary, drinking coffee 'makes the erection more vigorous', and the treatise *The Manner of Making of Coffee, Tea, and Chocolate* (1685) stated: 'it is evident that many find this drink to be very profitable, taken in the Morning fasting, with a little Sugar, in a moderate quantity'.[5]

Aphrodisiacs

Throughout history, humans have turned to aphrodisiacs to help them fan the flames of sexual passion and ignite arousal. Oranges were— and sometimes still are—believed to have aphrodisiac qualities. In *The Wandering Whore* (1660), the character Gusman states, 'Fine oranges, sweet lemons, the best in Checquer-Ally near Bum-hill, of so strange a quality as never came from Seville, Barbados, or Virginia, for provoking lust and lechery'.[6]

In a 1737 letter to Hans Sloane, William Byrd conveyed his opinion of the Ginseng that grows in the mountains of Virginia, which had 'merry effects...towards obliging the bashful sex'—a reference to its perceived aphrodisiac qualities. But he warned: 'man is so depraved...I'm afraid a very bad use would be made of it.'[7] Gervase Markham stated that 'Water of Radish drunk twice a day, at each time an ounce, doth multiply and provoke lust'.[8] Nicholas Culpeper suggested that nettle seeds not only 'provoke lust', but also 'open stoppages of the Womb'.[9]

Lubrication

Failure to achieve a satisfying vaginal wetness to aid penetration (be it from penis, finger, or sex toy) can occur for a number of possible reasons. Hormones can play a significant role—whether due to (the) Menopause, breastfeeding, or recent childbirth,[10] or the reason can simply be insufficient sexual arousal. Whatever the cause(s), a lack of natural lubrication can make sex painful and unpleasant, and whether their activity was illicit or legitimate, lovers in Stuart Britain sometimes sought further lubrication.

Sex manuals and erotic literature from the Stuart period suggest that people weren't very open to discussing the subject of foreplay—or acts that lead to sexual arousal. It would be extremely surprising, though, if Stuart-era lovers didn't engage in some form of foreplay prior to sexual intercourse—for example, kissing, petting, or stimulation of areas such as the nipples, buttocks and the genitals—and there is evidence that this was indeed the case.

From the *School of Venus*: 'Mournfully pulling out his Prick before me, he takes down a little Pot of Pomatum, which stood on the Mantle-tree of the Chimney, 'oh' says he, 'this is for our turn', and taking some of it he rubbed his Prick all over with it, to make it go in the more Glib'.[11] On the same page, the second narrator replies that he could have used his saliva as a lubricant. Of course, this makes sense, for if the couple were engaging in oral sex, saliva would have been the lubricant.

Modern-day sexual lubricants are generally based on water, silicone, or oil. The 'pomatum' mentioned above would have been an ointment probably made from animal fats, but would have worked in a similar manner and would have been used not only by heterosexual couples (on the man's penis, or on the woman's vulva and vaginal lips—*labia minora* and *labia majora*) but also by 'sodomites' and 'tribades'.

Impotence

Impotence was a frightening prospect for the average Stuart man. There are many examples of women marrying men considerably older than themselves and it wouldn't be surprising if some of these men suffered from erectile dysfunction from time to time, but this problem did not only affect older men. Earlier in the book, for example, we learned about Frances Howard and Robert, Earl of Essex's divorce on the grounds of his impotence. Unfortunately for Robert, his second marriage, this time to Elizabeth Paulet, proved to be yet another disappointment. He may, or may not, have been the father of his second wife's short-lived child.

Impotence, during the Stuart period, was sometimes believed to have been caused by magic;[12] a man may have had a spell cast upon him by another so he couldn't rise to the occasion. Referring once more to the scandalous union between Frances Howard and Robert Devereux, a part of Frances's defence was the claim that her husband may have been targeted by this kind of magical impotence.[13] Such cases of impotence attributed to sorcery were, however, much rarer in Stuart Britain than in other parts of Europe.[14]

Stuart-era ballads are full of references to cuckoldry and impotence. In one undated balled entitled, *'My Husband has no Courage in Him',* a sexually frustrated wife laments that despite all of her enticements, her handsome, tall, young husband simply can't, or won't, have sex with her. Finally, she states that if he keeps on in this manner, she's going to cheat on him with their neighbours![15]

In another late-seventeenth-century ballad, *'The Quaker's Wives Lamentation For the Loss of Her Husband's Jewels',* the husband has actually castrated himself, and the wife complains:

> 'You might as well have cut off all,
> As leave behind a thing so small,
> And thus to break your Wedlock band,
> to leave a Thing that cannot stand'.[16]

Satyriasis and 'The Frenzie of the Womb'

Satyriasis is a word which came into use during the seventeenth century and stems from the Greek word 'saturiasis', meaning a very high level of libido. In Greek mythology, satyrs were half-man/half-goat beings who had a very high sex drive and usually chased after a nymph or two! Men with this condition accordingly have an uncontrollable, compulsive sex drive, and want to have sex with as many people—usually women— as possible. Sinibaldi, however, applied the term 'satyriasis' to women, describing it as a powerful disease that forces women, against their own will, to entice men into bedding them to quell this insatiable need for copulation.[17]

Likewise, women were believed to be susceptible to a condition called 'the Frenzie of the Womb', whereby they would be driven mad with lust, or intense sexual desire. English apothecary and physician, Nicholas Culpeper (1616–54), blamed: 'hot meats spiced, strong wine, and the like, that heat the privities, idleness, pleasure, and dancing, and reading of bawdy Histories'.[18]

Masturbation

Masturbation has for hundreds of years, in the western world, been associated with a kind of moral uncleanliness, so it's not surprising that it is another aspect of sexuality that was frowned upon during the Stuart era. Masturbation often made many people feel sullied or ashamed. When Pepys, for example, became sexually aroused while reading *The School of Venus,* he masturbated and ejaculated, but after achieving his sexual release he felt a strong wave of shame wash over him, and burned the book.[19] When describing this incident Pepys could not even bring himself to do so entirely in English, electing to write partly in Spanish and French, too.

This shame surrounding masturbation and the notion that it was inherently wicked is also evident in scientist Leeuwenhoek's reassurance to the Royal Society that the ejaculate sample he had used to examine sperm cells was obtained following sex with his wife and not through 'sinfully defiling myself'.[20]

Masturbation with hands was called 'frigging' and, according to *The School of Venus*, genital stimulation of another person with a finger was known as 'digiting'.[21] *Advice to His Son* (1673) warns about 'unclean thoughts', since they could lead to masturbation: 'Leave your Bed upon the first desertion of Sleep: It being ill for the Eyes to read lying, and worse for the Mind to be idle: since the Head, during that laziness, is commonly a cage for unclean thoughts'.[22] And masturbate was precisely what Samuel Pepys did in a crowded, Catholic chapel during an interminable mass at which both his crush Barbara Palmer, Lady Castlemaine, and Queen Catherine were present.[23] While he enjoyed it at the time, Pepys was wracked with guilt afterwards when he reflected on how he had behaved in a house of God.

Female masturbation can be done just by clenching the muscles of the vagina, but can also involve massaging or stimulating the genitalia, including the clitoris, to experience sexual pleasure. Some Stuart-era writers believed that this could cause the clitoris to grow abnormally— especially if a given woman was a frequent masturbator. Bartholin, for example, suggested that in some women, 'it [the Clitoris] hangs out like man's Yard [the penis], namely when young women do frequently and continually handle and rub the same'.[24]

Sex toys

Those unfamiliar with the history of masturbatory toys may assume them to be a modern concept. In fact, not only were they available and in use during the Stuart period, but they date to ancient times! John Wilmot, 2nd Earl of Rochester's poem, *Signior Dildo*, written around 1673, is a bawdy piece about dildos and about how much women love to use them. Women without dildos resorted to masturbation with other objects, claimed Rochester, such as a 'candle, carrot, or thumb'.[25] Dildos were also depicted on the frontispiece of both 1680 editions of *The School of Venus* and *L'Académie des Dames*—in both artworks the sex toys are seen hanging from stalls and displayed upon tables, where they are carefully inspected by potential lady customers.

In the play *The Farce of Sodom, Or, The Quintessence of Debauchery* (often attributed to John Wilmot), there is a scene in which the characters Fuckadilla and Officina actively masturbate Queen Cuntigratia with a dildo, and complain about the short length of the sex toy: 'This dildo by a handful is too short', and 'short dildos leave the pleasure half behind'.

There were also poems that actively used the word 'dildo' to amusing and erotic effect, such as *Dildoides: A Burlesque Poem* by Samuel Butler, Thomas Nash's *The Choice of Valentines,* among others.

Bawdy poetry aside, the use of dildos—along with other kinds of masturbation—was generally disapproved of and held to be the preserve of 'bad women': 'Whiles to allay, not quench her wanton Fires, Sometimes she Dildoes, sometimes Stalion hires'.[26] After all, if women resorted to using inanimate objects to satiate their carnal appetites, where would that leave the men, who already had a wariness and fear regarding impotence and women's sexuality?

Henry Savile lamented to John Wilmot, 2nd Earl of Rochester, that a consignment of leather dildos had been destroyed by fire at the hands of 'barbarian farmers',[27] and in the aforementioned *The Women's Petition Against Coffee*, we find a striking warning: stop drinking coffee or 'run the hazard of being *Cuckol'd* by *Dildos*' by sexually frustrated wives!

Chapter 17

Stuart Love: Or, Ye Heart's Delighte & Torment

'Love, like a Burning-glass, contracts the dilated lines of Lust, and fixeth them upon one object'[1]
—Advice to a Son, 1673

We have now covered some of the most intimate aspects of the physical unions humans could share; but something that must certainly be included in any work about sexuality is the union of the emotions, of *souls*—for romantic love and sex are often entwined.

Love for another human being can transport us to heights of emotional bliss, and when love is spurned, this can take us down into the depths of despair. That has never changed, nor is likely to. Love is one of the most integral and beautiful aspects of our humanity and of the human experience: '...all the Gifts in the World, how excellent soever, are nothing worth without Love'.[2]

There are many examples of great romances during the Stuart period. Early in the seventeenth century, the marriage between Princess Elizabeth and Frederick V, Elector Palatine, took place on Valentine's Day 1613 with spectacular and sumptuous celebratory events.[3] Despite the fact that the bride's mother, Queen Anna, did not approve of the match, on the grounds that she thought Frederick of too low a station for her daughter, the young couple fell in love, and from that union came several prominent and dynastically-important children, including Prince Rupert of the Rhine and Sophia of Hanover. The latter's line became the Georgians—heirs to the British throne following the death of Queen Anne in 1714.[4]

A lesser-known, but very long-lasting love story was that of Alice (daughter of Francis Holland of Burwarton) and Henry Baugh of

Aldon Court in the county of Shropshire, England. The couple, according to the inscription on their tomb, were married for sixty years and two months—an incredible feat, especially given longevity in the seventeenth century. Alice died in January of 1662, followed by her husband in November of 1665, and both were laid to rest in St John the Baptist Church, Stokesay Castle, near Craven Arms, Shropshire.

One of the great Stuart romances was that between Dorothy Osborne and Sir William Temple, which began in the midst of the tumultuous Civil Wars. Love tokens were exchanged, including the gift of William's hair, which Dorothy cherished.[5] Such tokens were common throughout this period, and were even mentioned by Sir Francis Bacon: 'It is received, that it helpeth to continue love, if one wear a ring, or a bracelet, of the hair of the party beloved. But that may be by the exciting of the imagination: and perhaps a glove, or other like favour, may as well do it'.[6] They faced many obstacles, and at times it seemed likely that their story would end in tragedy, but ultimately love was triumphant.

Of course, many Stuart love stories did not have a happy ending—no wonder, bearing in mind the considerable upheavals and major calamities of the period such as plague, civil wars, fire, and rebellion. Following the Rye House Plot of 1683, in which the assassinations of King Charles II and his brother and heir, James, Duke of York were planned, William Russell, Lord Russell was arrested and incarcerated in the Tower of London. Soon enough, he was found guilty and sentenced to a traitor's death. His beloved and devoted wife, Rachel Lady Russell, fought for his life to the very end—she was by his side in the courtroom, and did everything she could to try to save him. Alas, despite her many endeavours, Lord Russell was beheaded in 1683. He was later granted a posthumous pardon, during the reign of William and Mary in 1694.[7]

Love in Art

Jacob Ochtervelt's painting *The Love Letter*[8] (1670–72) depicts a pretty, wealthy young woman dreamily reading a love letter while one maidservant arranges her hair and another walks away holding a pewter basin and ewer. In Godfried Schalcken's *Lovers Lit by a Candle* (1665–70), a beaming young man with one arm around an equally mirthful young woman and a lit candle in his other hand, stares out at the viewer, and we are filled with the happiness of the couple's love.[9]

Another great work depicting love is *Cupid and Psyche*, painted by Antony van Dyck between 1639–1640. The ultimately happy story of the god Cupid and his mortal love and wife, Psyche, was a popular subject for paintings during the Stuart period, and a number of high-profile artists made created their own depictions of this tale, including Luca Giordano and Abraham Bloemaert.

The Green-Eyed Monster

There are few things in life more painful than loving someone who does not reciprocate those feelings… and there's a common saying: 'Hell hath no fury like a woman scorned'. Some instances from Stuart Britain serve as examples of this! In June 1607, a case of Defamation was brought before a court by Richard Meredith against a widow, Alice Morgan of St. Michael's Parish near Bath.[10] She had claimed that Meredith had used her house as a meeting place to have illicit assignations with her sister-in-law. The court found that Morgan had concocted this tale out of jealousy because she believed Richard fancied her sister-in-law and not her.

In Barwick,[11] a man witnessed a shocking and tragic incident on a bridge[12] in which a soldier, carrying his toddler daughter, kissed her many times before throwing her into the water below—and then threw himself in shortly after. The girl miraculously survived, but the father's body was found the next day: 'Jealousy was the supposed occasion of this adventure; another soldier having maliciously told him, 'While you stand here on the guard, such as one is lying with your wife'.[13] This rumour of his wife's infidelity may have triggered his rash and violent actions, which would have resulted in a murder-suicide, had the child not survived.

To die for love

According to Anthony Wood, in October 1655, a 'handsome maid living in Catstreet, being deeply in love with Joseph Godwin, a junior fellow of New College, poyson'd herself with rats-bane'.[14] Wood was rather taken aback by this, for 'it made a great wonder that a maid should be in love with such a person as he, who had a curl'd shag-pate, was squint-ey'd and purblind, and much deform'd with the small-pox'.[15] Apparently Wood wasn't very familiar with Shakespeare's line: 'Love looks not with the eyes, but with the mind And therefore is winged Cupid painted blind'.[16]

Arbella Stuart and William Seymour married in a secret wedding in the early hours of 22 June 1610.[17] Both were descended from the Tudors and together could have been more politically and dynastically powerful than the then-king, James VI & I. Once the king learned of this forbidden union, which had probably already been fully consummated,[18] he sent William to the Tower and had Arbella held under house arrest.[19] The couple attempted a dramatic joint escape, but were apprehended. Arbella, utterly distraught, began to starve herself,[20] and she died on 25 September 1615.[21] Some time after Arbella's death, William—who had been thirteen years her junior—remarried, and this wife bore him a daughter who was named 'Arbella', no doubt in honour of his tragic first wife.[22]

Those who *didn't* want to die for love (unrequited or otherwise), sought remedies to rid themselves of it. *The Ladies Dictionary* (1694), provides several recommendations, such as: 'Exercise yourself in Walking or Running, do it vigorously...and the burning Flames of Love...may expire, or much abate of their vehemency'.[23] Another tip was to change one's diet, since it was believed that, just as some foods had aphrodisiacal properties, others had the opposite effect.

Chapter 18

Adultery & Divorce in Stuart Britain: Or, O Lamentable Sinne!

In May of 1650, *An Act for Suppressing the Detestable Sins of Incest, Adultery, & Fornication* was passed. Committing Adultery was, from that point onward, a criminal offence—and one that carried a life sentence. This meant that adultery was seen as tantamount to other crimes such as bestiality and incest.[1] Both parties would be found guilty, even if one (whether it was the man or the woman) was not married.[2] This law and subsequent punishment did not, however, apply to a married woman who was raped, and therefore had been 'carnally known' by a man other than her husband.[3] A decade later, with the Restoration of the monarchy, the draconian Adultery Act of 1650 was repealed by the English Parliament. The House of Lords was re-established, having been abolished in 1649 for being 'useless and dangerous to the People of England to be continued'.[4]

You might wonder whether social class affected sentencing. It depended: in the North American colonies, harsh punishments were meted out to both men and women quite equally, while in domestic aristocratic circles adultery—though commonplace—was rarely punished to the same degree, if at all.

According to the Quaker William Penn, 'if love be not thy chiefest motive, thou wilt soon grow weary of a married state, and stray from thy promise, to search out thy pleasures in forbidden places'.[5] This is quite reasonable advice, for many Stuart-era aristocratic persons married for reasons other than love, only to later find emotional and sexual solace in the arms of another. Matrimony means two people will have to bear life's joys and sadnesses, hardships and pleasures together—and while all relationships have their difficult patches, where there is love, these can be surmounted.

In an official court document held in the Lancashire Archives, an entry states that William Richardson of Brathwaite, Cumbria, was suspected of Adultery with Eliza Drydon in 1670. A male member of Eliza's family (probably her husband) named as Marmaduke Drydon of Harrington,[6] and a woman named Mary were expected to testify before the court on the matter.[7] The outcome is unknown, but it's fair to assume that, if found guilty, the two would have suffered punishment of some kind.

Isaac Ambrose warned readers to be on guard during 'natural actions' such as eating, drinking, visitations, and recreation because even in innocent diversions, sin—including adultery—could be waiting for them.[8]

Cuckoldry

> '…a Cuckold is no such strange thing in our Age'[9]
> —Aphra Behn, The Town-Fopp, Or Sir Timothy Tawdrey,
>
> Act I, Scene I.

A man who was being cheated on by his wife was usually referred to as a 'cuckold' during this period. The main problem with being cuckolded was that a husband couldn't be sure whether children his wife birthed were his own. This might cause his own family line to be replaced by his wife's lover's—at his own expense. Another problem was of course embarrassment: the wife would be seen to be making fun of the husband behind his back—making him into a fool. There are many ballads, poems and plays, among other literature, which feature a cuckolded man. In illustrations he is often depicted as having horns on his head.

Penelope, Lady Rich, née Devereux (1563–1607), was a noblewoman whose scandalous love life gave rise to litigation. The beautiful Penelope inspired the pen of several late Elizabethan poets, including Philip Sidney. In the early 1580s, she served as one of Queen Elizabeth I's ladies-in-waiting and, in 1581, she married Robert Rich, with whom she had five children. The marriage had its share of troubles, however, and by 1590 Penelope had fallen in love with Sir Charles Blount, the Earl of Devonshire. The two embarked upon a passionate adulterous relationship, which wrecked Blount's otherwise excellent reputation. Penelope even gave birth to no fewer than five children by her lover.

As for Robert Rich, divorce was sought—and granted—on the grounds of Penelope's adultery with Blount. Despite the fact that remarriage was not permitted, Charles Blount and Penelope Rich nevertheless married in 1605, and Blount's 1606 *Defence of His Marriage With Lady Penelope Rich* is a rambling, almost desperate, attempt to justify (with copious Biblical references) his marriage to Penelope.[10] Their marriage proved of short duration, however, for Blount died—aged forty-three—in 1606; Penelope followed him to the grave a little over a year later, in 1607.[11]

Cuckolds also made for interesting subject matter on the stage, with plays such as Nahum Tate's *Cuckolds-Haven* (1685) and Thomas Southerne's *The Wives' Excuse: or, Cuckolds Make Themselves* (1691). They were often the butt of jokes in comedies, for they were regarded as ridiculous and lacking in masculinity.

Astrology being quite popular during the Stuart period, it's no surprise to find some cheeky words concerning adultery and cuckoldry in *The Perpetual Almanack* from 1663: 'The fourth House, gives judgement...(of) when a man may lie with another man's wife, but not when another man lies with his own, for that the best astrologer could never yet tell'.[12]

There were several well-known cases of cuckoldry during this period, not least that of Roger Palmer, the husband of Barbara Palmer (neé Villiers)—a woman who very publicly was Charles II's mistress for many years, and who, both during and after this period, had affairs with many other men. On December 7 1661, Samuel Pepys recorded that he went to the Privy Seal and there 'was a patent for Roger Palmer to be Earle of Castlemaine and Baron of Limbricke (Limerick) in Ireland; but the honour is tied up to the males got of the body of his wife, the Lady Barbary: the reason whereof every body knows'.[13] The reason being all of his wife's children at that time were sired by King Charles II.

Although he had been compensated for being cuckolded with financial remuneration and status, Roger and his wife eventually reached so toxic a place in their relationship that, by July 1662, Barbara took her best things, left his house, and moved in with her brother in Richmond— where she would be conveniently situated for further assignations with her royal lover.[14] Her husband, understandably incensed and very much aware of so public a humiliation, left England and went to the Continent, where he became more deeply devoted to Catholicism and spent time in the study of languages.[15] He subsequently returned to England, where he faced further difficulties, including being tried for treason and imprisoned in the Tower of London. He died, without having another known relationship, in 1705. Barbara went to her own grave the following year.

Adultery was looked down upon not only by the law, but also by many writers of the day. There was, accordingly, a plethora of warnings against engaging in this sin—for example: 'To make love to married women doth not only multiply the Sin, but the danger',[16] and 'The corrupting of a man's wife, enticing her to a strange bed, is by all acknowledged to be the worst sort of theft, infinitely beyond that of goods'.[17]

The latter line indicates that a wife was considered something of a possession, and this attitude adheres to religious texts of the time such as William Austin's *Hæc Homo* (1639), which stated that a wife 'belongeth but to one husband-man; and ought, but by one alone to be ordered and disposed. So that, whosoever comes, either by craft or by force, to take any of the pleasures there, is but a thief'.[18]

Finally, a tongue-in-cheek 1608 work entitled *The Pennyless Parliament of Thread-bare Poets: Or, All Mirth and witty Conceits*, states: 'It is also thought necessary, that some shall suspect their Wives at Home, because they themselves play false abroad'[19]—some men may have projected their own guilt of having engaged in adultery onto their wives.

Adultery in the colonies

In an entry dated 4 September 1638 in the Plymouth Colony Records, one Francis Baver of Scituate, Massachusetts was presented before a court for 'offering to lie with the wife of William Holmes, and to abuse her body with uncleanliness'.[20] In 1641, another colonial example of a single man having a sexual relationship with a married woman was brought to court. Thomas Bray and Anne Linceford, 'committed the act of adultery and uncleanesse, and have divers tymes layne in one bed together in the absence of her husband'. Their punishment was soon meted out: both were 'severely whipt' in public and made to wear the two letters 'AD' on their clothing to publicly show that they were adulterers.[21]

English-born Boston colonist William Hudson left his wife, Anne, and his business in the care of his trusted servant, Henry Dawson, in 1645 to attend to things back in England.[22] Unfortunately for him, Anne and Henry seem to have embarked upon an illicit romance and were even caught in bed together. Despite this, they claimed they hadn't had sexual relations and were only charged with adulterous behaviour instead of the more serious charge of adultery. A flogging in public was part of their punishment, and Anne was welcomed back by her husband.[23]

Aristocratic adultery

Adultery among the Royal Stuarts is such a popular topic that it often eclipses important political and socio-economic matters of the time. Luckily, the express purpose of this book is to examine the Stuart-era person's love life—with all that it entailed!

Much is made of George Villiers, 1st Duke of Buckingham—and for good reason. His family conspired to marry him off to one of the great heiresses in the kingdom, and they were successful in this. But George isn't the only Villiers who deserves our attention. For example, George had an elder brother, John Villiers, who in late 1617, was married to fourteen-year-old Frances Coke—who was given away by King James VI & I himself.[24] This lady, who had been bullied and ultimately forced into the marriage, scandalously left her aloof, mentally-ill husband for her lover Sir Robert Howard, who went on to become the father of their illegitimate son, Robert.[25]

James Scott—the Duke of Monmouth and the eldest illegitimate son of King Charles II and his Welsh mistress, Lucy Walter—had a very dramatic life (and death). His love life was no exception, and Aphra Behn's poem *Young Jemmy, Or, The Princely Shepherd* undoubtedly is about this man: 'For he with glances could enslave each heart'.[26] Monmouth was considered exceptionally handsome, and he never lacked a comely bedfellow, despite having been wed to the Scottish heiress, Anna Scott, when both were very young (the bridegroom was only thirteen, and the bride twelve). The couple were married on a Tuesday, April 23 'at 5 of ye clock in the afternoon'.[27] Among Monmouth's many affairs, two were particularly significant: the first was that with Eleanor Needham, with whom he had two children, and the second was his affair with Lady Henrietta Wentworth—of all Monmouth's extramarital relationships, this was to prove to be the most emotionally-fulfilling, and the longest-lasting.[28]

The Repentant Adulterer

William Winstanley's 1687 collection of biographies of famous English poets includes a brief profile of the Late Elizabethan romantic Robert Greene (1558–1592), which describes how Greene married a 'virtuous gentlewoman, whom yet he forsook'[29]—in other words, he cheated on her. Although Greene technically belongs to the Tudor period, the repentance he displayed in a 'Letter written to his Wife' in his posthumously published book, *A Groatsworth of Wit*, merits mention here. After sharing his concerns that his son will grow up to be as lecherous as him, he ends with a moving penitence: 'For my contempt of God, I am condemned of men; for my swearing and forswearing, no man will believe me; for my gluttony, I suffer hunger; for my drunkenness, thirst, for my adultery, ulcerous sores'.[30] This letter was signed 'thy repentant husband for his disloyalty, Robert Greene'. Greene was clearly in a wretched state, his body tortured from one of the symptoms of a venereal disease (probably syphilis)—hence the 'ulcerous sores'—and we might wonder whether his repentance was truly sincere, or motivated at least in part by him knowing the end was near and fearing holy punishment in the hereafter.

Stuart Divorce

Divorce was extremely rare during the Stuart period and was usually only granted via a private Act of Parliament. It only became more common in Britain following the *Divorce and Matrimonial Causes Act* of 1857.[31]

John Rainolds (1549–1607) expressed his views on divorce as follows: 'Who so marrieth another as long as he is bound to the former, is an adulterer. The band then of marriage is loosed & dissolved between that man and wife who are put asunder and divorced for whoredom'.[32] Rainolds later states: 'It is lawful for him [the husband] who hath put away his wife for whoredom to marrie another'.[33] In short, Rainolds believed that a man had every right to divorce a woman who had been cheating on him, and marry another.

Although John Milton (1608–1674) is best known for his epic poems *Paradise Lost* (1667) and *Paradise Regained* (1671), he was also the author of many political writings, most notably *Eikonoklastes* (1649). In 1642, he married a young woman, but after a month, she left him and went back to her family home. What happened? In this case, we don't have the evidence to know, but whatever the cause of their separation, Milton controversially published a tract in favour of divorce the following year entitled, *The doctrine and discipline of divorce, restored to the good of both sexes from the bondage of canon law and other mistakes to Christian freedom.* There was something of a backlash from other Christians, most notably in the form of Herbert Palmer's condemnation of Milton's tract, published in 1644.

There were other forms of marital separation during the Stuart period. Although not a divorce, a *divortium menso en thoro* (separation from bed and board) meant a couple could live apart, but were not entitled to remarry.[34] This kind of separation was granted only following proof that the wife had committed adultery or that the husband was cruel. But for most Stuart-age people, divorce and separation simply weren't likely to happen. Instead, if a marriage completely broke down, a spouse would typically simply abandon the other, which led to other legal (and social) problems. In 1604's *An Act for the Due Execution of Diverse Laws and Statutes Heretofore Made Against Rogues, Vagabonds and Sturdy Beggars and Other Lewd and Idle Persons*, for example, people who deserted their families were considered rogues and this could lead to their punishment if caught.[35]

Chapter 19

Rakes & Rogues:
Or, Ye Stuart Libertine

'The Drunkard, Glutton, or Whoremonger.... have no higher end than Pleasure, and can give you no better account why they feed their lust, but because they Love it, and it's their delight'[1]

– Richard Baxter, 1675

What exactly was a 'libertine'? According to *The English Dictionarie* of 1623, it was 'one of a loose life'.[2] What characterises the libertine if not a tendency towards debauchery, the abandonment of morals, and a proclivity for hedonistic excesses of the flesh? 'Restoration rakes' were usually wealthy enough to be untroubled by the hardships most Stuart-era people had to face. Nonetheless, the majority of the most notorious Stuart libertines ended up meeting tragic ends: 'For albeit for a time they sleep in their sins and blindness, delighting in their pleasures, and taking sport in cruelties and evil deeds, yet they draw after them the line wherewith (being more ensnared than they were aware) they are taken and drawn to their final destruction'.[3]

Dying at the age of thirty-three, his body riddled with sexually transmitted diseases and the effects of alcoholism, John Wilmot, 2nd Earl of Rochester, is remembered for his hedonistic dissipations, his talented (though sometimes shocking!) literary output, and for his pathetic and tragic death. The 2nd Earl of Rochester remains to this day one of the best-known (and most notorious!) Stuart-era libertines because of his penchant for debauchery. Gilbert Burnet said of him, 'Wilmot...was naturally modest, till the court corrupted him',[4] and that 'he gave himself up to all sorts of extravagance, and to the wildest frolics that a wanton wit could devise'.[5] One of the wild stories of his life involved his abduction of the wealthy and beautiful heiress, Elizabeth Malet, in late May 1665—a rash act that led to his imprisonment in the Tower of London.[6] Miss Malet had been a highly-sought-after bride who had turned the heads of the likes of John, the son of the Duke of Ormond, and also James Scott, Duke of Monmouth.[7] Two years later, the twenty-year-old Wilmot successfully took the sixteen-year-old as his bride when they wed in secret on 29 January, 1666/67.[8]

Wilmot's friend and fellow debauchee, George Villiers, 2nd Duke of Buckingham, also had an eventful life and a lonely death. Buckingham, the son of the infamous first Duke of Buckingham, was a great childhood friend of King Charles II, fought for King Charles I during the English Civil Wars, and was later a member of the former's 'Cabal' government. His intimate circle of friends included some other great hedonists of the time; and, as Bishop Gilbert Burnet lamented, 'Buckingham gave himself up to a monstrous course of studied immoralities of the worst kinds'.[9] He married Mary Fairfax—the daughter of Parliamentarian general Thomas Fairfax and Anne de Vere—at Nun-Appleton, near York, in 1657.[10] Whilst his wife remained faithful to him, Buckingham was a prolific philanderer.

One of the major episodes of his love life was his entanglement with a married woman, Anna Maria Talbot, Countess of Shrewsbury— one of the great beauties of the Restoration court. Buckingham's doubly-adulterous liaison ultimately proved fatal for Anna Maria's husband, Francis Talbot, when the cuckolded husband challenged his wife's lover to a duel in 1668.[11] The Duke accepted, and in the resulting swordfight, killed his challenger. Buckingham, his wife Mary, and his mistress, Anna Maria, all lived together for some time until the flames of passion fizzled out between the adulterous couple. Their extraordinary relationship at an end, Anna Maria lived in a convent abroad for some time. The Duke of Buckingham died alone in 1688, aged sixty and in poverty. His long-suffering wife Mary outlived him by many years, dying in 1705.[12]

Harry Jermyn, the dashing nephew of Queen Henrietta Maria's favourite, Henry Jermyn, 1st Earl of St. Albans, was another major Restoration rake. Jermyn's reputation as a lothario was so firmly entrenched that when it became common gossip that he was trying to woo King Charles's sister, Mary, the Dowager Princess of Orange, Charles intervened, and Mary felt obliged to send Jermyn away.[13]

Reputedly possessing a large penis,[14] this seductive rake had a number of the most beautiful women at court to warm his bed. Among these, was Barbara Palmer, Lady Castlemaine, who, in 1667, had: 'fallen in love with young Jermin who hath of late lain with her oftener than the King'.[15]

Sir Charles Sedley (1639–1701), of whom John Evelyn said was 'none of the most virtuous, but a wit',[16] is most infamous for his bizarre and explicitly sexual behaviour atop a balcony at the Cock Inn at Covent Garden, which was an area known for brothels and other seedy establishments.[17] It was here that Sedley—probably blind drunk—stripped naked and pretended to sodomise a man while hurling sexually-explicit abuse at passers-by. According to Samuel Pepys, Sedley then thrust his penis into a glass of wine, rubbed and washed the organ, and then—*bottoms up!*—imbibed the wine.[18] He was fined £500 for his shocking behaviour.[19]

Other notable libertines include Sir George Etherege, and Charles Sackville, 6th Earl of Dorset (who was, for a time, known as Lord Buckhurst). Etherege was a playwright who enjoyed the lifestyle of a libertine and dedicated his 1664 play, *The Comical Revenge, Or, Love in a Tub* to Buckhurst. A debauched lifestyle wasn't enough for Buckhurst—he also set up a household with both Nell Gwynn and the aforementioned Sedley. Pepys lamented this situation: 'And to the town to the King's Head; and hear that my Lord Buckhurst and Nelly are lodged at the next house, and Sir Charles Sedley with them: and keep a merry house. Poor girl! I pity her'.[20] Given the hedonistic excesses for which these two libertines were known, it wouldn't be far-fetched to assume the three partook of the occasional *ménage à trois*. Pepys had been right to pity Nell: after only a few weeks of living with the young actress in this scandalous manner, Buckhurst broke up with her.[21]

Richard Jones, 1st Earl of Ranelagh (1641–1712), was an Irish peer and politician and, according to Bishop Burnet, was 'a young man of great parts, and as great vices'.[22] The same could have been said of many a young Restoration rake, for often these men were not just dissolute pleasure-seekers, but had a variety of talents, ambitions, and accomplishments.

Henry St John, 1st Viscount Bolingbroke (1678–1751), had a penchant for licentious activities, just like other libertines of his time.[23] According to his eighteenth-century biographer, he was spotted running naked through a park whilst intoxicated 'during this period, as all his attachments were to pleasure'.[24]

Another Stuart-era lady-killer was Henry Sidney, Earl of Romney (1641–1704). His drop-dead good looks enabled him to seduce many women, but his sense of responsibility was lacking. Absentee or irresponsible fathers are nothing new, and in typical rakish style, Sidney fathered several illegitimate children, then refused to provide for them.[25]

Some men managed to get in on some action with the ladies by pretending to be a well-known rake. According to a letter from one Mr Humfrey Wanley dated 25 August 1698, a man in Sussex went about pretending to be the Duke of Monmouth (who had, by that time, been dead for thirteen years). By doing so, this imposter (whose real identity is unknown) not only conned his easily-led followers out of money to support him, but also had sexual relations with around fifty women in the local area—no doubt attracted not only by his good looks but also by the romanticism associated with that tragic duke.[26]

Before the Restoration rake, however, there was the Cavalier of the Civil Wars. One of the most illustrious—and enduringly romantic—of these figures was Prince Rupert of the Rhine. Rupert was the son of Frederick V of the Palatinate and Elizabeth Stuart, who were known as the 'Winter King and Queen' due to their very short reign as rulers of Bohemia. Although he can't really be described as a 'libertine', the gorgeous Prince Rupert had more than his share of love affairs during his life (which was full of adventure)—even including an amour with his jailer's daughter, Susan, in Vlotho.[27] Following the Restoration came the 1660s, when Rupert met his two best-known loves: Frances Bard and Margaret Hughes. Frances' father, Henry Bard, had fought on the cavalier side during the English Civil Wars. Frances was a gloriously beautiful woman who soon captivated the dashing prince's heart. The couple had a son together, Dudley Bard. Frances claimed to be Rupert's wife, and even said as much in her later years when she lived at his sister Sophie's court. Rupert, however, always denied there had been any wedding. In his final years, he fell in love again—this time to Margaret Hughes, who was known affectionately by many as 'Peg'. Hughes was an actress who had previously taken Sir Charles Sedley as her lover (yes, he of the balcony-stunt!). Rupert and Peg moved in together, never married, and had one illegitimate child, a daughter named Ruperta.

George, Baron Goring (b. 1608) was a handsome but aggressive man, who, within four years of his marriage, frittered away his wife's dowry on whoring, gambling, and alcohol. During the British/English

Civil Wars, Goring was involved in a big argument with fellow Royalist Prince Rupert and ended up moving to the Continent, ultimately dying in Madrid, Spain, in 1657.

Sir Henry Blount (1602–1682) was another rake whose libidinous excesses took place mainly in the 1630s, during which time he 'was pretty wild when young, especially addicted to common wenches'.[28] He was so much inclined towards carnal pursuits, he apparently bragged that he had gone to a bordello without any money with his friend who did have money, and the prostitutes there preferred to have sex with him because he was so attractive.[29] He got himself into some legal trouble when he spread an 'abominable and dangerous doctrine that it was far cheaper and safer to lye with common wenches then with ladies of quality'.[30]

Some libertines hid behind the veneer of saintliness offered by the Church. One of the events described by Scottish traveller William Lithgow was the execution in 1609 of a forty-six-year-old Roman Catholic friar at St. Mark's Square, Venice. 'Mine associate and I, were no sooner landed, and perceiving a great throng of people, and in the midst of them a great smoke; but we began to demand a Venetian what the matter was? Who replied, there was a grey Friar burning quick at St. Mark's pillar, of the reformed order of Saint Francis, for begetting fifteen young noble nuns with child, and all within one year; he being also their Father confessor'.[31] Fifteen young nuns! The friar certainly paid the ultimate price for his lust.

In another case, Thomas Ward, Dean of Connor of Co. Antrim, Ireland, was supposed to be a respectable man of God, but he gained an unsavoury reputation as a fornicator with the women in his parish and for siring multiple illegitimate offspring.[32]

The erotic writer and Dutch philosopher Adriaan Beverland (1650–c.1716) developed a reputation for libertinism in his youth and was even expelled from university following his publication of a scandalous work on Original Sin, *Peccatum originale,* in 1673. One of the most striking portraits of the 1670s is by artist Ary de Vois, c. 1675, which depicts a handsome, periwigged, twenty-five-year-old Beverland sitting back casually, lace at his throat and wrists, smoking from a long clay pipe. There is a beautiful young woman sitting by his side, *en déshabillé,* who is often described as either a prostitute, a 'woman of light morals'[33] or a 'wanton woman'. Beverland seems content in this languid position, and satiated in every sense of the word. Beverland eventually moved to England during the reign of King William III and appears to have ended his days in repentance, writing and publishing *De fornicatione cavenda: admonitio sive adhortatio ad pudicitiam et castitatem* (1698), which, loosely translated from Latin, is: *Beware Fornication, Or, An Encouragement of Modesty and Chastity.* In this work, he wrote: 'I condemn the warmth of my imprudent youth; I detest my loose style and my libertine sentiments. I thank God, who has removed from my eyes the veil which blinded my sight in a miserable manner, and who would not suffer me any longer to seek out weak arguments to defend this crime'.[34] He explained that he had burned all copies of *Peccatum Originale* that he had in his possession, and urged readers to do the same. A nineteenth-century biography states that Beverland ended his days in madness—if this is true, perhaps it was due to yet another case of syphilis. Unlike his fellow libertine contemporaries, however, Beverland died in his sixties.

Some Stuart-era libertines also killed. In 1713, an English attorney named Richard Noble seduced and ran off with Mrs Mary Sayer, the wife of a wealthy gentleman. Sayer's husband followed the adulterous pair, only to be murdered by Noble, who was later hanged for his crimes.[35]

If you asked a Stuart-era person their opinion about the inhabitants of Port Royal, Jamaica, you would probably be told not that some libertines lived there, but that the whole village was infested with debauchery. Thus, few were surprised when this area suffered a terrible earthquake in 1692. According to a French merchant resident there at the time, this was a 'punishment from Heaven'[36] for the enormity of sins committed by Port Royal's inhabitants—sins which included fornication, sodomy, and piracy. Not much changed by 1698, for Ned Ward wrote:

> 'Virtue is so Despis'd, and all sorts of Vice Encourag'd, by both Sexes, that the Town of Port Royal is the very Sodom of the Universe'.[37]

Broken promises

> 'What we love, we will hear; what we love, we will trust; and what we love, we will serve, aye, and suffer for too'[38]
> —William Penn (1644–1718)

Aristocratic men would sometimes seduce a woman while dangling the carrot of matrimony before her eyes—only to satiate their lust then walk away, consequences be damned. But occasionally they were not allowed to simply get away with this.

Over in the Dutch Republic, at the court of William & Mary, Prince and Princess of Orange, one of Mary's ladies-in-waiting found herself in this kind of situation. By 1681, Jane Wroth, daughter of Sir Henry Wroth, had formed an attachment to the Prince of Orange's good-looking cousin, William Hendrik of Nassau, Lord Zuylestein. He had promised to marry Jane; she had sex with him…and (surprise, surprise) became pregnant.[39] Zuylestein reneged on his promise, but once Princess Mary found out about this, she took matters into her own hands. She effectively forced Zuylestein to marry Jane, having her own chaplain, Thomas Ken, perform the wedding ceremony in secret (Mary knew the union was going to anger her husband, who wanted a more politically-advantageous marriage for his cousin).[40] When William discovered what had happened, he was as angry as Mary had feared he would be—but, tough grits, he had to accept it. Zuylestein eventually regained favour and was made Master of the Robes and Earl of Rochfort in 1695.[41]

Predatory suitors

In 1690, the pretty and outgoing widow, Lucy Hooper, became the prey of a fifty-two-year-old predatory suitor by the name of Jean-Jacques Fazas. The penniless French refugee was attracted not solely by her comeliness but also by the fact she was left in possession of a handsome fortune by her late husband. After attempts at wooing Mrs Hooper failed, Fazas resorted to dastardly means of making her his wife: with the help of several others, he managed to spike her dish of hot chocolate with a powerful drug which rendered her incapable of defending herself. She was then spirited away to another house, wherein a clergyman married her to Fazas, who then 'consummated' the union by raping the drugged woman. When she became aware of what had happened, Lucy took Fazas to court for forcible marriage. With the help of eyewitness testimony and other damning evidence, she won, and the forced marriage she had endured to Fazas was declared null and void.[42] It appears that no further action was taken against Fazas.

140

Chapter 20

Interracial & Interethnic Unions:
Or, Exotick Sex

'For who's he, that's not ravished with delight,
Far Countries, Courts, and Cities, strange to see?'[1]

Stuart sex in foreign lands

Today, those who take a DNA test to determine their ethnic background
often thereby also receive a stark indication of the historical events that
have occurred over the past 500 years or more. The Spanish, Portuguese,
Dutch, French, and British conquered considerable territory in foreign
lands after the late 1400s and invariably, a lot of sex took place, whether
with willing participants or not, as Europeans sired mixed offspring with
the native inhabitants of the areas they invaded.[2]

What drove the intrepid Stuart-age man to sail from the British Isles to
far-flung lands? Perhaps the words of William Lithgow (1582–1645)—a
Scottish adventurer—will help us understand:

'the nature of man, by an inward inclination, is always
inquisitive of foreign news; yea, and much more affecteth
the sight and knowledge of strange, and unfrequented
kingdoms, such is the instinct of his natural affection'.[3]

Indeed, Stuart people *were* inquisitive about foreign news; and for the
literate in Stuart Britain, there were many travel books full of thrillingly
exotic lands and peoples.[4] A section of the travel book *The New Atlas*
(1698) discusses Turkish seraglios[5] and the roles of the eunuchs
and women who inhabited such places,[6] while in Johan Albrecht de
Mandelslo's *Travels to the East Indies* there's an overtly erotic element

141

to the author's written account of his 1639 observations of the women: *'[They]...do all they can to appear lovely, and attract the men, covering their privy parts only with a thin piece of linen, which fits not so close, but the least wind shows all they have'.*[7]

We can imagine how striking this must have been for Mandelslo—especially considering the much more conservative garments worn by European women at the time!

George Psalmanazar, who claimed to be a native of Formosa (modern-day Taiwan) wrote, in his 1704 work, *An Historical and Geographical Description of Formosa*, that the strict law against adultery in that faraway land 'does not extend to Foreigners, to whom the natives are wont to offer virgins or whores, to be made use of at their pleasure, with impunity'.[8] However, Psalmanazar wasn't from Formosa at all: he was a fraudster from France, whose book merely promoted a stereotype of the wanton sexuality of foreign women—women of whom he had no personal knowledge.

These texts, no doubt, whetted many a European's appetite for Orientalism and exoticism—occasionally in Stuart-era plays there would be a token character for this flavour, such as the character of Abnidaraes Quixot in *Hans Beer-Pot, His Invisible Comedie* from 1618. Aphra Behn's *Abdelazar: Or, The Moor's Revenge* (1676), music for which was composed in the early 1690s by Henry Purcell, was a revenge tragedy with exotic characters and places.[9]

Sir John Chardin noted his observations of Mingrelia (which is part of modern-day Georgia, by the Black Sea):

'Neither is their discourse any better among the women: for they are pleas'd with all sorts of Love-Tales, let 'em be never so obscene, or never so Lascivious: and their children learn their filthy words and phrases, as soon as they can speak: insomuch that by that time they come to be ten years of age, all their discourse with the women, is the most beastly that a Brothel-House can utter'.[10]

He was rather gushing when it came to the physical attributes of the Mingrelian women: 'Nature having bestow'd upon the Women of that Country Graces and Features, which are not other where to be seen...'tis impossible to behold 'em without falling in Love'.[11]

Sir Robert Shirley, a Sussex-born English diplomat, travelled to Persia with his brother, Sir Anthony Shirley. The latter spoke highly of his younger brother's qualities to the King of Persia, and stated that Robert possessed an 'excellent spirit, which in his younger years he bettered with higher studies' and that he genuinely sought to improve himself, unlike others in their highborn circle who 'under a magnificent title, love slothful idlenesse'.[12] It was whilst he was in Persia in 1607 that Robert married a Christian Circassian woman, Sampsonia. She later had a Carmelite baptism and was thereafter known as Lady Teresa Shirley.[13] The couple travelled extensively together as part of Shirley's political missions, visiting places such as Goa and Spain.[14, 15]

The famous foreign noblewoman Pocahontas also adopted an English name. In 1614, Matoaka (Pocahontas), princess of the Algonquian nation of Virginia, was baptised as a Christian, and she took the name 'Rebecca'. She married the English settler and widower John Rolfe in the same year of her conversion, and gave birth to a son the following year.[16] There is some disagreement in the academic community as to whether she willingly converted and married Rolfe or was forced to do so as a captive. Either way, the Rolfe Family journeyed to England together in 1616. The portrait of her by Simon de Passe, dated from the year of their arrival, depicts Rebecca Rolfe dressed in sumptuous Jacobean clothing with a tall sugarloaf hat, and holding a feather fan in her hand. She died in 1617, probably of pneumonia, and was buried in St George's Chapel, Gravesend, England.

During the Stuart period, foreign cultures (including those on the Continent) were thought to be vice-ridden. For example, in his entry on the poet George Sandys, William Winstanley tellingly wrote, 'He [Sandys] was not like to many of our English travellers, who with their breath suck in the vices of other nations'.[17]

Jamestown, created in 1607, was the first successful attempt at establishing an English colony since the failure of the Roanoke Island colony in the previous century.[18] It was named Jamestown 'in honour of the King's most excellent Majesty',[19] King James I. The aristocratic settlement of Virginia (named after the 'Virgin Queen' Elizabeth), found itself lacking in women. In 1621, a group of fifty-six young women travelled from England to this colony in a plan concocted by Sir Edwin Sandys to bring brides to their colonists in the New World.[20]

Tales of the punishment meted out to foreign sexual offenders were of almost as much interest to Stuart readers as tales of exotic and sensual women. In Adam Olearius' *The History of Muscovy, Tartary, & Persia*, translated into English and published in London in 1669, one of the accounts includes an observation of horsemen. All these men were very capable riders, but on closer inspection, it transpired that one of them had no hands or feet; for these had been cut off as punishment for his strange debauches and extravagances, even to the 'ravishing of maids and women in their houses'.[21] Reportedly, the stumps were boiled in butter to 'stop the blood'.[22]

The Royal African Company was established by the Royal House of Stuart in 1663. It traded valuable raw materials such as gold and silver ore, but also participated in the burgeoning trade in black slaves from West Africa to the plantations of the New World.[23]

In the French colony of Haiti—ruled by King Louis XIV, a cousin to the royal Stuarts—white masters were permitted to marry their black or native Haitian women as long as they had a Catholic marriage, at which point, the woman and any children would no longer be slaves.[24] A decree called *Le Code Noir*, devoted to slavery, was passed in 1685.

In the English colony of Maryland, however, things were very different. Maryland legalised slavery in 1663 and, a year later, unions between white women and black slaves made the white woman and any children of that union slaves.[25] Interracial procreation was even mentioned in Robert Hooke's *Micrographia*: 'We find by relations how much the *Negro* Women do besmeer the off-spring of the *Spaniard*, bringing forth neither white-skinn'd nor black, but tawny hided *Mulattos*'.[26] Hooke continued, neither particularly for nor against race-mixing, but rather fascinated by its natural result.

The poem, 'A Fair Nymph scorning a Black Boy courting her', by John Cleveland (1613–1658), depicts a dialogue between a black man and the white nymph he is sexually pursuing:

> 'our curl'd Embraces shall delight
> To checker Limbs with black and white'.[27]

When the nymph states she will not have him because of his colour, he says he will 'strive to wash it off with Tears', to which she replies:

'Tears can no more affection win,
Than wash thy Aethiopian Skin'.

Although fictional, William Shakespeare's *Othello* centres upon Othello, a Moor, who ends up killing his white wife, Desdemona, in a fit of jealous madness. Shakespeare has the villain Iago make incendiary, racially-charged, and sexually-explicit comments to Brabantio, Desdemona's father:

'Even now, now, very now, an old black ram
Is tupping your white ewe...[28]
I am one, sir, that comes to tell you your daughter and the
Moor are now making the beast with two backs.[29]

Stuart-era explorers thought nothing of using foreign women to satiate their sexual needs, since they had an inherent sense of racial superiority, but Iago's comments to Brabantio would have hit a nerve with many audience members, who would have been uncomfortable with the idea of a black man (whom they thought of as being inferior) having sexual relations with a white woman.

There is also evidence that European pirates thought little of non-Caucasian women.[30] The English buccaneer William Davis, for example, apparently had no qualms about trading his black African wife for a drink.[31] During this period, all women were generally regarded as being inferior to men, but white women were regarded as superior to women of other races.

In Chester County, Pennsylvania, one John Powell was brought to court for swearing oaths and drunkenly 'attempting to ride over several Indian [Native American] women and being withheld drew his knife [and] threatened to rip them up'.[32] Powell was fined for his swearing and for his other offences, but what became of his intended victims is unknown.

In a letter from Roger Williams to John Winthrop dated October 26, 1637: 'there is now at Pequat with the Monahiganeucks one William (Baker I think his name is) who was pursued, as is said, by the English of Qunnihticut for uncleanliness with an Indian Squaw, who is now with child by him'.[33] This William Baker, the letter continues, was shacked up with a new 'Squaw'.

Native American women were not the only targets. In September 1639, Mary Mendame of Duxburrow, a married woman, was found guilty of committing adultery with Tinsin, a Native American man. The court was much more severe on her than on Tinsin because it concluded that he had been hounded by the sexually-aggressive Mary into having sex with her. As punishment for this, she also was whipped and made to wear a badge. She was further warned that if she was ever seen thereafter without the badge, she would be branded on the face with a hot iron.[34]

Stuart-era aristocratic portraiture (for example from Britain and the Netherlands) often depicts a white nobleman or noblewoman with a black African servant. This was done partly for aesthetic reasons, since it was believed a dark-skinned person would emphasise the whiteness of the sitter's skin, and also to demonstrate affluence, as generally only the wealthiest could afford these exotic servants.[35]

European sailors to Africa would have sex with the native women there. Describing his time serving with the Spanish Navy, English chirurgeon (surgeon) Richard Wiseman made observations regarding fornication and infection:

> I have seen the frequent experiment during the three years I served in the King of Spain's Navy, where our Mariners as soon as their pockets were full of money would be getting ashore to the Negroes and other common Woman, that usually attended their Landing, and served their pleasures in the neighbouring Broom which grew very plentifully on some of those shores. I have known, and dare say, more than twenty men lay with one and the same woman the same day, and only some of them infected, the rest going free, though they all equally deserved it.[36]

Again we see the belief that bad behaviour—particularly of the sexual variety—ought to be punished.

The English author of the aforementioned *The New Atlas,* T.C., wrote in his chapter on Mexico, that 'the Spanish women are here very beautiful, and take a greater liberty than allowed in Spain, in Gaming, Drinking, and making Visits'.[37] He then observed that 'many of the Spanish Marry with Indian [Native American] women, and beget a race called Mollotos,[38] of a Tawny Complexion'. He goes on to write disapprovingly of the Spaniards and their sexual liaisons with Native American women, and of the rather gaudy manner in which some of these women dressed: '...and these sorts of wenches are allowed or winked at to be Curtizans or Common Women, to satisfy the Spaniards' Venery, to which they are insatiably given'.[39]

We should note, however, that not all Stuart-era sex between Europeans and foreign peoples involved the Europeans being in the dominant position. Although the transatlantic slave trade of Africans was taking place during this time, another slave trade was also occurring: that of white Europeans. Coastal towns and villages throughout Europe lived in fear of the notorious Barbary pirates, who would attack these areas and either kill the inhabitants or abduct them with the intention of selling them into slavery (sometimes sexual slavery) at North African coastal towns and cities such as Salé and Tunis.

A relation of the whole proceedings concerning the redemption of the captives in Argier and Tunis (1646), details the names of British men, women, and children who were kidnapped and sold into foreign slavery. They came from a variety of coastal towns: Ursula Corlion of Falmouth, Daniel Piper of Plymouth, William Dunster of Dover, Sarah Leeds of Chatham, John Case of Bristol, Mary Weymouth 'and her two sons', Thomas Underhill of London... the list goes on.

Just as many African slaves were denied their native religion and forced to convert to Christianity, Christian European slaves often received the same treatment at the hands of their Muslim masters. Some enslaved European men were beaten severely until they renounced Christianity and converted to Islam. These men would then be forcibly circumcised.[40] Since (as previously mentioned) circumcision was not a cultural norm in Stuart Britain, this would have caused not only excruciating physical pain but also psychological and emotional trauma. The white women who ended up in North African harems were often selected from markets which were stocked from these piratical raids on coastal European towns and villages.[41]

The pirates, and their practice of capturing people as slaves, became a major problem for many European nations, some of whom responded with force. The French Minister of State, Marquis de Louvois, wrote that:

> the example of Tripoli and Morocco showed we were unable
> to overcome the brutality of the Algerians...Your Majesty
> sent, in the end of the year 1682, a fleet to Algiers which has

thrown so many bombs, ruined so many buildings, damaged so many mosques, and made so many people perish, that these barbarians were charmed with their insolence... and at last they were abated and submissive, and were content to let you buy [the freedoms of] more than four hundred Christian slaves, which were returned to you, among whom were also your own subjects, all the foreigners whom these pirates had taken under your banner.[42]

In Stuart Britain, people were no less concerned about the situation. The MP John Jones (c.1610–1692) left £100 in his will to go towards the recovery of English slaves in Africa,[43] while Daniel Defoe, author of such famous works as *Robinson Crusoe* and *A Journal of a Plague Year,* penned *A General History of Pyrates*.

In 1631, Barbary pirates also attacked the village of Baltimore in Ireland, seizing men, women, and children. The women and children tended to be treated better than the men (many of whom were beaten), as unharmed women and children would fetch higher prices at market, but women who refused to convert to Islam were likely to face torture and death.[44] The most notorious sultan was one Moulay Ismail, who forced his black and white slaves to have sex in order to breed mulattos[45] and had one young English girl whipped when she refused to convert and let him have sex with her. The girl was treated so badly that she ultimately yielded, the sultan impregnated her, and that was that.[46]

PART TWO

The Sexy Stuarts

Now that we have explored the whole spectrum of sex and sexuality in Stuart Britain, it's time to take a much closer look at the monarchs who ruled during this period, one by one. The sex lives and sexual preferences of the Royal Stuarts have been the subject of much speculation, rumour, and plain old fabrication for political gain. In this section, we'll have a look at the seven reigns—and one Interregnum—in more detail.

REIGNS OF STUART KINGS & QUEENS
James VI of Scotland & I of England: 1603–1625
Charles I: 1625–1649
Interregnum: 1649–1660
Charles II: 1660–1685
James II & IV: 1685–1688 (deposed)
William III & II & Mary II: 1689–1694 (her death)
William III: 1694–1702
Queen Anne: 1702–1714

Chapter 21

James VI & I, Swinging Both Ways?
(1603–1625)

Rex fuit Elizabeth, nunc est regina Iacobus
(Elizabeth was King, now James is Queen)[1]

Why did the Scottish royal family become the rulers of Scotland, England (including Wales), and Ireland? The Royal House of Stewart—or Stiùbhairt—dates back to the 1300s with Robert the Bruce. Although they experienced their fair share of upheavals, the Stewarts retained control of Scotland for hundreds of years. In March 1603, the English queen Elizabeth I, the last of the Tudors, died—without issue. For years, there had been speculation as to who would succeed her. That person ultimately turned out to be her cousin, King James VI of Scotland.

James was descended from the Tudors, however, as his great-grandmother was Margaret Tudor, a sister of Henry VIII. Margaret had married the Scottish James IV in 1503 with whom she had a son and heir, James V. This king, in turn, left only one heir by the time of his death aged only thirty: Mary. This woman, more popularly known as Mary, Queen of Scots, was James VI's mother.

James's own conception and birth actually sprung from a misguided union between Mary, Queen of Scots, and her cousin, Henry Stuart, Lord Darnley. Mary had returned home to Scotland from France in 1561, a teenaged widow and a Dowager Queen of France (her husband, King Francis II, died in 1560, aged only sixteen[2]). Following her first husband's death, she had received the interest of several suitors for her hand, to no avail. Things changed, however, when she met her English-born cousin, Henry, in 1565.

Darnley was descended from the same grandmother as Mary, Margaret Tudor, but via the latter's second marriage to the Earl of Angus.[3]

What turned out to be a poor choice of husband may have been due to Mary's intense passion and sexual attraction for him;[4] for when she saw him 'she said that he was the lustiest and best-proportioned man she had ever seen'.[5] Henry was almost effeminately beautiful, and his height of over six feet was a major attraction for a woman who was herself 5 ft 11.[6]

Henry, however, proved to be a cruel, jealous, violent, and unfaithful husband prone to excessive drinking. He was murdered at Kirk o' Field in 1567, aged only twenty-one. By then, the unhappy couple's only child and heir, the future James VI, was around eight months old. After Darnley's assassination—an event which remains mysterious today[7]—Queen Mary ended up marrying James Hepburn, 4th Earl of Bothwell.

Around this time, a myth was propagated by Mary's enemies that she was sexually promiscuous. This became a potent mark upon her character that helped to justify her overthrow—as had been the intention.[8] It was ruinous for a woman—especially a woman with power—to have a reputation for wantonness. Scurrilous and incendiary sketches of Mary were also made, wherein she was depicted as a mermaid (at this time a symbol of prostitution).[9] Following nearly two decades of house arrest, Elizabeth finally had her rival cousin and queen executed at Fotheringhay Castle in Northamptonshire in 1587.

During the tumult surrounding his mother's flight and house arrest, what became of Mary's child, James? He was, for all intents and purposes, an orphan, and was cared for by the Earl and Countess of Mar and was crowned King of Scots. Political intrigues and plots abounded—including the Raid of Ruthven (1582) and the Gowrie Conspiracy (1600).

What of the young king's amorous inclinations? Esmé Stuart, 1st Duke of Lennox, was an early favourite of James VI, and Scottish court observers wrote of 'the carnal lust' he inspired in the king, and how the king would passionately 'kiss' him.[10] Indeed, the then-teenaged James was so openly demonstrative and tactile with the older Esmé that it is no surprise that some assumed the king to be in love with him.[11] James's preference for Esmé set a precedent for his subsequent favourites: James made him the Duke of Lennox, with all the power that such a position entailed.[12] Unlike the case of some of his descendants (for example William III and Queen Anne), who are often rumoured to have been both physically and emotionally attracted to their own sex, there is good evidence that this was true of James.

Whilst James VI/I's sexual tastes appear to have inclined principally towards other men, he nevertheless had no aversion to bedding and impregnating his wife, Anna of Denmark. Upon their first meeting, after their proxy wedding, Anna was taken aback by James's kiss. The young King James married Anna in 1589, when she was fifteen.

The royal couple's sex life must have been active, for Anna conceived many times and gave birth to seven children—Henry, Elizabeth, Margaret, Charles, Robert, Mary, and Sophia—but only Henry, Elizabeth, and Charles survived childhood.[13] Shortly after giving birth to her eldest son, Henry Frederick, Anna was again pregnant. This child, however, she miscarried (possibly due to the great stress she was suffering when her eldest baby was taken away to his own household in Stirling).[14]

There is no evidence that King James had extramarital affairs with other women, though he may have visited a Southwark brothel from time to time with some of his courtiers.[15]

When Queen Elizabeth I died in 1603, her successor was named and James decided to move with his family down to London. England was by far the wealthier of the two kingdoms, and James eventually developed a reputation for lavish spending.[16] The court of King James VI of Scotland/I of England was very different from those which preceded and followed it, for among other things, the new king had a lavatorial sense of humour and an eye for pretty young men.[17] Besides being uncouth and vulgar, he also had a tendency to lose his temper and this sometimes manifested itself in physical violence.[18]

Lucy Hutchinson didn't mince her words when she wrote, 'The court of this king was a nursery of *lust* and intemperance; he had brought in with him a company of poor Scots, who, coming into this plentiful kingdom, were surfeited with riot and *debaucheries*, and got all the riches of the land only to cast away'.[19] Hutchinson continued, 'The honour, wealth, and glory of the nation, wherein Queen Elizabeth left it, were soon prodigally wasted by this thriftless heir; and the nobility of the land was utterly debased by setting honours to public sale…for the maintenance of *vice* and *lewdness*'.[20]

The favourites

The king, whilst more intellectual than some other monarchs, was rather louche, and rumours of his sexuality abounded. One Robert Carr was, by all accounts, a very handsome young man whose good looks immediately attracted King James I during a court joust in 1607.[21] Four years later, in a similar vein to Esmé Stuart's rise, James made

Carr Viscount Rochester and the young man became the first Scot to sit in the English House of Lords.[22] Carr's affair with the already-married Frances Howard caused a stir, but it was their subsequent marriage and involvement in the Overbury Poisoning Scandal which really made things difficult for the favourite. The couple was imprisoned in the Tower of London in 1616 and released in 1622.[23] A couple of years before Carr's imprisonment, however, James's head had already been turned by a younger, and even more exceptionally handsome young man who had completely taken his heart...

George Villiers rose from being virtually unknown to being one of the most important and powerful men in the realm, and in doing so he inspired both great admiration and intense hatred in those around him. James, twenty-six years older than his new love interest, nicknamed George 'Steenie' after Saint Stephen, because he was so very beautiful. Even his critics such as the puritan historian Sir Simonds D'Ewes conceded that Villiers had an 'effeminate' beauty.[24] Not only did he possess this attribute—and enjoyed the status of being the great favourite of King James—but he was also shrewd when it came to the king. Given the intimate content of the many letters from King James to 'Steenie' (whom the former referred to as 'sweet child and wife'[25]) it seems likely that these two men were lovers, as they seem to indicate a close familiarity with each other's bodies,[26] but there was a sort of father-son dynamic as well. However, as mentioned in the introduction to this book, we will probably never know whether they were lovers with certainty, and if so, for how long.

Surely such a relationship would have aroused jealousy in Anna of Denmark? Surprisingly, it doesn't seem to have—and, what's more, she appears to have got on well with her husband's great intimate.[27] Her letters to him are affectionate, she even addressed him as 'my kind dog'.[28] The king's relationship with Villiers was, however, regarded negatively by most of James's subjects, especially because of the latter's powerful hold upon the monarch and his political interference.[29] James heaped titles upon his great love: the Earl of Buckingham in 1617, a Marquess two years later, and then, finally, the 1st Duke of Buckingham in 1623.[30]

Buckingham's own sexual preferences suggest that he favoured women to men, and it is possible that he welcomed the king's love mainly, if not exclusively, in order to advance his own fortunes and those of his family. Buckingham was, for example, romantically linked to (and perhaps physically intimate with) the likes of Lucy Hay, Countess of Carlisle, and Anne of Austria, the queen consort of Louis XIII of France.[31] He also attracted other, less famous, women such as Frances Shute—the mistress of the Earl of Sussex—who was so enamoured with Buckingham that she hired a magician with the purpose of making him reciprocate her affections.[32]

Sexual dalliances aside, Buckingham ultimately needed an advantageous marriage to secure his family's fortunes. Sixteen-year-old Lady Katherine Manners, of plain looks and unremarkable personality, and from a Catholic family, would not have been considered remotely suitable for so dashing and powerful a man as George Villiers now was—were it not for the fact she was one of the wealthiest heiresses in the country and possessed excellent connections and pedigree. With the magnetic Villiers after her hand, young Katherine didn't stand a chance. The most striking portrait, c. 1620, of George and Katherine is by Anthony van Dyck, in which they are depicted half naked as Venus and Adonis. It is a sensual painting: whilst George gazes lovingly at her, his hand gently lying over his naked chest, her eyes are on the viewer, a knowing look upon her face, her breasts exposed, her nipples erect.

The couple had several children together, including Charles, who did not survive infancy, George, who later became the dissipated 2nd Duke of Buckingham, Mary, who became the Duchess of Richmond and Lenox, and Francis, who was born after his father's murder.[33] The letters between Buckingham and the King reveal a playful, yet vulgar and dismissive regard for the women in Buckingham's life: his wife, mother, and sister were referred to as 'the cunts'.[34]

Next to his own romantic pursuits, King James took a keen interest in the those of the nobles of his kingdoms and presided over the weddings of a few of the biggest names of the Jacobean period. In 1607, he attended the nuptial ceremonies of Honoria Denny and James, Lord Hay—whose union he had brought about.[35]

But all things come to an end. King James died in 1625. Rumours spread that he had been poisoned by his lover, Buckingham, and by the mid-1620s, Buckingham was almost universally reviled. He was stabbed to death at the Greyhound Inn in Portsmouth in 1627. Almost three decades later, in 1655, diarist John Evelyn observed that York House, situated on the River Thames, was once 'belonging to the former great Buckingham, but [was] now much ruined through neglect'.[36] Indeed, visitors to present-day London's Embankment Gardens can still see the York Water Gate—all that now remains of York House.

Chapter 22

Charles I, Lusty but Loyal (1625–1649)

The disdain with which Henry Stuart, Prince of Wales, viewed the debauched and loose morality of his father's court is clear from the way he ruled over his own, satellite, court. In perhaps a reaction to what he saw in his father's conduct, he appears to have had a dislike of effeminacy in men.[1] Swearing was punishable by a fine, which would be collected and then given to charity. Henry was dynamic, learned, cultured, and accomplished. He was a prince who had a glorious future before him and who was entertaining thoughts of finding a suitable bride. He abhorred sexual indiscretions, and is believed to have spurned the Jacobean femme fatale, Frances Howard, Lady Essex, who was rumoured to be sleeping with his father's favourite, Robert Carr.[2]

All that came to naught, however, when Henry was eighteen years old, for at this age he sickened and died (probably from Typhoid). In a death which sent shockwaves throughout the lands, the golden boy was no more, but there was yet hope as the royal family had another son who would inherit the throne.

Prince Charles, like his elder brother, Henry, was a very different animal to their father, King James. Born in Scotland in 1600, Charles—who was very much treated as the 'spare' he was—faced personal challenges including a speech impediment and rickets—but the latter he managed to overcome through a regimen of consistent, regular exercise.[3] Henry had enjoyed collecting art, and Charles did as well, eventually procuring some of the most beautiful works of art that can be seen in today's Royal Collection.

In 1616, four years after Henry's untimely death, *The Workes of the Most High and Mightie Prince, James, by the grace of God, King of Great Britain and Ireland*, was published. In this, there is a preface dedicated to Charles—the 'onely sonne of our soveraigne lord the king'. This features numerous compliments of Charles's virtues and talents and ends with the line: 'God grant together with the length of many good and happy days'.[4] If only the author knew that his subject's life was to end with an executioner's axe.

One of the greatest (mis)adventures of Charles's life was his secret journey into Spain in 1623 (accompanied by George Villiers), on a rather idealistic and romantic quest to woo and marry the Spanish Infanta Maria Theresa. Along the way, the duo stopped at the French court in Paris where they were entertained in the company of the French royal family. Among the party were Princess Henriette Marie, the youngest daughter of the deceased Henri IV of France, a king who survived the infamous St Bartholomew's Day Massacre of 1572, and his second wife, Marie de' Medici, of the powerful Italian family. Charles paid neither much attention, for his mind was on his goal: his Spanish bride.

Although there had been considerable antipathy between Charles and Buckingham early on, their relationship improved significantly as a result of this Spanish adventure. Their personalities were quite different: Charles was serious and formal, whilst Buckingham was more laid-back and flashy. There is an oft-regurgitated myth that Charles shared the Duke of Buckingham as a lover with his father, but there is scant evidence to support this claim. Indeed, Charles, just like his brother Henry (as mentioned earlier) was very different to his father and wanted to maintain a moral and formal court—such behaviour would have been entirely out-of-character for him.

Finally, the two nobleman from Stuart Britain arrived in Madrid, where they finally revealed their true identities. The King of Spain, Felipe IV, proceeded to entertain his foreign guests with wolf-hunting, feasting, *juego de cañas*,[5] and fencing, among other activities.[6] The Spanish court was extremely formal and abided by a rigid system of etiquette, and when Charles met the Spanish Infanta, he and the Duke of Buckingham were received 'with much curtsey'.[7] The young prince's quest to win the hand of the Infanta proved ultimately unsuccessful, however it was while at the Spanish court that he briefly spoke with the former French princess, Elisabeth de Bourbon, now Queen Isabel of Spain, the wife of Felipe IV. She suggested that her little sister, Henriette Marie, would be a suitable wife for him.[8]

Charles took Elisabeth's advice. It was not to a Spanish princess of the House of Habsburg that he was wed, but to that little French princess of the House of Bourbon who had been in attendance during his brief visit to Paris. Whilst she was known as Queen Mary during her time in England, history has since remembered her as Henrietta Maria.[9]

Henrietta Maria was the youngest child of King Henri IV of France and his second wife, Marie de' Medici (his first having been Marguerite de Valois). Henri IV was stabbed to death by an assassin in May 1610, when his daughter was only a few months old.

When all negotiations with the Spanish had come to an end, he began proceedings with the French for her hand. In an extremely sumptuous wedding ceremony in the Cathédrale de Notre-Dame de Paris on the Île de la Cité in May 1625, the fifteen-year-old Princess Henrietta Maria married the new King Charles I via a proxy, the duc de Chevreuse (as the intended proxy, George Villiers, Duke of Buckingham, had been delayed).[10] Villiers' behaviour was a source of embarrassment, however, for he tried to make love to Louis XIII's wife, Anne of Austria.[11]

By 22 June of that year, a very seasick Henrietta Maria had arrived on English soil, in Dover.[12] On the night of their consummation, Charles shooed the servants away and bolted the door—breaking with the tradition of the bedding ceremony, so typical of Stuart-era weddings.[13] The following morning, the king looked to be very pleased, but his young bride was not as content.[14] Charles and Henrietta Maria spent their honeymoon at Hampton Court Palace.[15]

Their early married life was difficult and filled with rows and misunderstandings. Henrietta Maria, from the very beginning of their marriage, proved to be a somewhat volatile young woman inclined towards temper tantrums. Her youth and her situation in a new country, combined with the antipathy against her beloved Roman Catholicism and the obligation to adopt a new language and culture might have contributed to this behaviour. Her devout faith, combined with her strict priests, meant that she was not permitted to engage in sexual activity on holy days—and lusty Charles became very annoyed with this unwelcome restriction upon his conjugal rights.[16] The lusty monarch abhorred the meddlesome priests who got in the way of his sexual gratification. One of the other great arguments between Charles and Henrietta Maria occurred in 1626 and was to do with her French retinue, whom Charles had disliked since they had arrived the year before.[17]

Despite these hiccups, the couple grew closer in time, particularly following the Duke of Buckingham's assassination in 1627 (many believe he had always been something of a 'third wheel' in their relationship). Charles was heartbroken at the loss of his friend, a man whom he had genuinely admired, and in his grief he turned to his young wife. The couple's love flourished from then onward, although it would later face much greater troubles.

The marriage of Charles and Henrietta Maria was sexually passionate and loving. Furthermore, unlike some of the other royal women—including, later, her own granddaughters—Henrietta Maria proved to be wonderfully fertile and had no difficulty conceiving.[18] Nonetheless, she and Charles did endure some heartbreak: for the first couple of years there was some concern because Henrietta failed to get pregnant, leading to rumours that she was barren. Following the tragic birth and death of a premature son in May of 1629, the couple welcomed a healthy son, Charles on 29 May 1630.[19] A year later, their eldest daughter, Mary Henrietta, Princess Royal (later, Princess of Orange) was born.[20] Mary was followed a couple of years later by James, Duke of York, Elizabeth in 1635, Anne in 1637, and Henry in 1640.[21] Their last child, Henrietta Anne (Minette) was born in Exeter in June 1644.[22]

Charles and Henrietta Maria also had a shared enjoyment of the arts, had exquisite taste in art, and together amassed a stunning collection of artwork.[23] The royal couple also found excitement in going hunting together, and enjoyed producing court masques with the multi-talented Inigo Jones.[24]

But political troubles soon came to their door, paving the way to civil war. As the flames of discord began firmly taking root, the couple's personal lives took another painful blow. Young Princess Anne, who had been suffering from tuberculosis, died at the age of four at Richmond Palace.[25] After this bereavement, civil war broke out when the king had his standard raised at Nottingham in 1642.

The letters Charles and Henrietta Maria sent to each other, particularly during the volatile 1640s, are filled with love. In them, Henrietta Maria addresses Charles as 'my dear heart'.[26] During one of many difficult times, she wrote: 'I hope God will bless our pains; it is the only reward I ask for them, and that you will always love me'.[27] Their family, by this time, had been torn apart. His wife often ended her letters with,

'Absolutely yours', and at one parting in Dover, the couple were seen to take leave of one another with a multitude of kisses and embraces.[28]

Charles I, in contrast to his eldest son Charles II, is not known for having had extramarital affairs. He was, for the most part, loyal to his wife, despite being targeted in the early 1630s by the seductive Lucy Hay, Countess of Carlisle, who was herself being positioned by others to become his mistress.[29] The king's only known adulterous liaison took place with one Jane Whorwood while he was imprisoned in Carisbrooke Castle in 1648. Whorwood was a devoted Royalist spy who became Charles's follower, friend, and then mistress. It seems that she both physically and emotionally comforted an increasingly doom-laden monarch who, by this time, had been separated from his wife for more than four years. He had a strong sexual drive, and the brief sexual fling with Jane Whorwood was what he needed.[30]

Henrietta Maria, by this time, had already taken refuge in her native France, and was eventually joined by some of her children, Henrietta Anne, James, Charles, and finally, Henry. Henrietta Maria was also rumoured to have taken her favourite, Henry Jermyn, 1st Earl of St. Albans, as her lover.[31]

Years of house arrest at various sites plus further political machinations from both sides eventually led to the king being put on trial for treason. He was found guilty and sentenced to death. Charles I met his fate when he was publicly executed outside the Banqueting Hall of Whitehall Palace on 30 January 1648/9, and was buried in St. George's Chapel, Windsor Castle. When told the shocking news that her husband had been beheaded, Henrietta Maria went into a sort of catatonic state.[32] Her grief and shock consumed her, and her profound heartbreak over the violent and untimely death of her beloved husband lasted for the rest of her life.

Eleven years later, in October 1660, Henrietta Maria returned to England, as described by John Evelyn: 'Arrived the Queen-Mother in England, whence she had been banished for almost twenty years; together with her illustrious daughter, the Princess Henrietta, diverse princes and noblemen, accompanying them'. The now Queen Dowager returned to France with her long-time favourite, Harry Jermyn, living in Colombes, where she died from an opiate overdose on the tenth of October 1669.[33]

Chapter 23

Interregnum Intimacies (1649–1660)

With the execution of Charles I, Parliament abolished the monarchy and the House of Lords. The period sandwiched in between the Caroline court of Charles I (1625–1649) and Charles II's Restoration court (1660) is known as the 'Interregnum' or Commonwealth during which the Three Kingdoms was a republic.

Puritans[1] have generally been portrayed over the centuries as rather severe, prudish, and devout. This is not without good reason: under the rule of the Parliamentarians, the 1640s and 1650s saw considerable destruction of stained-glass windows and altars in churches, the closure of theatres, the banning of traditional pastimes such as maypoles,[2] and the tearing down of monuments such as the Cheapside Cross in 1643. In 1647 Christmas was actually banned—by Parliament, not by Oliver Cromwell—and some people rebelled against this, most notably in Ipswich and Canterbury.

Heavy-handedness against sexual immorality during this period, however, centred mainly on *premarital* sex, general fornication, and adultery (and indeed some well-known figures of the time had their own share of sexual scandal). Sex within the holy bonds of matrimony was regarded as an entirely different matter, and was welcomed.

The Parliamentarian commander Edward Montagu, 2nd Earl of Manchester (1602–1671), married an astonishing five times. Tragically, he was bereaved four times, before his last wife, Margaret, survived him by five years.[3]

Andrew Marvell (1621–1678), was an English politician and an acclaimed Metaphysical poet whose poem *To His Coy Mistress* remains one of the most popular of the seventeenth century. He never officially married, but following his death, his housekeeper, Mary Palmer, claimed she had married him secretly in 1667.[4] Marvell's sexual inclinations remain a source of contention and interest among researchers.

William Walwyn (1600–1681), was a major figure in the radical Leveller movement, writing and publishing *The Bloody Project* in 1648. In his love life, he appears to have been a most amorous husband—he was married to Anne and the couple had twenty children![5]

In 1652, Gregory Clements, an English politician and a regicide of Charles I, found himself embroiled in a sex scandal when it was claimed he was having an illicit sexual relationship with a maidservant.[6] There is some speculation that this was trumped-up, however, as by this time Clements had made enemies among more radical politicians. Nonetheless, he was forced to resign and kept a low profile until the Restoration, at which point he was sent to the Tower of London for High Treason, and was executed by hanging, drawing, and quartering at Charing Cross in October 1660.[7]

Colonel Henry Marten (b. 1602) was a notorious womaniser, and had developed such a reputation for his sexual escapades that the sexually straight-laced Charles I dismissed him from his service, allegedly referring to him as a 'whore-master'.[8] Following the Restoration, Marten was sent to the Tower (being another of King Charles I's regicides). There, he wrote letters to his mistress—the mother of his three daughters, Mary Ward. These letters were published in 1662 as *Coll. Henry Marten's Familiar Letters to his Lady of Delight* and are largely about mundane everyday things, but there are some expressions of love in them. For example: 'So for this time I bid thee good morrow, and rest, my sweet Soul, thy own every day that goes over my head, every night too, whether I talk to thee or no, whether I dream of thee or no'.[9] At one point, Marten even affectionately refers to his mistress as 'Monkey-Face'.[10] Having successfully avoided the traitor's death that befell so many of his fellow regicides, Marten died in 1680 from choking on his dinner.[11]

The Ranters were a radical group who emerged during the Civil Wars and developed during the 1650s. The sexual freedoms allegedly espoused by the group were previously unheard-of in Stuart Britain; they were said to reject societal views on morality.[12] Although there is continuing debate amongst researchers as to whether or not the Ranters actually existed,[13] Laurence Clarkson (1615–1667) —the man most associated with the movement—certainly did exist and was notorious for his sexual promiscuity. He went so far as to make a sort of commune in London where he had sex with willing virgins who believed in his ideology of free and pure love without sin.[14] In his 1660 work,

The Lost Sheep Found, he described how he seduced one of the young women (probably a virgin) who was starry-eyed by his rantings, and she—not knowing he was already married—expected to marry him after he had carnally known her. Having been thus deceived, she ended up marrying another in his sect.[15] Preston-born Clarkson, who married twice and fathered at least five children, eventually died in debtor's prison in 1667.

Sir John Gell, a Parliamentarian during the English Civil Wars, is known for his harassment of Sir John Stanhope over a disagreement about Charles I's controversial Ship Money tax. Stanhope died in 1638. According to Lucy Hutchinson, Gell was 'so revengeful, that he pursued his malice to Sir John Stanhope... with such barbarism after his death, that he, pretending to search for arms and plate, came into the church and defaced his monument that cost six hundred pounds, breaking off the nose and other parts of it.'[16]

In 1644, Gell's wife Elizabeth died. Three years later—and very surprisingly—Gell then married Stanhope's widow, Mary. Hutchinson wrote that Gell 'wooed that widow, who was by all the world believed to be the most prudent and affectionate of womankind, till, being deluded by his hypocrisies, she consented to marry him, and found that was the utmost point to which he could carry his revenge, his future carriage making it apparent he sought her for nothing else but to destroy the glory of her husband and his house'.[17]

Oliver Cromwell is often portrayed as a cold-hearted villain, especially with regard to his admittedly stomach-turning dealings with the Irish, but there are some aspects of his life that reveal him to have been a passionate man. When he was a teenager in Huntingdon, Oliver gained a reputation for enjoying carnal pursuits and other sinful activities, such as gaming.[18] Shortly after he came of age, he married Elizabeth Bourchier in August of 1620,[19] and the couple went on to have several children: Bridget (b. 1624), Richard (b. 1626), Henry (b. 1628), Elizabeth (b. 1629), Mary (b. 1636), and Frances (b. 1638). When one reads the surviving letters between Cromwell and his wife Elizabeth, their love and devotion to each other is evident.

Although there have been rumours that Cromwell had a sexual relationship with Elizabeth Murray, Countess of Dysart, this is highly improbable given his attitude towards such things.[20] In another probable attempt to discredit Cromwell, his wife Elizabeth was the subject of scurrilous gossip which claimed she had been bedded by officers and soldiers in her husband's regiment.[21] Similar Royalist propaganda accused the wives of other prominent Parliamentarians, such as Mary Corbet, as being sexually promiscuous.[22] Indeed, these rumours of female unchastity were similar to those previously faced by Henrietta Maria during her husband's reign.

The Cromwell children had interesting lives, too. Bridget Cromwell married two major Parliamentarian officers. Her first husband was Henry Ireton—one of the first men to sign Charles I's death warrant in 1649. Ireton became his father-in-law's second in command during the Irish campaign, then Lord Deputy of Ireland in 1650, dying a year later. Bridget's second husband was Major-General Charles Fleetwood— another army radical.

Elizabeth, or 'Bettie', Cromwell is considered to have been her father's favourite child. She married John Claypole, and the couple had three children, including a son named Henry. According to Lucy Hutchinson, 'Claypole, who married his (Oliver's) daughter, and his son Henry, were two debauch'd ungodly cavaliers'.[23] It's widely believed that the death of Bettie in 1658 contributed to Oliver Cromwell's own decline and eventual death one year later.

During the 1650s, government and society at large lay firmly under Puritan control,[24] but in the years following the Restoration of the monarchy in 1660, the pendulum of societal mores thundered away from repression and towards a more licentious age.

Chapter 24

Charles II & the Sexually Ravenous Restoration (1660–1685)

'His sceptre and his prick are of a length,
And she may sway the one who plays with th'other'
             – *A Satyr on Charles II*, John Wilmot, 2nd Earl of
                                                  Rochester

Of all the royal Stuarts, none other captures the sexual imagination as much as King Charles II, the man so often referred to as 'the Merry Monarch' because of the poem cited above and the randy and debauched flavour he and his courtiers brought to late-seventeenth-century Britain. Although some truly tragic personal events, and many important political events, occurred during Charles's life and reign, his steamy and promiscuous love life tends to overshadow these. Indeed, numerous books have been written on this subject alone.

Born on 29 May 1630, Charles Stuart was the eldest surviving son of King Charles I and Henrietta Maria. He was soon joined by several other siblings, and the Stuart family had a loving and happy existence... until the storms clouds of rebellion and civil war rolled in.

It was during this time of political turmoil that Charles, aged fourteen, lost his virginity to Christabella Wyndham—a woman in her late-thirties who had been both his wet-nurse and one of his governesses until he was five![1] Charles was so smitten with his lover (who was the wife of Sir Edmund Wyndham) that the prince's governors decided they had better remove him to another place, just to get him away from her.

Whilst he was in exile Charles had a major romantic liaison which would have significant ramifications later on. The young woman was Lucy Walter (aka Lucy Barlow), and she gave birth to the first of Charles's many illegitimate children: James, whom Charles later made the Duke of Monmouth. A portrait of Lucy, attributed to Peter Lely, at Scolton Manor Museum, Wales, depicts a woman whom even today we would call beautiful.[2] Yet John Evelyn, one of the Stuart period's great diarists, once rode in the same carriage as Lucy, and was not very complimentary of her: 'I went to St. Germains, to kiss his Majesty's hand; in the coach, which was my Lord Wilmot's, went Mrs. Barlow, the King's mistress and mother to the Duke of Monmouth, a brown, beautiful, bold, but insipid creature'.[3] The passion between Charles and Lucy soon died down, and she went on to have two more children by different men.[4] Things between the former lovers became so difficult, in fact, that Charles eventually had their son kidnapped from Lucy as her promiscuous lifestyle was becoming well known.[5] He placed the boy under the care of the Crofts family, and young James was known as James Crofts for some time.

Gilbert Burnet writes that, 'With the restoration of the King, a spirit of extravagant joy overspread the nation, which was soon attended with all manner of profaneness and immorality'.[6] In contrast to the clampdown on certain forms of enjoyment in the 1650s, things went decidedly the opposite way when Charles reclaimed the throne, and arguably the example set by Charles trickled down to general society during the sexually ravenous Restoration.

The mistress who held the most sway over King Charles, particularly during the early years of his reign, was Barbara Palmer (née Villiers). At a time when modesty, faithfulness, and gentleness were valued qualities in the female sex, Barbara was the opposite. Notoriously volatile, a true bitch, and possessing an apparently insatiable sexual appetite, her antics have passed almost into legend. Among her lovers was her cousin, John Churchill, while he was still young and impoverished, with his days of glory as the Duke of Marlborough still far into the future. On one occasion, Charles is believed to have turned up when Barbara was having sex with John in her bedchamber.[7]

In *The Present State of England* (1675), Charles's surviving brother, James, and his cousin, Prince Rupert, are listed as the only two 'Dukes of the Royal Blood'—despite the fact that three of the nine dukes 'not of the Blood Royal' were his bastards:[8] James Scott Fitz-Roy, Duke of Monmouth, Charles Fitz-Roy, Duke of Southampton, and Henry Fitz-Roy, Duke of Grafton.

A single king with no fortune would be desirous of obtaining a wealthy bride and ensuring the continuation of his dynasty by siring a legitimate heir with her. Many women were considered, but the search finally centred upon the Portuguese Infanta, Catherine of Braganza. While her Catholicism might present a problem in her prospective country, which was overwhelmingly Protestant, she would bring with her an impressive dowry, including the port towns of Bombay and Tripoli. She and Charles wed in 1662.

In May of 1662, John Evelyn described the arrival of the new queen:

> The queen arrived with a train of Portuguese ladies in their monstrous farthingales...their complexions olivader and sufficiently unagreeable. Her Majesty in the same habit, her foretop long and turned aside very strangely. She was yet of the handsomest countenance of all the rest, and, though, short of stature, prettily shaped, languishing and excellent eyes, her teeth wronging her mouth by sticking a little too far out: the rest, lovely enough.[9]

Catherine's introduction to Charles's court along with her Portuguese entourage was at first rather embarrassing for her, since there was a great gulf fixed between the two royal courts with regard to fashion. She soon, however, adopted the clothing and hairstyles of the Restoration court and began to settle into her new life and role. One difficulty, however, was that Barbara Palmer (now Lady Castlemaine) was pregnant by the King at the time, and quite brazenly chose to have her lying-in at Hampton Court Palace—where the new Queen would soon arrive!

Samuel Pepys had kinder things to say about Catherine than Evelyn did, although he had not yet seen her in person himself:

> The Queene is brought a few days since to Hampton Court: and all people say of her to be a very fine and handsome lady, and very discreet; and that the King is pleased enough with her: which, I fear, will put Madam Castlemaine's nose out of joynt.[10]

But Castlemaine had no need to worry, for poor Catherine's charms proved to be insufficient to keep Charles faithful—or interested—for very long. Charles was a very lustful—and virile—man, who sired countless children with his numerous lovers. The new consort soon had

166

to face the insulting and humiliating fact that her husband was a prolific philanderer—and that the identity of his main squeeze was public knowledge. Even worse, Barbara insisted on becoming Catherine's Lady of the Bedchamber.[11]

The following year, 1663, saw the marriage of Charles's eldest—and favourite—bastard son, James, Duke of Monmouth, to the Scottish heiress, Anna Scott. Although we earlier mentioned the very young ages of the bride and groom, we have not examined what Charles himself thought of this. As he related to his sister Minette in a letter dated 20 April 1663, the couple would enjoy all the traditions associated with a wedding, include a bedding ceremony, but they would not be allowed to have sex nor spend the night together, because they were simply too young.[12] This indicates that Charles's views on the subject of age and marital consummation were the same as those of most other people in Stuart Britain.

Although his liaisons were for the most part shameless, the king did had a soft spot for his Portuguese wife, and she certainly had fallen in love with him quite quickly. During this period, any wife's primary role was to bear her husband children; this was doubly so when that wife was a royal, whose duty it was to bear the sovereign's heir for the sake of the country's stability and the continuity of the royal line. Catherine was under enormous pressure, and eventually, with no heir in sight, was assumed to be 'barren'.

After six years of marriage, Catherine still hadn't had a baby. When she miscarried a foetus one morning, this of course saddened her husband, but also gave him some hope. As he again confided to his sister in a letter from Whitehall, dated 7 May 1668, the tragedy proved that Catherine not only *had* conceived, but mainly that she *was* capable of conceiving—something which he had begun to doubt.[13] Yet, for some reason, Catherine was never able to bring a child to term. In the following century, Catherine of Braganza found a defender in the form of David Hume, who, in his *History of England, Vol. II*, noted that 'the report … of [Catherine's] natural incapacity to have children, seems to have been groundless; since she was twice declared to be pregnant'.[14]

Charles showed compassion towards Catherine when she was delirious from a particularly severe illness (probably smallpox), and asked after their children: although they had none, he told her they were well.[15]

Frances Stuart, one of Charles's cousins, came to England in 1662, having been raised at the French court with the exiled British royal family. She was, by most accounts, extremely beautiful—so much so that her nickname was *La Belle Stuart*. By November 1663, Pepys observed that 'the King is now become besotted upon Mrs Stewart, that he gets into corners, and will be with her half an hour together kissing her to the observation of all the world'.[16] The Count de Grammont stated, 'at this time the King's attachment to Miss Stewart was so public, that every person perceived, that if she was but possessed of art, she might become as absolute a mistress over his conduct as she was over his heart'.[17]

The pressure to succumb to the king's advances must have been great, but to Frances' credit, she stayed true to her own heart. Pepys wrote that 'she could no longer continue at Court without prostituting herself to the King, whom she had so long kept off'.[18] She instead fell in love with her cousin, another Charles Stuart, the twice-widowed 3rd Duke of Richmond and 6th Duke of Lennox. The pair secretly eloped, leaving the king angry, sexually frustrated, and nursing a wounded ego. Although Frances had a reputation for being childish and of low intelligence,[19] in married life she proved to be a good wife who was economical with the household finances.[20]

Hortense Mancini, one of the Mazarinettes, or nieces of the Italian Cardinal Mazarin of France, was next on Charles's radar. Her cross-dressing, exotic beauty, and her daring and scandalous ways made her the subject on everyone's lips. From 1676, Hortense was the king's mistress and held popular *salons*, or intellectual social gatherings.[21] Her relationship with Charles, however, had fizzled out by 1678, though the two remained on friendly terms.[22]

Another of the king's lovers was the popular and witty actress Nell Gwynn. Nell was probably born in a brothel that her mother ran in 1650s London.[23] Her rags-to-riches/bawdy-Cinderella story is a favourite (indeed, in one poem she was referred to as 'Cinder Nell' because of her impoverished background). Her knock-out looks combined with her fun, salt-of-the-earth nature made her an endearing and attractive woman. It's recorded that when she was fourteen, she performed the role of Cydaria opposite her real-life lover, Charles Hart, who played Cortez in the 1665 play, *The Indian Emperour, or The Conquest of Mexico*.[24]

In *A Panegyrick Upon Nelly* (1681) whose authorship is attributed to an anonymous writer, or John Wilmot, 2nd Earl of Rochester:

> E'en while she Cinders rak'd, her swelling
> Breast With thoughts of glorious
> Whoredom was possess'd
> Still did she dream (nor did her Birth withstand)
> Of dangling Scepters in her dirty Hand...[25]

One of Nell's rivals was another actress, Moll Davies. According to one anecdote, Nell made sure Moll wouldn't spend the night with Charles by lacing her food with a herb which produced a strong laxative effect.[26] So instead of being mounted upon on a Stuart for a night of carnal pleasure, she was perched upon her chamber-pot.

Moll 0, Nell 1.

As for children, Nell gave birth to a son, Charles, in May 1670—adding yet another to Charles's illegitimate brood,[27] while Moll gave birth to a daughter by the king who was named Mary Tudor.[28]

Around 1668, Nell Gwynn sat as Venus for a nude portrait by Peter Lely. This painting was hung in Charles II's private chambers at Whitehall Palace, and was for his eyes only: it was hidden behind a landscape painting! Nell was shrewd: she sought and obtained the freehold of her property in St James's Square (a dream for many in London even today). She also obtained a property in Windsor, Burford House, which was very close to Windsor Castle. Her descendants, the Beauclerks, owned this until the late eighteenth century.

The aforementioned Louise de la Kerouaille—arguably the most fortunate of all of Charles's mistresses—first came to England as part of Henrietta Anne, Duchesse d'Orleans' retinue (Henrietta Anne is probably best known as 'Minette', the youngest sister of Charles II).[29] Louise, perhaps the plumpest and the most baby-faced of Charles's mistresses, was affectionately nicknamed 'Fubbs' by him in reference to what he saw as her attractive pudginess.[30] Back in her native France, she became the talk of the town. Take, for example, Madame de Sévigné's letter to Madame de Grignan, dated Sunday 12 January 1676: 'Mademoiselle de Kerouaille has not been disappointed in anything she proposed; she desired to be a mistress to the King, and she is so. He lodges with her almost every night in the face of all the court: She has had a son, who has been acknowledged, and presented with two Duchies'.[31]

Louise's main rival was Nell, who, again according to Madame de Sévigné, constantly insulted Louise and childishly made faces at her. Nell was not alone in her animosity towards the Frenchwoman: legend states that on one occasion an angry mob who disliked foreigners with popish religious leanings mistook her for Louise, and Nell stuck her head out of the window and cried, 'Good people, you are mistaken, I am the *Protestant* whore!'[32]

Although he is perhaps most famous (or infamous) for his sex life, King Charles II had many other interests. Among these was science: he was a founding member of the Royal Society, and historians such as J.D. Davies have shown that Charles took a keen interest in naval and military matters.[33] His interest in natural philosophy and alchemy may have led to his death, for he may have died from mercury poisoning.[34]

It was the winter of 1685, and the 'Merry Monarch' lay dying following a stroke and after suffering the horrid treatments administered to him by his physicians. Charles summoned his brother, James, his heir, to his side and requested him to 'be kind to the Duchess of Cleveland, and especially Portsmouth, and let not poor Nelly starve'.[35] Nell Gwynn followed her royal lover to the grave only three years later, having suffered a stroke.[36]

Upon Charles's death, his widow Catherine became the Queen Dowager and moved into Somerset House—but by the time William and Mary ascended the throne, she no longer felt welcome. According to the Jesuit Father Petrie, 'her resolve [was] to retire into Portugal, to pass the remainder of her days in Devotion'[37]—and so it was, for she lived the rest of her life in her native Portugal. When she died in 1705—some twenty years after Charles—her body was interred in the *Panteão da Casa de Bragança* in the Monastery São Vicente de Fora, Lisbon.

Chapter 25

James II: Or, 'The Most Unguarded Ogler of His Time' (1685–1688)

James VII of Scotland & II of England was in many respects the opposite of his saturnine elder brother, Charles II. Where Charles was dark-set and famously said of himself 'Odd's fish, I am an ugly fellow',[1] James was fair and handsome, with blue eyes; where Charles had been fun-loving, James came across as rather dour and humourless. When it came to sex, however, he certainly had the famed Stuart appetite. As Gilbert Burnet put it, 'the Duke...was even to his old age of an amorous disposition![2] He was, according to the Count of Grammont, 'the most unguarded ogler of his time'.[3] Samuel Pepys was wary when his own wife, Elisabeth, found herself on the receiving end of that steely, ogling gaze.

James was arguably the most strikingly attractive of his brothers. While portraits—particularly those of royalty—were often painted in such a way as to flatter the subject, a pattern develops when there are a variety of portraits of the same person. James had several facial characteristics generally associated with the stereotypical aesthetically-pleasing male: a well-defined jaw, sensual lips, a cleft in his chin, and a penetrative air. His resplendent portrait of 1672–73 by Henri Gascar depicts James, then Duke of York, in ostentatious classical garb, and thus attired, we see more of his body than usual. This portrait, which now hangs in the Queen's House, Royal Museums Greenwich, shows a slim, slightly muscular, man who had well-shaped, athletic legs.

Anne Hyde, the daughter of Edward Hyde, Earl of Clarendon and the Chancellor of England, was probably the last woman in the world who James's family ever thought he'd marry. She was a commoner; rather attractive but by no means a 'stunner', she was also a mere lady-in-waiting. Whilst his family may have turned a blind eye to his liaisons, he apparently was so besotted by Anne that he pledged—in writing—to marry her. That settled, she welcomed him to her bed, where James proved to be a regular and active lover. Anne was soon pregnant.

That's when the trouble started, and James's ill-thought-out love affair with Clarendon's daughter was soon out in the open. James's family, particularly his mother, Henrietta Maria and his sister Mary, Princess Royal and Princess of Orange, under whom Anne had been a lady-in-waiting, were aghast, outraged, and utterly opposed to his entanglement with Anne. James's younger brother Henry, Duke of Gloucester, apparently found her rather physically repugnant.[4] Even Clarendon himself was angered by his daughter's actions and threatened to have her jailed in the Tower of London for her behaviour. In October of 1660, John Evelyn, another great English diarist stated, 'There dined with me a French count, with Sir George Tuke, who came to take leave of me, being sent over to the Queen-Mother [Henrietta Maria], to break the marriage of the Duke with the daughter of Chancellor Hyde. The queen would fain have undone it'.[5]

Under such pressure, it's no wonder that James tried to back out of his promise to Anne. On the same day that Evelyn wrote his entry, Samuel Pepys wrote, 'the Duke of York hath got my Lord Chancellor's daughter with child, and that she do lay it to him, and that for certain he did promise her marriage, and had signed it with his blood'.[6] James managed to smuggle this signed document away from Anne and promptly destroyed it, but that did little good. 'And that the King would have him to marry her, but that he will not. So that the thing is very bad for the Duke, and them all; but my Lord do make light of it, as a thing that he believes is not a new thing for the Duke to do abroad'.[7] From this sentence, we can gather that James may have done this sort of thing before with others. Had he offered other women marriage as a means to enjoy their sexual favours? It's impossible to say, but the intelligent and authoritative Anne wouldn't let him break his promise.

It seems James had a change of heart, since he married the by-then heavily pregnant Anne secretly in September of 1660. The child, a boy named Charles Stuart, Duke of Cambridge, was born a few weeks later, in October of that year. By then, rumours of Anne's past sexual profligacy began to circulate, with men such as Charles Berkeley and Richard Talbot coming forward to claim that they had also bedded her, thus casting the child's paternity—and therefore, legitimacy—into question.

The subsequent damage to Anne's reputation, and the fact that James appeared to have been hurt by it, caused Berkeley to admit that he had actually lied: he hadn't had sex with Anne.[8] Neither had Talbot, who probably lied out of his strong sense of loyalty to the Stuart family. During this whole fiasco Henrietta Maria travelled to England from France to sort out the mess her son had made—to no avail. King Charles II stood by the couple, and in December James made his marriage to Anne public. Sadly, baby Charles died a little over six months after his birth.

Despite this loss, the Duke and Duchess of York would conceive several times again: Anne gave birth to a daughter, whom they named Mary, in 1662, a son, James, in 1663 (who died aged three), Anne in 1665, Charles in 1666 (who didn't make it to age one), Edgar (who also died aged three), Henrietta (1668–1669), and Catherine (1670–1671).[9] The only children who survived infancy from their union were their two daughters, Mary and Anne. Despite the troubles surrounding his marriage to their mother, James proved to be a very loving father and more directly involved with their care than were many others of his rank.

James, however, was not a faithful husband, and his choice of mistresses was considered poor. Bishop Burnet, in conversation with the Duke of Buckingham, was told that James was perpetually in one amour or other, without being very discerning in his choice, and that the king 'believed his brother had his mistresses given to him by his priests for penance![10] Indeed, according to the Count of Grammont's memoirs, James made his preferences clear one evening when Frances Stewart rather boldly showed off her legs up to the knees. Whilst the other men present—including his brother, King Charles II—eagerly admired her pins, James apparently fell to criticising them and remarked that her legs were 'too slender', and that for himself he 'would give nothing for a leg that was not thicker and shorter...and no leg worth any thing without green stockings'[11]. This is credible, given that he was sexually aroused by Anne Hyde—who, by all accounts, became a rather plump woman. Did James have a kinky preference for green stockings? Or, rather, was a recent sexual encounter with a lady in green stockings still enticingly playing in his mind's eye?

According to the Count of Grammont, the Duke of York took his pleasures with several court women, including Lady Robarts,

Miss Brooke (later Lady Denham), and Lady Chesterfield.[12] We'll never know the identities of all his sexual partners, nor how many mistresses he took to his bed.

Samuel Pepys recounted how his friend Mr Povy told him that, 'the Duke of York hath not got Mrs. Middleton, as I was told the other day: but says that he wants not her, for he hath others, and hath always had, and that he hath known them brought through the Matted Gallery at White Hall into his closet; nay, he hath come out of his wife's bed, and gone to others laid in bed for him: that Mr. Brouncker is not the only pimp, but that the whole family are of the same strain, and will do any thing to please him'. It's clear that, although less well-known than his brother when it came to sexual exploits, James had a very strong sex drive.

Although he likely had many mistresses, two are principally associated with James. Arabella Churchill was the eldest sister of John Churchill, the man who would later become the first Duke of Marlborough. She was yet another odd choice, for she was too slender to be considered attractive at that time. She may never have caught his attention were it not for an incident in which she was flung off her horse and landed with her legs in the air, probably accidentally flashing her genitalia (remember, no knickers!). James was stirred by what he saw, and so began their affair. Arabella proved faithful to her royal lover and bore him several children, including James FitzJames, Duke of Berwick—who became one of the most talented cavalry leaders of his time.[13] Eventually, however, Arabella married Colonel Charles Godfrey.[14]

Catherine Sedley, the only daughter of the notorious libertine Sir Charles Sedley, was skinny and plain, but very witty—if a little crude. Oddly enough for a staunch Catholic man (who, as it happens, was also the last Catholic monarch of Britain) both of these mistresses, Catherine Sedley and Arabella Churchill, were Protestants.[15] Neither woman was considered particularly physically attractive, but both were intelligent and evidently sexually compatible with James.[16]

With the death of his first duchess from breast cancer in 1671, James was back on the market, and having made a pig's ear of his first marriage in terms of his wife's social status, this time he looked for a lady of similar rank to himself. His chosen bride was a young woman who was completely different to his first wife in terms of both looks and personality: Maria Beatrice Anna Margherita Isabella d'Este (popularly known as Mary of Modena). Mary was slim, with a good figure, dark brown hair and almond-shaped dark eyes set within a very pretty face;[17] she was highly educated as well. Born in 1658, Mary of Modena was twenty-five years James's junior and only four years older than his eldest daughter, Mary of York.

Members of Parliament were not enthusiastic about the proposed match, and 'when the duke applied to a princess of the house of Modena, then in close alliance with France; this circumstance, joined to so many other grounds of discontent, raised the commons into a flame; and they remonstrated with the greatest zeal against the intended marriage'.[18]

James didn't let this stop him, and in 1673, he married the Italian princess by proxy. The fifteen-year-old Mary of Modena arrived in Dover on 21 November 1673, where she married James in person and they had sex the same night.[19] She was apparently revolted by him, and cried often in his presence.[20] Although James was quite taken with her, it took a bit of time for her to fall in love with him.

Maria of Modena, whilst seen more as James' equal due to her aristocratic heritage, was a Roman Catholic, with family connections to the Pope. Worse, she was an Italian—a foreigner. Italians having a somewhat unsavoury reputation at this time, scurrilous rumours spread and some rather lewd pamphlets were published. John Wilmot's crass *Signior Dildo* was written following Mary of Modena's arrival:

> The Duchess of Modena, though she looks so high,
> With such a gallant is content to lie,
> And for fear that the English her secrets should know,
> For her gentleman usher took Signior Dildo.

James—true to his reputation—continued to ogle other women, and cheated on his new bride. He suffered for his pleasures with a guilty conscience, though, and might possibly have corporally punished himself with a rod.[21]

Following the miscarriage of their first child in the summer of 1674, Mary of Modena then gave birth to a daughter, Catherine Laura, in January 1675—this child died of 'convulsions' only nine months later. Her parents were devastated, and this was made worse by the fact that Mary was pregnant again and the loss of Catherine Laura, in turn, seems to have caused her to miscarry a day later.[22] A subsequent pregnancy resulted in the birth of Isabella in 1676, and a year later, marked the birth of their first son, Charles, who lived only a month until his death from smallpox.[23] To his credit, James was unlike other royal men in that he wasn't much bothered by the sex of his children— most of whom were girls.[24]

In 1676, three years after his wedding to Mary of Modena, James made the ill-advised decision to openly convert to Roman Catholicism. This had long-lasting effects that impacted not only upon himself and Mary, but also upon their descendants for generations to come.[25] In the political tumult following the Popish Plot and the Test Acts, the Duke and Duchess of York were sent to Scotland. Their daughter, Princess Isabella, had been left in London, where she died aged only four.[26] Another daughter, Charlotte Mary, born in 1682, died two months later from 'convulsions', and two more miscarriages followed.[27]

Even after becoming king in 1685, James's continued infidelities were not hidden away from his young wife. Indeed, she was made acutely aware of them, particularly when, in January of 1686, he bestowed upon his mistress, Catherine Sedley, the title of Countess of Portsmouth. Sedley was the mother of two of James's illegitimate children.[28] John Evelyn observed Mary of Modena's sadness following Sedley's investiture, and her inability to eat much at table.[29] Stress clearly put her off her food, and having her husband so publicly indicate his betrayal of her must have been deeply humiliating and emotionally distressing.

Mary of Modena's succession of ill-fated pregnancies had made many Protestants complacent; they were confident that she would not bear an heir and that instead James's daughter, Mary, would become the next monarch. Imagine their shock, then, when Mary of Modena conceived, and subsequently was delivered, of a very healthy son in the summer of 1688. The birth of James Francis Edward Stuart heralded the start of what came to be known as the 'Glorious Revolution'.[30]

Protestants were alarmed that James' arrival represented the beginning of a Catholic Stuart line. Soon enough, scurrilous rumours about the child's origins began circulating, particularly a story which came to be known as the 'warming-pan baby': Mary of Modena had never been pregnant, or had given birth to a dead child, who had been stealthily removed out and replaced with another newborn who was smuggled into the birthing chamber inside a warming pan. It was a ludicrous story, entirely lacking in grounds, but it suited those who did not want to believe the truth. Princess Anne became convinced that the baby was not her half-brother, and through her correspondence with her sister Mary, in Holland, also managed to convince William and Mary of this.[31] The wheels had been set in motion against King James and his young family.

Forced to flee Stuart Britain in 1688, James's new family sought refuge with King Louis XIV and finally settled in the Château de Saint-Germain-en-Laye, France. It was there that Mary gave birth to a daughter, Louisa Maria Theresa Stuart, in 1692, whom James referred to as his consolation, or, 'La Consolatrice'.[32] James died in exile in September of 1701 after two weeks of extremely poor health, and his 'consolation' died from smallpox—that killer of so many Stuarts—in 1712.[33] Mary of Modena, having survived the deaths of most of her children and her husband, succumbed to breast cancer in 1718.[34]

James Francis Edward Stuart, the only surviving child of their union, was denied his birthright as king due to his being Roman Catholic, married Princess Maria Clementina Sobieska.[35] This couple had two sons: Charles Edward Stuart and Henry Benedict.[36] The latter became a Cardinal in the Roman Catholic Church, the former—known by his enemies as 'The Young Pretender' and by his supporters as 'Bonnie Prince Charlie—was the figurehead for the Jacobite movement which would end in defeat at the Battle of Culloden in 1746.[37]

Chapter 26

William & Mary: Or, Marriage between First Cousins (1689–1702)

'Love me whatever happens, and be assured I am ever entirely yours till death'[1]

— Mary II to William III

Some hold that William and Mary were usurpers who took James II's throne, others that they saved the nation from a Catholic autocrat. Following what some at the time thought was the licentious nature of the Restoration court, the much-more austere and religious William and Mary certainly brought about change—indeed, social/moralistic movements were established, such as the Society for the Reformation of Manners, in 1691.

There were nonetheless rumours that chipped away at the moral edifice William and Mary created. A strange fact is that all the Protestant Stuarts who ascended the throne as either sovereign or consort following James II's exile were rumoured to be sexually attracted to their own sex.[2] The chances of this being true are very low, and these rumours (unlike those associated with James VI & I) have little or no evidence to support them.

But let's not get ahead of ourselves. William and Mary's story started long before William controversially invaded England in 1688. First, we need to have a look at *another* William and Mary: William's parents, William II of Orange, and Mary, Princess Royal of England. Mary was not the only daughter of King Charles I to be considered as a bride for William: her younger sister, Elizabeth, was a candidate for a while.[3] The couple married on 2 May 1641 as tensions were escalating on the road to civil war. At first, the bride stayed in England, due to her being only nine years old, but as the political situation steadily worsened, she was sent to her husband in the Dutch Republic with the firm instructions that the newlyweds were not allowed to physically consummate the marriage.[4] Unfortunately for Mary, three years after their wedding, her young husband gained entry into her chamber and had sex with the twelve-year-old girl.[5] Mary's first conception occurred when she was fifteen, but this child was miscarried.[6]

The next pregnancy was successful, but tragedy accompanied it. The boy who would become King William III was born in early November 1650—a week after his father's death from smallpox at the age of twenty-four. Despite his many sexual infidelities, Mary nevertheless loved and missed her husband, William II.[7] Already cast into the world with an all-encompassing gloom of tragedy, William wasn't expected to survive. His mother, a teenaged widow, was not even permitted to name her own son. She would have chosen 'Charles', but her formidable mother-in-law, Amalia van Solms, insisted he be named 'Willem' (the Dutch version of William) in keeping with the House of Orange.[8] William's mother was very unhappy in the Dutch Republic, yet would not consider remarriage unless it was for her son's benefit. Despite being the target of some rather persistent wooing by George Villiers, 2nd Duke of Buckingham, and there being rumours associating her with Harry Jermyn—nothing came to fruition and Mary never remarried.[9]

Orphaned at the age of ten, it is perhaps no surprise that William's personality left much to be desired; he was then, and still is, regarded as a 'cold and calculating'[10] type. He was wary of letting people get close to him, but the few who knew him well found him to be amiable. Later, as King William III, a foreigner, he kept his Dutch friends, rather than Englishmen, as his favourites. This automatically irritated the English at his court, most of whom disliked and distrusted foreigners only slightly less than they did Catholics. William's closest friend was Hans Bentinck—a childhood friend from the Dutch Republic. When William was stricken down with smallpox, Bentinck slept in the same bed. This was not necessarily due to any sexual motivation, however, since at the time it was believed that if a person afflicted with a disease shared a bed with a healthy person, this would draw the evil humours away from the patient. What actually happened, predictably, is that Bentinck contracted smallpox as well—but both men recovered. While their friendship remained strong until the late 1690s, given their personalities and Bentinck's clear sexual preference for women, it is highly unlikely that their relationship was sexual.[11]

William's wife Mary was born to James, then Duke of York, and his first wife, Anne Hyde. Samuel Pepys mentions her birth in his Diary: 'the Duchesse of York is brought to bed of a girle, at which I find nobody pleased'.[12] Though some people may not have been pleased at her arrival, Mary's temper was 'naturally sweet and cheerful', her judgment 'deep and correct', and her heart was filled with 'sincere piety and religion'.[13] She was maternal and ebullient, beautiful and graceful. In other words, she was a perfect seventeenth-century lady. Mary was a naturally bright girl, but—in common with other girls of the time— was not formally educated. She and her sister, Anne, grew up with the Villiers girls, Sarah Jennings, and Frances Apsley.

Frances, several years older than Mary, was attractive and kind, and Mary developed a sort of girl-crush on her, as did several other girls in their small group, for Frances was a lovable young lady with many admirable qualities. Mary was an intensely affectionate person by nature and her letters to Frances reveal her fantastical and ebullient sentimentality.[14] The two girls used pen names: Mary was 'Mary Clorine', and Frances was 'Aurelia'.[15] Were Mary's feelings towards Frances more than friendship? According to William Wake's 1695 *Sermon Preach'd before the Honourable Society of Grayes-Inn: Upon the Occasion of the Death of our late Royal Sovereign Queen Mary*: she was a 'queen so virtuous, that her very example was enough to convert a Libertine, and to reform an Age'.[16] Mary was an extremely devout person and afraid of sinning; any acts of same-sex physical love would have conflicted with her deeply-entrenched views on morality. Her relationship with Frances Apsley was probably, therefore, no more than an adolescent role-playing game.

In September of 1677, William requested—and obtained— permission to be a suitor to his first cousin, Mary of York. William was twenty-six years old, while Mary was fifteen. The two met, William apparently liked her immediately (she was considered, at this time, very beautiful) and he speedily pressed King Charles II for her hand. The king had reservations about the match, and this prompted William to declare that if Charles forbade him to marry Mary then William would become his enemy.[17] Observing his nephew's sincerity, Charles quickly relented, apparently saying, 'Well, I never yet was deceived in judging a man's honesty by his looks…and if I am not deceived in the Prince's face, he is the honestest man in the world'.[18]

While the bridegroom was very keen, Mary was less so: she was a highly romantic girl, and William wasn't exactly a dreamboat! He was frail, slightly hunched, of average height (but short for a Stuart), he had a hook nose, was unfashionable, and suffered from terrible asthma. In fact, Mary wept for over a day on learning of her upcoming nuptials. The two were nevertheless married on 4 November 1677 in St. James's Palace. The bride cried throughout the wedding.

The bedding ceremony took place that night, and William and Mary slipped between the sheets together. Charles II is believed to have said 'Now, nephew, to your work! Hey! St George for England!'[19] It is likely that William did perform his 'work' and physical consummation of the marriage occurred that night. What Mary thought of her first sexual encounter, though, we can only imagine.

Following this, away they went to William's country, accompanied by Mary's household with three Villiers girls—Anne, Katherine, and Elizabeth—amongst her ladies-in-waiting. After settling into life in the Dutch Republic, William and Mary grew to love one another, both physically and emotionally. All the playful passion that Mary had only previously been able to release in her letters to Frances Apsley was now directed towards her increasingly-beloved husband. And, despite the somewhat difficult, taciturn, nature of his personality, Mary had fallen deeply in love with him. William had gone to battle and she was worried about him losing his life, stating in her letter to Frances, 'what can be more cruel in the world than parting with what one loves, and not only common parting, but parting so as may never to meet again'.[20] Now sexually-experienced, Mary must have giggled as she set quill to paper to inform her 'dear husband' Frances that 'I have played the whore a little'.[21] Indeed, the newlyweds had wasted no time: Mary was soon pregnant, and William was excited at the prospect of becoming a father.

Sadly, only a few months into her pregnancy in early 1678, Mary suffered a miscarriage. Her father, James, Duke of York wrote to William 'I was very sorry to find…that my daughter has miscarried; pray let her be carefuller of herself'.[22] In Mary's case it seems likely that some foetal tissue remained within her uterus and led to infection. This could be why she later suffered a further miscarriage and was ultimately unable to bring a child to term.

This misfortune was a terrible blow to Mary, and it caused her grief for the rest of her life. As previously noted, during the Stuart period a woman's identity was closely associated with her role as a begetter of children, but this was especially so for a princess, whose duty required her to bear heirs. Mary felt this pressure acutely.

Tragedy having sullied his relatively new—and fragile—union with Mary, William now turned to one of her ladies-in-waiting, Elizabeth Villiers. His attachment to this mistress lasted throughout the remainder of his marriage to Mary, ending only after her death. Mary II's early-twentieth-century biographer, Nellie M. Waterson suggested—quite plausibly—that 'William never loved anyone but his wife, but to deny that he had illicit relations with Elizabeth Villiers would be impossible'.[23]

If we grant that mistresses, particularly those who bed royalty and aristocracy, are usually physically attractive, Elizabeth Villiers is not what one would expect. Ungainly, and with a cast in her eye which caused her to 'squint like a dragon',[24] she was not considered a beauty at the time. But William already had a stunning wife; what he needed was someone who met his intellectual needs, and this sharp Villiers woman fitted the bill perfectly. Not only was she cerebral, but, according to her great friend and admirer, the satirist Jonathan Swift, 'she is perfectly kind, like a mother'.[25] Since William had lost his mother at the age of ten, this may have been a point of attraction, too. In yet another link, Elizabeth was a sister of Anne Villiers, who had married Hans Bentinck in 1678. Ladies-in-waiting throughout history have been the go-to women for royal adultery, and Elizabeth's close proximity to William through her position in Mary's household and her being his best friend's sister-in-law simply sealed the deal.

William and Elizabeth's adulterous relationship was carried out with the utmost discretion and secrecy—so much so that Mary was unaware of it until she was told about it by four members of her household staff.[26] The princess lay in wait outside the doors to the bedchambers of her ladies-in-waiting, and, sure enough, caught William as he made what he hoped was a stealthy exit. There then ensued a tremendous domestic argument between the royal couple, complete with the accusations, tears, anger, pain and embarrassment that such proof of betrayal would usually elicit. Mary sacked Elizabeth as her lady-in-waiting and sent her back to England, but Elizabeth decided to stay with her sister, Katherine, in The Hague—still in the Dutch Republic—where she continued her relationship with William, who also had a residence in that city.[27]

But what of Mary? Did she, too, find solace in the arms of a lover? It is unlikely. She may have flirted with her cousin, the Duke of Monmouth, during his visit in early 1683, but she would not have taken him to her bed. There is no evidence that Mary ever had sexual or romantic relationships with anyone (man or woman) other than her husband; despite discovering his infidelity, she remained faithful and loving to him for the remainder of her life.

The 'Glorious Revolution' of 1688 is often mistakenly referred to as a 'bloodless' revolution. Its direct and indirect consequences in fact included the Battle of Killicrankie (1689), the Battle of the Boyne (1691), the Glencoe Massacre (1692), and even the royal succession itself—paving the way for the Hanoverians in 1714. During this period, William was often separated from Mary, and his frequent, necessary, absences deeply saddened her.[28] Mary's letters to William are full of impatience to see him again and declarations of her love for him.[29]

There had previously been rumours about William's sexuality during the time of his long friendship with Hans Bentinck (most likely fuelled by the relentless Jacobite propaganda machine). But the rumour mill went into overdrive with the arrival of Arnold Joost van Keppel around 1685. Keppel, who was twenty years younger than William, rose from being a lowly page to Earl of Albemarle and Knight of the Garter 'by a quick and unaccountable progress'.[30] His later portrait shows a damned good-looking man with an almost feminine face—the kind of look that remains popular with dreamy-eyed teenagers. His lips were luscious and full, his nose refined and his cheekbones pronounced. Especially in William's post-Elizabeth Villiers days, the presence of this Dutch (and, therefore, 'foreign') young man was certainly sufficient to set gossips' tongues wagging.

The question of King William III's sexuality remains a contentious subject which is sometimes cited by political and social advocacy groups.[31] Historians themselves are divided upon the matter.[32] William was an intensely private individual, but also very religious, and his sexual (and, therefore, adulterous) liaisons were not something of which he would have been proud. Furthermore, it is likely that with the poor nature of his health (in particular, haemorrhoids, chronic asthma, among others things) he had a lower sex drive than other Stuart royals.

When William was a teenager visiting his uncle's licentious court, his uncles got him so drunk that he ended up breaking into the apartments of the ladies-in-waiting intent on having a sexual encounter with one of the women there but was pulled away before anything truly reprehensible occurred.[33] *In vino veritas,* he indicated that he was sexually attracted to women.

There is gossip, but there is no proof, that William was sexually attracted to other men, and not even any reliable evidence that he and van Keppel were lovers.[34] Meanwhile, there is the credible suggestion that van Keppel was a serial womaniser and 'was so much given up to his own pleasures that he could scarcely submit to the attendance and drudgery that were necessary to maintain his post'.[35] The relationship between William and van Keppel most likely fulfilled the loving 'father/son' dynamic that William had never been able to enjoy—not with his own father, whom he never knew, and because his marriage to Mary had ultimately been childless. William clearly had a paternal streak, as indicated by his kindness to Anne's ill-fated son, William Henry, Duke of Gloucester (b. 1689)—indeed, losing Gloucester at the tender age of only eleven in 1700 dealt yet another blow to the Stuart monarch.

In the background of all these rumours, Mary's love for William remained steadfast: 'I love you more than my life, and desire only to please you', she wrote to him in a letter in 1690.[36] Four years later, in December 1694, Mary was struck down by a severe illness which was given several different diagnoses, including smallpox and measles, but she certainly had haemorrhagic smallpox. Mary had harboured a macabre fascination with her own death for some time, and when she was in her final illness, she calmly and methodically went through her private papers and burned some letters, journal entries and more, destroying material that would undoubtedly have afforded us much greater insight into her feelings and her life.[37]

William ultimately realised the depth of his love for Mary and slept near her on a camp-bed so he would not miss a single moment of her remaining time. Political strategy, personal ambition, and private sufferings had taken a toll upon their relationship, and William was in despair. Finally, Gilbert Burnet wrote that the normally-cold King broke down in tears before him, 'and cried out, that there was no hope of the Queen; and that, from the happiest, he was now going to be the miserablest creature upon Earth'.[38]

When the thirty-two-year-old Mary died in the early hours of 28 December 1694, William fainted. He was beyond devastated, and his grief was sincere and all-consuming. The following day, Narcissus Luttrell wrote that 'the king is mightily afflicted'.[39] Thrown, as he was, into such a pit of misery, many courtiers expected him to soon follow Mary to the grave—and many of his enemies, in particular the Jacobites, certainly would have liked that to happen. But it was not yet William's time to exit the stage.

One of the most tragic aspects of William's relationship with Mary is surely his apparent failure to fully realise how much he loved and valued his wife until her final days. She had been devoutly loyal to him throughout all the years of their marriage, including the crucial turning-point of 1688/1689.

Mary's death, and her concerns over his soul, motivated William to break up with Elizabeth Villiers finally, and permanently. According to the English theologian and historian William Whiston:

> There was a court lady, the lady Villers, with whom it was well known king William had been too familiar, and had given her great endowments. Upon the queen's death, the new archbishop, whether as desired by the queen before her death or of his own voluntary motion, I do not know; took the freedom, after his loss of so excellent a wife, to represent to him, the great injury he had done to that excellent wife by his adultery with the lady Villers.[40]

Whiston continued that although William didn't deny having committed adultery with Elizabeth, it was at this moment that he vowed to break up with her for good. She was not, however, cast aside without remuneration: William arranged for her to marry her cousin, Lord George Hamilton, in 1695, whom he had created the Earl of Orkney a year later.[41] As a result, Elizabeth became Lady Orkney, and after her wedding she produced several children. If she had enjoyed full sexual relations with William III, would this not have produced offspring? The English historian, Thomas Birch (1705–1766), suggested that Elizabeth provided William with fellatio throughout their relationship.[42] It is possible that, like some later figures, William believed (or tried to convince himself) that engaging in sexual acts such as mutual masturbation and oral sex—but not vaginal intercourse—with Elizabeth meant he wasn't really committing adultery.

Meanwhile, van Keppel's power was on the rise, and in 1697, he was created the Earl of Albemarle. By 1698, Bentinck, whose wife Anne had died a decade before,[43] had become increasingly fed up with Albemarle's rise and quit his post. He also took the time to inform William of the scurrilous rumours about the king and the young earl and, from his letters, he appears to have had doubts about his lifelong friend's behaviour.[44] William's response is direct: 'It seems to be very extraordinary that it should be impossible to have esteem and regard for a young man without it being criminal'.[45] The king was shocked that anyone could have misconstrued his friendship for van Keppel as being romantic and sexual—a kind of relationship which he himself regarded as criminal.

Although William was cold and reserved with Mary, especially in front of others, his genuine love for her was once again proven at the end of his own life. Early one February morning, he went for a ride on his horse near Hampton Court Palace. The animal stumbled upon a molehill, causing its royal rider to be thrown into the air. He hit the ground violently and broke his collarbone, which was later set by a physician. Having always been plagued with bad lungs, William developed pneumonia, which led to his death. William died at Kensington Palace on the 8 March 1702, and when his body was inspected there was discovered upon it an item of jewellery containing Mary's likeness and a lock of hair—which belonged neither to Bentinck, nor Keppel, nor even Elizabeth, but to Mary.[46] He was buried in Westminster Abbey, his coffin beside that of his dear wife.

So what became of the Countess of Orkney, previously known merely as Elizabeth Villiers? Well, there were several mentions of her in later years, including one by Jonathan Swift, who wrote in 1712: 'Lady Orkney, the late King's Mistress, who lives at a fine place 5 miles from hence called Cliffden,[47] and I are grown mighty Acquaintance. She is the wisest woman I ever saw'.[48]

Chapter 27

Queen Anne Probably Wasn't a Lesbian (1702–1714)

Queen Anne, the last Stuart monarch to sit on the throne, is often overlooked.[1] She was obese, shy, stubborn, and short-sighted, with low self-esteem, and she had one of the most tragic gynaecological histories of the entire Stuart family.

Anne was born in 1665, three years after her elder sister, Mary, to Anne and James, the Duke and Duchess of York. From her birth, she was eclipsed by her ebullient and more aesthetically appealing elder sister. Dissimilar to her sister in many respects, Anne was no social butterfly and did not thrive in the midst of societal entertainments as Mary did.[2] Like two little girls squabbling over the same toy, Anne and Mary bickered over a mutual friend, Frances Apsley. As you may recall from the chapter on Mary, there is much scurrilous speculation surrounding her relationship with Frances. *Anne's* correspondence with Frances, however, was just as fervent—confirming that the three girls all enjoyed romantic role-playing: Frances used the name 'Semandra' whilst Anne used the male name 'Ziphares'.[3] It was around this time, however, that Anne became friends with another young woman at court, one Sarah Jennings.

Sarah, who was born into an impoverished aristocratic family, had an elder sister, Frances, who later became the titular Duchess of Tyrconnell and a famous Jacobite. Both sisters were renowned beauties. Frances successfully avoided becoming mistress to James, Duke of York, and in 1666 married George Hamilton, an Irish army officer.[4] From an early age, Sarah possessed a wilful, strong character, and it was posthumously reported that 'no passion gratify'd except her Rage'.[5]

Anne's romantic associations were very few—despite her being a princess, many who might otherwise have been suitors were put off by her common-stock maternal ancestry.[6] Lord Mulgrave pursued a teenaged Anne, sending her love letters, which she apparently received with some enthusiasm,[7] but this potential relationship was thwarted by members of her family, particularly by Charles II, her uncle. Another, more prestigious alliance, was proposed: that of Anne with her cousin, Prince Georg Ludwig, the man who would eventually succeed her to become King George I. This too fizzled out into nothing following the potential couple's first meeting and Georg Ludwig ended up marrying another cousin, Sophia Dorothea of Celle, who would come with a more bounteous dowry.[8] That royal marriage would prove to be extremely unhappy, leading to adultery on both sides, divorce, the murder of Sophia's lover (the handsome Swedish Philip von Königsmarck) in 1694—and Sophia's house arrest for the remainder of her life.[9] Perhaps Anne had unknowingly made a lucky escape, after all.

The eighteen-year-old Princess Anne eventually married Prince George of Denmark, on 28 July 1683, after some months of negotiations and only five days getting to know one another.[10] George, 'of the Danish countenance, blond, of few words',[11] proved a good husband for Anne, and they enjoyed a loving and faithful marriage; their tragedy stems from the fates that befell their many children. It is rarely mentioned that Anne's husband was rumoured to have been a 'sodomite'—but, as previously mentioned, every Stuart following James II & VII's exile was made the subject of this kind of rumour. George, who was twelve years older than Anne, is very often overlooked in histories of this time period, possibly because of his personality, which was considered rather boorish. Some historians have dismissed him as having 'impenetrable stupidity',[12] and Charles II famously said of him, 'I've tried him drunk and I've tried him sober and there's nothing in him'. But there is much more to this man than such a comically dismissive analysis might lead us to believe. In a letter from the Reverend Father Petre, a Jesuit, to the Reverend Father la Chese: 'Luther was never more earnest than this Prince'.[13] George was a very handsome man, good-natured, and loyal, but his perceived over-friendliness with Elizabeth (wife of his Secretary, Edward Griffith) made Anne fume with sexual jealousy.[14] She complained to Sarah that she would not be surprised if, given the opportunity, the flirtation between the two led to something else.[15]

Sarah Jennings began to be pursued romantically by one John Churchill who, as a young page in the household of the Duke of York, is traditionally held to be depicted in the Gascar portrait previously mentioned.[16] This striking young man was 'tall and handsome, of a noble and graceful appearance, with a very obliging address', and although he wasn't well read, he possessed a sharp mind and 'seldom failed of success in any thing he undertook'.[17] Churchill was beguiled by Sarah's good looks, and her spirited nature meant she was no wilting flower; she had strong opinions about how their relationship was going to proceed. For one thing, she wasn't going to let her suitor bed her and then leave. She had seen what had befallen other women at court who had allowed this to happen: loss of virtue, their good name run through the mud, pregnancy and birthing illegitimate children. No, that was not how Sarah would do things, despite her strong sexual and romantic attraction to John Churchill. If he wanted to have sex with her, he would have to marry her first—and this he did, secretly, sometime in 1677.[18]

A couple of years after the 'Glorious Revolution' of 1688, Anne and Sarah began to use pen names in their correspondence with each other: Sarah took the name of 'Mrs Freeman', whilst Anne took the name of 'Mrs Morley'—this was due to Anne's wish that they would have less formal communications.[19] William and Mary conferred upon Churchill the Earldom of Marlborough, while his wife became the Countess of Marlborough. Then, in 1692, things came to a head between Anne and William and Mary. The sisters had not been on the best of terms for some time, and the Queen was wary of Sarah's complete control over her younger sister. She ordered Anne to dismiss the Marlboroughs from her household—but Anne refused.[20]

In the winter of 1702, Anne's brother-in-law William III (for whom she had no affection) died from pneumonia. Anne now ascended the throne, aged thirty-seven, and her friend Sarah Churchill simultaneously reached the zenith of her power, for she was as manipulative and controlling as ever.[21] By 1706, Sarah, now Duchess of Marlborough, was referred to by Richard Hearne as 'an insatiable covetous proud woman'.[22]

Like her chronically asthmatic brother-in-law, William III, Anne was plagued with a myriad of health problems. She had between sixteen and eighteen pregnancies, and none of her children survived to adulthood. Whether by miscarriage, stillbirth, or killed in childhood by illnesses such as smallpox, all of them died. Her longest-surviving child was her son, William Henry, Duke of Gloucester, who was sickly and suffered from hydrocephalus, ultimately perishing shortly after his eleventh birthday in the summer of 1700. And so, despite Anne having had this many pregnancies (the precise number is uncertain), her marriage with Prince George of Denmark resulted in childlessness. The Act of Settlement in 1701 automatically excluded any Catholics from the line of succession, including Anne's own half-brother, Prince James Francis Edward Stuart.

As many women would, Anne—in her immense grief—turned to her best friend, Sarah. But Sarah was not always the most sympathetic and understanding person. Indeed, as one biographer of Queen Anne wrote, Sarah's impatience and unkindness towards her royal friend grew to a whole new level following the Duke of Gloucester's death.[23] It is often said—unfairly—that Queen Anne was a weak woman, but to lose so many children and not lose one's reason as well arguably shows great strength and resilience.

The death of young William Henry—the Protestant heir—impacted William III, too, and it had political repercussions. *The Act of Settlement (1700)* stated: 'The Princess Sophia, Electress and Duchess Dowager of Hanover, Daughter of the late Queen of Bohemia, Daughter of King James the First, to inherit after the King and the Princess Anne, in Default of Issue of the said Princess and His Majesty, respectively and the Heirs of her Body, being Protestants.' Some courtiers, such as John Evelyn, lamented the state of the line: 'the unhappy family of the Stuarts seems to be extinguishing'.[24]

Blenheim Palace was commissioned by Queen Anne as a gift to the first Duke of Marlborough following his victory at Blenheim in 1704 during the War of the Spanish Succession. Sir John Vanbrugh and Nicholas Hawksmoor designed the extravagant English Baroque building, but the notoriously difficult Sarah ended up falling out with Vanbrugh and blaming him for everything and anything she didn't like about the construction.[25]

The most well-known rumour about Queen Anne is that she was a lesbian who had two lovers: Sarah Jennings and, later, Abigail Hill. Queen Anne probably was not sexually attracted to her own sex, although she yearned to be loved all her life. The same as for her predecessors, William and Mary, Anne's reign is often overshadowed in the modern age by this rumour about her sexuality. From whence does it come? Sarah, Anne's bosom friend of nearly two decades, made some insinuations in her writings and in pamphlets she had commissioned. But what of Sarah? She was disgusted with the extramarital liaisons which were so commonplace at the Restoration court, and for all the difficulties inherent in her nature, she never wavered in her loyalty to her husband.[26]

Abigail Hill (b. 1670) was Sarah's first cousin, whose family was hit hard financially, obliging her and some of her siblings to go into service in order to survive. When Sarah became acquainted with this situation, she decided to do her poor relations a good turn by obtaining employment for some of them in the royal household.[27] Alice Hill, Abigail's sister, had been given a job as a laundress for Anne's son, the Duke of Gloucester. When Anne was still a princess, during the reign of Charles II, she had a governess, four dressers, one laundress, one seamstress, and a necessary woman. This staff was of course expanded when she became queen. As a Lady of the Bedchamber, Abigail was in close proximity to the queen. She would not have obtained this position had she not been connected to Sarah, but once there, this resourceful young woman did her job well, and the queen noticed.

The early 1700s saw new figures appear on the political scene, including the Tory politician Robert Harley. By this time, Anne had become increasingly displeased with her old favourite's domineering behaviour. It is no coincidence that Harley became more powerful around the same time as his cousin, Abigail Hill, was becoming more firmly entrenched as the new royal favourite.

Then, in 1707, during one of Sarah's frequent absences from court, the queen attended the marriage of Abigail Hill to a Samuel Masham, at Kensington Palace. Masham, who, although a rather poor Baronet, was still considered to be above Abigail in station, and was nine years her junior.[28] When Sarah found out, some considerable time later, that this had taken place without her knowledge, she was livid and made a tremendous scene at Windsor Castle.[29]

Sarah continued to treat Anne like a silly little girl, notoriously telling her to 'be quiet!' outside St. Paul's Cathedral.[30] Anne was being regularly disrespected by her best friend and it's not surprising that she began to gravitate towards another person who was kinder to her. Abigail, although a mere bedchamber woman, increasingly provided the compassionate and deferential treatment that Anne needed. It is easy to become cynical and regard Abigail's different manner as a tactical manoeuvre in order to win the queen's favour, but she does seem to have provided Anne with a refreshingly different friendship to that which the Queen had known with Sarah.

Anne's emotions received yet another massive blow when her beloved husband of twenty-five years died in 1708. She repeatedly kissed him amidst her tears as he lay on his deathbed at Kensington Palace.[31] Her grief at losing George was profound—yet Sarah maliciously implied that she was feigning such feelings and even cruelly remarked that Anne had eaten a great deal that day.[32] Most people who saw Anne in the days following George's death had no doubt that she sincerely mourned her great love, but Sarah went so far as to have George's portrait removed from the queen's wall, which brought the widow a fresh wave of emotional pain.[33] By contrast, Abigail's behaviour around this time was the exact opposite of Sarah's: she genuinely pitied Anne.[34]

Bizarrely, despite knowing that if her power over Anne waned, this would have negative repercussions on her family's fortunes, Sarah continued to be grossly unkind to Anne. Sarah is believed to have, at this point, commissioned Arthur Maynwaring to write a scurrilous pamphlet which hinted at Queen Anne having a lesbian relationship with Abigail Masham—this being done for political reasons.[35] Masham and the rise of the Tories had to be stopped and the best way to do that was by discrediting them completely with tales of 'unnatural' sexual deeds between women.

Then, in 1708, further propaganda in the shape of a bawdy poem called *A New Ballad* appeared: 'When as Queen Anne of great Renown Great Britain's Scepter sway'd, Besides the Church, she dearly lov'd a Dirty Chamber-Maid.'[36] (The talk of swaying sceptres is nothing new—a more memorable allusion to royal sex and power is to be found in the Earl of Rochester's poem about Charles II: 'His sceptre and his prick are of a length, and she may sway the one, who plays with t'other.') The next verse arrogantly disparages Abigail's menial work, 'O! Abigail – that was her Name, She starch'd and stitch'd full well'.[37] Another swipe at her background: 'Her Secretary she was not, Because she could not write [...] But had the Conduct and the Care of some dark Deeds at Night'.[38] All of this work expresses contempt for Abigail due to her low station. Similarly disparaging comments about Abigail being a 'chambermaid' were later made in the 1715 piece, *King-Abigail: or, The secret reign of the she-favourite'*.[39]

Also in 1708, *The Rival Dutchess; or, Court Incendiary* was published. This work was even more explicit and took the form of a dialogue between Louis XIV's morganatic wife, Madame de Maintenon, and Abigail Masham, Queen Anne's supposed lesbian lover. In the dialogue, the French lady asks whether the 'female vice which is the most detestable' occurs in England. Mrs Masham replies, delightedly, that 'we have arriv'd to as great perfection in sinning that way' as could be imagined. It is in fact very likely that both this piece and *A New Ballad* were written by Arthur Maynwaring, a close friend of Sarah Churchill, Duchess of Marlborough. In *The Rival Dutchess,* as in *A New Ballad*, there are subtle and not-so-subtle indications of contempt for Masham because she was not of the same social class as Sarah.

But Sarah wasn't the only one to dish it out. In 1709, *Secret Memoirs and Manners of Several Persons of Quality* was published in London, creating quite a sensation. Although the author used fictitious names, a thinly-veiled Duke and Duchess of Marlborough were alluded to several times, as was Churchill's past sexual relationship with Barbara Villiers.

The 1710s saw the Marlboroughs' power over Anne deteriorate rather rapidly. The ballad, 'Sarah's Farewell to Court, Or, A Trip from St. James's to St. Albans' (1710) was unrelentingly hostile to Sarah:

> Farewell Queen, my once kind Mistress,
> To thy Royal Love Farewel,
> For thou didst raise me to a Duchess,
> But for what I ne'er cou'd tell[40]

This same ballad gives a nod to the ironic fact that Abigail, the Queen's new favourite, was initially employed in Anne's household because of Sarah's recommendation:

> Farewel to Intriguing M(asham),
> There I recommended thee;
> But thou hast play'd thy Cards so wisely,
> Now thou hast Supplanted me.[41]

In January of 1710, Sarah had to give up her key of office, which was delivered by hand to the queen by Marlborough.[42] According to

Jonathan Swift, in December 1711, John Churchill, the Duke of Marlborough, hadn't seen Queen Anne for some time and 'Mrs Masham is glad of it, because she says, he tells a hundred lies to his friends of what she says to him: he is one day humble, and the next on the high ropes'.[43]

A variety of works were printed celebrating the fact that the Marlboroughs had been ousted from power. *The Queen's and the Duke of Ormand's New Toast* (1712): 'Here's a Health to the Queen, who in Safety…truly now Reigns in Great Britain: Since those are dismiss'd from her Presence and Court Who her Rights and her Titles made their Jest and their Sport'.[44] By summer, construction at Blenheim Palace ended due to the cessation of payments from the Treasury.[45] Anne wasn't prepared to give Sarah any more money.

Some researchers claim that Sarah Churchill had sexual relations with Queen Anne, but there is no evidence—only speculation—to support this claim.[46] Furthermore, it is not necessary to posit a motive of sexual jealously in order to explain Sarah's actions: she could be vindictive to those with whom she fell out, and she fell out with a good many people (including members of her own family), for a variety of reasons.

Rumours and misinformation continued to spread like wildfire. Jonathan Swift, writing in a letter in 1712, lamented that:

> The Queen, Lord Treasurer, Lady Masham, and I, were all ill together, but are now all better; only Lady Masham expects every day to lie in at Kensington. There was never such a lump of lies spread about the town together as now. I doubt not but you will have them in Dublin before this comes to you, and all without the least grounds of truth.[47]

Queen Anne—having fallen into a coma—died on the morning of 1 August 1714 at the age of forty-nine. Her reign included some of the greatest military successes in British history, and the formal union of Scotland and England; and despite her personal tragedies, she was seen as a mother figure for the nation, thoroughly English unlike her Dutch brother-in-law. There are always political and social machinations around monarchs, and this was certainly true in Anne's case. She may have been unambitious, rather unlearned, stubborn, shy, and sometimes indecisive, but for most of her life she never expected to be queen. She gravitated to Sarah because of the latter's strength of character, and then to Abigail for her kindness. Her marriage to George for political reasons led to their great and life-lasting love.

The Marlboroughs outlived Queen Anne and found favour with the Hanoverians. Sarah's relationship with her husband John had always been intensely passionate and highly-sexed. An oft-repeated tale is that he would race back home and make fervent love to her without even bothering to first remove his boots. Even Sarah's children knew to stay away when their parents were together because they were such an amorous pair. In a letter to Sarah, written between 1703–4, her daughter Mary states that although she wants to spend time with her mother, she knows that she ought not to because her father was with her mother.[48] This suggests that even after twenty years of marriage, and several children, John and Sarah were still sexually desirous of one another— and the children had learned to give them their space.

Following Marlborough's death in 1722, his widow Sarah—still beautiful and wealthy—refused to remarry, despite romantic overtures from the likes of Charles Seymour, 6th Duke of Somerset. The widower, or 'Proud Duke', as he was called, sent many letters to Sarah after 1722 which conveyed not only his love for her, but also his desire to make her his wife.[49]

When Sarah Churchill, 1st Duchess of Marlborough, died, further works were published about her. 'Verses Upon the Late Duchess of Marlborough' (1746), stated—quite understandably, given her behaviour—that: 'who breaks with her provokes Revenge from Hell'.[50]

Chapter 28

Conclusion—Or, 'Parting is such sweet sorrow'

'Soft, Cupid, soft, there is no haste
For all unkindnesse gone and past,
Since thou wilt needs forsake me so,
Let us parte friendes, before thou goe'[1]
—Robert Jones (c.1575–1617)

With the death of Queen Anne, the Protestant Stuart line came to a quiet shudder of an end. The following year, however, a Jacobite uprising sought to install James II & VII's Catholic son and heir, James Francis Edward Stuart (whom the Jacobites regarded as King James III and VIII) upon his father's throne. Alas for them, the 1715 uprising failed.

As the reader will have observed, the love lives of the Stuarts easily gave the Tudors a run for their money! It is sometimes said that morality swings like a pendulum from one extreme to the other. In this work we've examined this pendulum as it swung from permissive, to strict, and back again. We've seen how the sexual mores at the top of society had a 'trickle-down' effect upon society at large.

We've encountered the whole gamut of human sex and sexuality: from the romantic to the depraved, and everything in-between. We've seen examples of true love, heartbreak, lust, disease, and betrayal, and learned of the sometimes grisly and cruel punishments that were meted out to those who strayed from acceptable behaviour in Stuart-era society. We have explored accusations of sexual impropriety levelled by those who sought to gain from another's fall. We have come across horrifying deeds, scintillating literature, and amusing anecdotes.

Conclusion—Or, 'Parting is such sweet sorrow'

What became of some of those royal mistresses? An oft-recounted story is that, during the reign of George I, Catherine Sedley (James II's mistress), Louise de Kerouaille (Charles II's mistress), and Elizabeth Villiers (William III's mistress) came to be in the same room together. Sedley, in her characteristically crass yet witty way, was said to have exclaimed, 'Well, well, well! Who would have thought to find three old whores like us in the same house?'[2] These ladies played their sexual cards to their advantage, obtained financial security, and lived to ripe old age—but whether they were happy is another matter.

Any sexual preference which deviated from the traditional man-and-woman coupling was widely regarded in Stuart Britain as unnatural, and often criminal. We have seen how some lives incorporated various circumstances which were viewed as immoral and deviant. Recall the pirate women Anne Bonny and Mary Read, for instance, illegitimate children who were both made to cross-dress from an early age and who behaved in a manner which fell outside acceptable norms (including their falling in love with each other).

Whilst homosexual relationships have become largely accepted in our own time, there are other sexual unions which remain illegal, for good reason. We approve of consensual, loving sexual relationships between adults, because these will benefit, not harm, the participants, but we regard sexual proclivities such as paedophilia and bestiality as sexual perversions: in these cases consent is not given and one or more of the participants can be hurt and traumatised. Perhaps this is the most striking aspect of the sexual morality of Stuart Britain that we retain today.

Some people in Stuart Britain gave in to sexual temptation, and sometimes they paid dearly for doing so. Whether through contracting an STD such as syphilis, giving birth to an illegitimate child, and/or being punished and humiliated in public, satiating one's desires could lead to unmitigated disaster. Imagine being branded with a hot iron on your face—marked for life—for a transgression. The permanence of this is difficult to fully comprehend in the twenty-first century.

That said, those who stayed loyal to their matrimonial bonds and conformed to the accepted lifestyles of the time would often face sorrows as well—for example in the loss of a beloved spouse or child. No matter which sexual road a Stuart-era person chose to take, the myriad of political and social upheavals of their age would affect them in some way. The Stuart period was a very religious time and we have seen the great solace that Christianity brought to those suffering the loss of others they held dear. Their religion was the bedrock of their society, a balm that helped soothe the often bitter trials and tribulations of life. For others, however, the deeply religious nature of the time was more of a curse.

We have witnessed how the sexual lives of those in power could have significant repercussions for 'ordinary' people—who constituted the vast majority of the population of Stuart Britain—but the lives of the ruling elite had consequences for everyone. Had Henry Stuart, Prince of Wales, not died in 1612, the bloodshed of the Civil Wars might have been avoided, and perhaps his line (had there been one) would have been more reproductively successful. If Catherine of Braganza had been able to bear Charles II's heirs, things again would have been different. If Mary of Modena hadn't given birth to James in 1688, the throne would have passed without issue to Mary II (maddeningly, her legitimate son, who had his own legitimate line, was denied his birthright due to his religion). If William and Mary could have had children, things again would be different. Had any of Anne's children survived, the Protestant Stuart line could have continued directly. Limitless 'what if's arise when we contemplate history, but it is fascinating how many of these have to do with sex and the bearing of children, of heirs, to continue a line.

If we were to somehow miraculously transport the average Stuart man or woman into our time, they would more than likely be deeply confused, frightened, and shocked by our present society, including our mainstream views on sex and sexuality. What would the average Stuart think about the fact that many more children are born to single mothers or unmarried parents than was normal in their time? Or that effective contraception is so readily available? We still have gonorrhoea, syphilis, pubic lice and herpes, which were common in the seventeenth century—we just have far more effective ways to treat them. We also have HIV, AIDS, and drug-resistant Gonorrhoea. Our Stuart time-traveller would likely interpret these new, horrific diseases as punishment from God.

We are animals, and our sexuality is an innate part of our being, an integral part of the human experience—but it isn't everything. We learn from the past. The lives and circumstances of people we encounter when we examine history stay with us, for they are our ancestors, and they live on through us and our children. We can never truly understand a time and a people until we take their own word for it.

The great Stuart-era philosopher Thomas Hobbes famously wrote that 'the life of man [is] nasty, brutish, and short'[3]. Whilst this is a fitting description for many in Stuart Britain, their lives were not entirely joyless. Then, as now, there was solace and companionship to be found in one's family, friends, and community. And, even in a time of civil war, plague, poverty, and social and religious upheaval, one thing remained constant: there was always love.

Bibliography

The following libraries and archives were used:

The British Library: (Add MS 11600, Sloane MSS 4224, ff. 56v-64v, 113.1.6, 9930.gg.33, 1141.a.37.(3).

British History Online/Institute for Historical Research, London.

Cornell University Library (F229. B9696 1901).

English Broadside Ballad Archive.

Early English Books Online.

Emory University's Emory Women Writers Resource Project.

The Grub Street Project.

Lancashire Archives, England (ARR/1/2/17a, Folio 2).

The Metropolitan Archives, London (LMA, DL/C 218).

The National Archives, TNA, Kew (ADM 106/414/316, ADM 106/427/196, C 7/451/88, C 86/1, C 9/27/136, C 9/27/136, SP 119/342, SP 16/207, SP 34/38/42, SP 119/342, STAC 8/49/21, STAC 8/102/16).

The National Library of Scotland (MS.1954, Crawford.EB.1318).

Newberry Library, Chicago (Luttrell Broadsides).

The Seventeenth Century Lady Archives.

Shropshire Archives, England (LB/14/800, P357/W/3/7/1–35).

Suffolk Archives (SA 194/F1/1).

Wellcome Library.

Primary Sources (Books, Pamphlets, and Periodicals):

A Complete Collection Of State-Trials And Proceedings For High-Treason And Other Crimes and Misdemeanours: From The Reign of King

Richard II. To The End of the Reign of King George I: In Six Volumes, Volume III.

A Continuation of a former Relation concerning the Entertainment given to the Prince His Highnesse by the King of Spaine in his Court at Madrid (John Haviland for William Barret, London, 1623).

An Account of Marriage, Or The Interests of Marriage Considered and Defended against the Unjust Attacques of this Age (B.G., London, 1672).

Adams, Jack, *Jack Adams, His Perpetual Almanack, with Astrological Rules and Instructions* (London, 1663).

Adams, Thomas, *The Diuell's Banket* (Thomas Snodham for Ralph Mab, London, 1614).

Addison, Joseph, *The Spectator*, No. 129, July 28, 1711.

Ady, Thomas, *A Candle in the Dark: or, A Treatise Concerning the Nature of Witches and Witchcraft: Being Advice to Judges, Sheriffes, Justices of the Peace, and Grand-Jury-men, what to do, before they passe Sentence on such as are Arraigned for their Lives as Witches* (R.I., London, 1656).

Allestree, Richard, *The Ladies Calling, In Two Parts, Part I* (James Glen, Edinburgh, 1675).

Ambrose, Isaac, *Media; The Middle Things* (Archibald Ingram, James Dechman, John Hamilton, and John Glasford, Glasgow, 1737).

Ancillon, Charles, *Eunuchism Display'd: Describing all the different Sorts of Eunuchs* (E. Curll, London, 1718).

A true and impartial relation of the informations against three witches, viz., Temperance Lloyd, Mary Trembles, and Susanna Edwards (Freeman Collins, London, 1682).

A True Relation of Four Most Barbarous and Cruel Murders Committed in Leicester-Shire by Elizabeth Ridgway (George Croom, London, 1684).

A True Relation of the Most Horrid and Barbarous murders committed by Abigall Hill of St. Olaves Southwark, on the persons of foure Infants (F. Coles, London, 1658).

Quack Doctors' Advertisement 'Without Offense...', (London, 1650). British Library. Shelfmark: 1141.a.37.(3).

The Men's Answer to the Women's Petition, vindicating their own performances (London, 1674).

State-Trials and Proceedings Upon High Treason, Volume 3, (London, 1730).

Atkins, Sir Robert, *A Defence of the Late Lord Russel's Innocency, by way of Answer of Confutation of a Libellous Pamphlet, Intituled, An Antidote Against Poyson* (Timothy Goodwin, London, 1689).

Austin, William, *Haec Homo: Wherein the excellency of the creation of woman is described* (R.O. for R.M. and C.G., London, 1639).

Bacon, Sir Francis, *The Works of Francis Bacon: Baron of Verulam, Viscount St. Albans and Lord High Chancellor of England, In Five Volumes, Volume I* (A. Millar, London, 1765).

Banks, John, *The History of John, Duke of Marlborough* (James Hodges, London, 1755).

Baptista, Mantuanus, *Mantuan English'd, and Paraphras'd, Or, The Character of A Bad Woman,* Broadside (London, 1679).

Barker, R.A., *Populaidias, A Discourse Concerning the Having of Many Children, In Which the Prejudices against a Numerous Offspring Are Removed* (W. Rogers, London, 1695).

Barret, Robert, *A Companion for Midwives, Child-bearing Women, and Nurses Directing them how to Perform their Respective Offices* (Thomas Ax, London, 1699).

Bartholin, Thomas & Caspar, *Bartholinus Anatomy: made from the precepts of his father, and from the observations of all modern anatomists* (Peter Cole, London, 1665).

Baylie, Robert, *Errours and Induration, Are The Great Sins and the Great Judgements of the Time* (R. Raworth for Samuel Gellibrand, London, 1645).

Baxter, Richard, *A Treatise of Self-Denial* (Robert White, London, 1675).

Beaumont, Francis and John Fletcher, *The vvoman hater As it hath beene lately acted by the Children of Paules* (Robert Raworth, London, 1607).

Beard, Thomas & Thomas Taylor, *The Theatre of God's Judgements* (S.I & M.H., London, 1648).

Behn, Aphra, *The Town-Fopp, Or, Sir Timothy Tawdrey, A Comedy* (Roger L'Estrange, London, 1677).

Behn, Aphra, *Young Jemmy, Or, The Princely Shepherd* (P. Brooksby, London, c. 1681).

Belchier, Dabridgcourt, *Hans Beer-Pot, His Invisible Comedie, Or, See me, See me not* (Bernard Alsop, London, 1618).

Bell, John, *Witch-Craft Proven, Arreign'd, and Condemn'd in its Professors, Profession and Marks...*(Robert Sanders, Glasgow, 1697).

Bentley, Thomas, *The Sixt Lampe of Virginitie* (Thomas Dawson, Henry Denham, William Seres, London, 1582).

Boursier, Louise Bourgeois, *The Complete Midwife's Practice Enlarg'd: With instructions of the Queen of France's midwife [Louise Bourgeois]* (O. Blagrave, London, 1680).

Bradford, William, *Of Plymouth Plantation* (Massachusetts Historical Society, Boston, 1856).

Brémond, Gabriel de, *The Amorous Abbess: Or, Love in a Nunnery* (R. Bentley, London, 1684).

Brevint, Daniel, *The Depth and Mystery of the Roman Mass* (London, 1672).

Brewer, Thomas, *The bloudy mother, or The Most Inhumane Murthers, committed by Jane Hattersley vpon diuers infants, the issue of her owne bodie: & the priuate burying of them in an orchard with her araignment and execution* (John Busbie, London, 1610).

Brown, Thomas and Edward Ward, *A Comical View of London and Westminster; Or, The Merry Quack* (Sam Briscoe, London, 1705).

Brown, Thomas, *A Legacy for the Ladies, Or, Characters of the Women of the Age* (H. Meere, London, 1705).

Browne, William Hand (ed*.*), *Judicial and Testamentary Business of the Provincial Court 1649/50–1657* (Maryland Historical Society, Baltimore, 1891).

Burnet, Gilbert, *History of His Own Time, Volumes I & II* (Thomas Ward, London, 1724).

Burnet, Gilbert, *A Thanksgiving Sermon Preached before the House of Commons* (John Starkey, London, 1689).

Butler, Samuel, *Hudibras* (D. Appleton & Co, New York, 1864)

Byrd II, William *Letters of William Byrd II and Sir Hans Sloane Relative to Plants and Minerals of Virginia.*

Calendar of State Papers.

Chamberlayne, Edward, *Angliæ Notitia: Or, The Present State of England, The First Part* (T.N. for J. Martin, London, c.1679).

Chardin, Sir John, *The Travels of Sir John Chardin* (The Argonaut Press, London, 1927).

Chardin, Sir John, *Travels of Sir John Chardin into Persia and Ye East Indies* (Moses Pitt, London, 1686).

Chorier, Nicolas, *Satyre sotadique de Luisa Sigea sur les arcanes de l'amour et de Vénus en sept dialogues* (Bibliotèque des Curieux, Paris, 1910).

Churchill, Sarah, *An Account of the Conduct of the Dowager Duchess of Marlborough* (London, 1742).

Clarkson, Laurence, *The Lost Sheep Found: Or, The Prodigal Returned to his Father's house* (Laurence Clarkson, London, 1660).

Cleveland, John, *The Works of Mr. John Cleveland containing his poems, orations, epistles, collected into one volume, with the life of the author* (Obadiah Blagrave, London, 1687).

Cockeram, Henry, *The English Dictionarie of 1623* (Huntington Press, New York, 1930).

Coke, Edward, *The Third Part of the Institutes of the Law of England: Concerning High Treason, and other Pleas of the Crown, and Criminal Causes: The Fourth Edition* (A. Crooke, W. Leake, A. Roper, et al, London, 1669).

Collier, James, *A Short View of the Immorality, and Profaneness of the English Stage, Together With the Sense of Antiquity upon this Argument* (S. Keble, R. Sare, and H. Hindmarsh, London, 1698).

Courtenay, Thomas Peregrine, *Memoirs of The Life, Works, and Correspondence of William Temple* (London, 1836).

Crowne, John, *Calisto: Or, The Chaste Nymph. The late Masque at Court, as it was frequently presented there, by Several Persons of Quality* (Magnes & Bentley, London, 1675).

C., T., *The New Atlas: Or, Travels and Voyages in Europe, Asia, Africa, and America, Thro' the most Renowned Parts of the World* (J. Cleave and A. Roper, London, 1698).

Culpeper, Nicholas, *Culpeper's Directory for Midwives: Or, A Guide for Women* (Peter Cole, London, 1662).

Culpeper, Nicholas, *The English Physitian Enlarged* (John Streater, London, 1669).

Culpeper, Nicholas, *Pharmacopœia Londinenseis: Or, The London Dispensatory* (Nicholas Boone, Boston, 1720).

Dalrymple, Sir John, *Memoirs of Great Britain and Ireland, Volumes I, II, & III* (W. Strahan and T. Cadell, London, 1771).

Dalton, Michael, *The Countrey Justice: Containing The Practice, Duty and Power of The Justices of the Peace* (Henry Lintot, Savoy [London], 1746).

Dauncey, John, *The History of the Thrice-Illustrious Princess Henrietta Maria de Bourbon, Queen of England* (E.C. for Philip Chetwind, London, 1660).

Defoe, Daniel, *A Treatise Concerning the Use and Abuse of the Marriage Bed* (T. Warner: London, 1727).

Defoe, Daniel, *The Fortunate Mistress: Or, A History of the Life and Vast Variety of Fortunes of Mademoiselle de Beleau, Afterwards Call'd The Countess de Wintselsheim, in Germany, Being the Person known by the Name of the Lady Roxana, in the Time of King Charles II* (T. Warner, London, 1724).

De La Rivière, Mary (aka Delarivier Manley), *Secret Memoirs and Manners of Several Persons of Quality, of Both Sexes, from the new Atalantis* (John Morphew, London, 1709).

Dekker, Thomas, *The Magnificent Entertainment: Given to King James, Queen Anne his wife, and Henry Frederick the Prince, upon the day of his Majesties triumphant passage (from the Tower)* (Thomas Man the Younger, London, 1604).

Dekker, Thomas, *Villanies discouered by lanthorne and candle-light* (Aug. Mathewes, London, 1620).

Digby, Kenelm, *The Closet of Sir Kenelm Digby Knight Opened* (Philip Lee Warner, London, 1910).

Downes, John, *Roscius Anglicanus, Or, An Historical Review of the Stage from 1660 to 1706* (J.W. Jarvis & Son, London, 1886).

Dufour, Philippe Sylvestre, *The Manner of Making of Coffee, Tea, and Chocolate* (William Crook, London, 1685).

Dugard, Samuel (attributed), *The Marriages of Cousin Germans, vindicated from the censures of unlawfulnesse, and inexpediency. Being a letter written to his much honour'd T.D.* (Hen: Hall, Oxford, 1673).

Dunton, John, *The Night-Walker: Or, Evening Rambles in search after Lewd Women* (J. Orme, London, 1696).

E.M.A.D.O.C, *Novembris Monstrum: Or, Rome Brought to Bed in England, with the Whores Miscarying* (John Burroughes, London, 1641).

Evelyn, John, *The Diary of John Evelyn* (M. Walter Dunne, New York & London, 1901).

Falloppio, Gabriele, *Gabrielis Falloppi Medici Mutinensis Observationes Anatomicæ* (Marcum Antonium Ulmum, Venice, 1561).

Felltham, Owen, *Resolves: Divine, Moral, Political* (J.G. & T.C. Brown, Leicester, 1840).

Garfield, John, *The Wandring Whore, Continued: A Dialogue* (London, 1660).

Gardiner, Ralph, *England's Grievance Discovered, in Relation to the Coal Trade* (D. Akenhead and Sons, Newcastle, 1796).

Gouge, William, *Of Domesticall Duties* (William Bladen, London, 1622).

Greene, Robert, *Greene's Groatsworth of Wit, Bought With a Million of Repentance: Describing the Folly of Youth, the Falshood of Make-shift Flatterers, the Miserie of the negligent, and mischiefes of deceiving Curtezans* (Henry Bell, London, 1629).

The Guardian, Number III, Saturday, March 14, 1713, Periodical (J. Tonson, London, 1713).

The Life of Epicurus, (London, 1712).

The School of Venus, Or The Ladies Delight, Reduced into Rules of Practice, being the Translation of the French L'Escoles des filles (London, 1680).

N.H., *The Ladies Dictionary, Being a General Entertainment for the Fair-Sex: A Work Never attempted before in England* (John Dunton, London, 1694).

Halifax, George Savile, Marquis of, *The Lady's New-Year's Gift: Or, Advice to a Daughter* (Matt Gillyflower, London, 1688).

Hall, T., *The Queen's Royal Cookery* (S. Bates, London, 1709).

Hamilton, Count Anthony, *Memoirs of Count Grammont* (A.H. Bullen, London, 1903).

Hammond, H., *The Whole Duty of Man* (E. Pawlet, London, 1657).

Haughton, William, *English-men, For my Money: Or, A pleasant Comedy called A Woman will have her Will* (W. White, London, 1616).

Hearne, Thomas, *Remarks and Collection of Thomas Hearne, Vol. I* (Clarendon Press, Oxford, 1885).

Henrietta Maria, *Letters of Queen Henrietta Maria, edited by Mary Anne Everett Green* (Richard Bentley, London, 1857).

Herrick, Robert, *Selections from the Poetry of Robert Herrick with Drawings by Edwin A. Abbey* (Harper & Brothers Publishers, New York, 1882).

Hobbes, Thomas, *The English Works of Thomas Hobbes of Malmesbury* (J. Bonn, London, 1839).

Hooke, Robert, *Micrographia: Or, Some Physiological Descriptions of Minute Bodies made by Magnifying Glasses* (Royal Society, London, 1665).

Hutchinson, Lucy, *Memoirs of the Life of Colonel Hutchinson, Governor of Nottingham Castle and Town* (Henry G. Bohn, London, 1863).

James VI & I, *A Counterblaste to Tobacco* (London, 1604).

James VI & I, *Dæmonologie* (Robert Walde-Grave, 1597).

James VI & I, *The Workes of the Most High and Mightie Prince, James, by the grace of God, King of Great Britain and Ireland* (James, Bishop of Winton, London, 1616).

Johnson, Charles, *A History of the Pyrates, from their first rise and settlement in the Island of Providence, to the present time. With the remarkable actions and adventures of the two female pyrates Mary Read and Anne Bonny* (T. Warner, London, 1724).

Jonson, Ben, *Plays and Poems by Ben Jonson* (George Routledge & Sons, London, 1895).

Kirk, Thomas, 'An Account of a Tour in Scotland', *Tours in Scotland, 1677–1681* (David Douglas, Edinburgh, 1892).

Le Clerc, Monsieur, *A Description of Bandages and Dressings* (W. Freeman, J. Walthoe, T. Newborough, J. Nicholson and R. Parker, London, 1701).

Lemnius, Levinus, *The Secret Miracles of Nature* (Jo. Street, London, 1658).

Lithgow, William, *The Totall Discourse of the Rare Adventures & Painefull Peregrinations of Long Nineteen Yeares Travayles from Scotland to the Most Famous Kingdomes in Europe, Asia and Affrica* (Glasgow University Press, Glasgow, 1906).

Louvois, Marquis de, Testament Politique du Marquis de Louvois, Premier Ministre D'Etar sous le regne de Louis XIV, Roy de France (Cologne, 1695).

Luttrell, Narcissus, *A Brief Relation of State Affairs, from September 1678 to April 1714, Vol. III* (The University Press, Oxford, 1857).

Markham, Gervase, *The English House-wife* (Nicholas Okes for John Harison, London, 1631).

Marten, Henry, *Coll. Henry Marten's Familiar Letters to his Lady of Delight* (Edmund Gayton, Oxford, 1663).

Mathews, Tobie (editor), *A Collection of Letters, Made by Sr Tobie Mathews, Kt. With a Character of the Most Excellent Lady, Lucy Countess of Carlisle* (Tho. Horne, Tho. Bennet, and Francis Saunders, London, 1692).

Middleton, Thomas and Thomas Dekker, *The Roaring Girl, Or, Moll Cutpurse* (Thomas Archer, London, 1611).

Milton, John, *Paradise Lost: A Poem in Twelve Books* (S. Simmons, London, 1674).

Newcome, Henry, *The Compleat Mother, Or An Earnest Perswasive to all Mothers (especially those of Rank and Quality) to Nurse their own Children* (J. Wyat, London, 1695).

Newton, John, *The penitent recognition of Joseph's brethren a sermon occasion'd by Elizabeth Ridgeway, who for the petit treason of poysoning her husband, was, on March 24, 1683/4, according to the sentence of the Right Honourable Sir Thomas Street ... burnt at Leicester* (Richard Chiswel, London, 1684).

Olearius, Adam, *The Voyages and Travells of the Ambassadors sent by Frederick Duke of Holstein to the Great Duke of Muscovy, and the King of Persia...Containing a Compleat History of Muscovy, Tartary, Persia and other adjacent Countries* (John Starkey and Thomas Basset, London, 1669).

Osborne, Francis, *Advice to a Son* (R.D., London, 1673).

Peacham, Henry, *Minerva Britannia: Or, A Garden of Heroical Devices, Furnish'd, and adorned with Emblems and Impresa's of sundry nature* (Wa. Dight, London, 1612).

Peña, Juan Antonio de la, *Relacion de las fiestas reales, y juego de cañas, que la Magestad Catolica del Rey nuestro señor hizo a los veynte y uno de Agosto desde presente año, para honrar y festejar los tratados desposorios del serenissimio Principe de Gales, con la señora Infanta doña Maria de Austria* (Juan Gonzalez, Madrid, 1623).

Penn, William, *Fruits of Solitude: Reflections and Maxims relating to the conduct of Human Life* (Benjamin Johnson, Philadelphia, 1792).

Pepys, Samuel, *Diary* (George Bell & Sons, London, 1893).

Petre, Edward, *Three Letters* (London, 1688).

Phil-Porney, *A Modest Defence of Publick Stews, Or, An Essay Upon Whoring* (T. Read, London, 1740).

Pickering, Danby, *The Statutes at Large, From the First Year of K. William and Q. Mary, to the Eighth Year of K. William III, Vol. IX* (Charles Bathurst, Cambridge, 1764).

The Post Boy: With the Freshest Advices, Foreign and Domestick. Periodical. Number 2095. From Saturday October 16 to Tuesday October 19, 1708.

The Post Boy With the Freshest Advices, Foreign and Domestick. Periodical. Number 1238. From Tuesday November 1 to Thursday November 3, 1709.

Prade, Jean Le Royer, *Histoire du tabac, ou il est traité particulierement du tabac en poudre* (M. Le Prest, Paris, 1677).

Prynne, William, *Healthes, Sicknesse: Or, A Compendious and briefe Discourse, prouing, the Drinking, and Pledging of Healthes, to be Sinfull, and utterly Unlawfull unto Christians* (London, 1628).

Prynne, William, *Historio-Mastix: Or, The Players Scourge, Or Actors Tragedie* (E.A. and W.I. for Michael Sparke, London, 1633).

Psalmaanazaar, George, *A Historical and Geographical Description of Formosa* (Dan. Brown, London, 1704).

Rabelais, François, *Gargantua* (London, 1693).

Rainolds, John, *A defence of the judgment of the Reformed churches* (George Walters, Dordrecht, 1609).

Record of the Courts of Chester County, Pennsylvania, 1681–1697 (Colonial Society of Pennsylvania, Philadelphia, 1910).

Salmon, William, *Pharmacopaeia Londinensis: Or, The New London Dispensatory* (J. Dawks, London, 1702).

Savile, George, Marquis of Halifax, *The Lady's New-Year's Gift, Or, Advice to a Daughter* (Matt. Gillyflower, London 1688).

Sermon, William, *The Ladies Companion, or The English Midwife* (London, 1671).

Sevigne, Madame de, *Letters of Madame de Rabutin Chantal, Marchioness de Sevigne, to the Countess de Grignan, Her Daughter, In Two Volumes* (J Hinton, 1745).

Shadwell, Thomas, *The Virtuoso: A Comedy, Acted at the Duke's Theatre* (T.N. for Henry Herringman, London, 1676).

Shakespeare, William, *The Works of Mr. William Shakespear, Volumes 1 & 5* (Jacob Tomson, London, 1709).

Shakespeare, William, *The Tragicall Historie of Hamlet, Prince of Denmark, Act III, Scene I* (I.R. for N.L., London, 1604).

Sherley, Sir Antony, *Sir Antony Sherley: His Relation of his Travels into Persia, etc* (Nathaniel Butter and Joseph Bagset, London, 1613).

Shurtleff, Nathaniel B. (ed.), *Records of the Colony of New Plymouth in New England. Court Orders: Vol. I, 1633–1640,* (William White, Boston, 1855).

Sinibaldi, Giovanni Benedetto, *Rare Verities: The Cabinet of Venus Unlocked, and Her Secrets Laid Open* (P. Briggs, London, 1658).

Smith, John, *The Voyages and Discoveries of Captaine John Smyth in Virginia* (Joseph Barnes, Oxford, 1612).

St. John Bolingbroke, Henry (Viscount) & Dr Goldsmith, *The Works of the Late Right Honourable Henry St. John, Lord Viscount Bolingbroke: Volume 1, With the Life of Lord Bolingbroke by Dr Goldsmith* (J. Johnson, Otridge & Son, Foulder & Son, T. Payne, Wilkie & Robinson, et al, London, 1809).

Sorbière, Samuel, *A Journey to London, In the Year 1698* (A. Baldwin, London, 1698).

Suckling, John, *The Poems of Sir John Suckling* (White, Stokes, & Allen, New York, 1886).

Suckling, John, *The Tragedy of Brennoralt: Presented at the Private House in Black-Friars, By His Majesties Servants* (London, 1694).

Swift, Jonathan, *The Journal to Stella* (Methuen & Co., London, 1901).

Talbot, Charles, Duke of Shrewsbury, *Private and Original Correspondence of Charles Talbot, Duke of Shrewsbury, with King William, The Leaders of the Whig Party, And Other Distinguished Statesmen,* editor William Coxe (Longman, Hurst, Rees, Orme, and Brown, London, 1821).

The Life and Death of Damaris Page, That Great, Arch, Metropolitan (Old-Woman) of Ratcliff High-Way (R. Burton, London, 1669).

The Life and Death of John Atherton (J. Barker, London, 1641).

Thornton, Alice, *The Autobiography of Mrs. Alice Thornton, of East Newton, Co. York* (Andrews & Co., Durham, 1875).

Unknown, *Lettre d'un Marchand À Un De Ses Amis Sur l'Eppouvantable Tremblement de Terre, qui est arrivé au Port-Royal de la Jamaïque, Isle d'Angleterre, le 17 Juin 1692* (Paris?, 1692).

Unknown, *The wonderful discouerie of the vvitchcrafts of Margaret and Phillip Flower, daughters of Ioan Flower neere Beuer Castle: executed at Lincolne, March 11. 1618 Who were specially arraigned and condemned before Sir Henry Hobart, and Sir Edward Bromley, iudges of assise, for confessing themselues actors in the destruction of Henry L. Rosse, with their damnable practises against others the children of the Right Honourable Francis Earle of Rutland. Together with the seuerall examinations and confessions of Anne Baker, Ioan Willimot, and Ellen Greene, witches in Leicestershire* (G. Eld for I. Barnes, London, 1619).

Unknown, *The Women's Petition Against Coffee* (London, 1674).

Wake, William AND/OR Hickes, George, *A Defence of the Missionaries Arts* (London, 1689).

Wake, William, *Sermon Preached before the Honourable Society of Grayes-Inn: Upon the Occasion of the Death of our late Royal Sovereign Queen Mary* (R. Sare, London, 1695).

Wallis, John, *An Eighth Letter Concerning the Sacred Trinity* (Thomas Parkhurst, London, 1692).

Wallis, John, *The Doctrine of the Blessed Trinity, briefly explained in a letter to a friend* (Thomas Parkhurst, London, 1690).

Wallis, John, *Three Sermons Concerning the Sacred Trinity* (Thomas Parkhurst, London, 1691).

Ward, Edward, *A Trip to Jamaica: With a True Character of the People and Island* (London, 1698).

Ward, Edward, *The History of the Grand Rebellion* (J. Morphew, London, 1713).

Ward, Edward, *The London-Spy Compleat* (J. Howe, London, 1703).

Wilmot, John (attrib.), *The Farce of Sodom, or The Quintessance of Debauchery* (1684).

Wilmot, John, *The Works of John Earl of Rochester: Containing Poems on Several Occasions* (Jacob Tonson, London, 1714).

Willughby, Percival, *Observations in Midwifery, as also The Countrey Midwifes Opsculum, or Vade Mecum* (Shakespeare Print Press, Warwick, 1863).

Winstanley, William, *The Lives of the Most Famous English Poets, Or The Honour of Parnassus* (Samuel Manship, London, 1687).

Winthrop, John, *Winthrop Papers, Volume III: 1631–1637* (The Merrymount Press, Boston, 1943).

Wiseman, Richard, *Eight Chirurgical Treatises* (Benjamin Tooke and John Meredith, London, 1705).

Wood, Anthony, *The Life and Times of Anthony Wood, antiquary, of Oxford, 1632–1697, described by Himself: Vol. I* (Oxford Historical Society, Oxford, 1891).

Woodward, Josiah, *An Account of the Progress of the Reformation of Manners* (Joseph Downing, London, 1704).

Woolley, Hannah, *The Gentlewoman's Companion: Or, A Guide to the Female Sex* (A. Maxwell for Edward Thomas, London, 1675).

Wycherley, William, *The Country Wife: A Comedy as it is Acted at the Theatre-Royal* (C. Bathhurst, London, 1751).

Yonge, James, *An Account of Balls of Hair Taken from the Uterus and Ovaria of Several Women, Royal Society of London* (London, 1705).

Secondary Sources:

Articles:

Anderson, A. L., & Chaney, E. (2009). Pubic lice (Pthirus pubis): history, biology and treatment vs. knowledge and beliefs of US college students. *International journal of environmental research and public health*, 6(2), 592–600.

Bergeron, David M. 'Court Masques about Stuart London.' *Studies in Philology*, vol. 113, no. 4, 2016, pp. 822–849. *JSTOR*, www.jstor.org/stable/44329617. [Accessed 26 January 2019].

Cummings, Megan, 'What urinating after sex does and does not prevent in women', My Med, https://www.mymed.com/health-wellness/sex-and-relationships/what-urinating-after-sex-does-and-does-not-prevent-in-women [Accessed 1 February 2020].

Davies, Owen, 'The War on Witches', *The Life and Times of The Stuarts,* BBC History Magazine, p. 68.

Gaimster, David, Peter Boland, Steve Linnane, & Caroline Cartwright (1996) 'The Archaeology of Private Life: The Dudley Castle Condoms'. *Post-Medieval Archaeology*, 30:1, 129–142, DOI: 10.1179/pma.1996.003 [Accessed 17 December 2018].

McClain, Molly, 'Love, Friendship, and Power: Queen Mary II's Letters to Frances Apsley'. *Journal of British Studies*, vol. 47, no. 3, 2008, pp. 505–527. doi:10.1086/587720.

Oaks, Robert F., '"Things Fearful to Name": Sodomy and Buggery in Seventeenth-Century New England.' *Journal of Social History*, vol. 12, no. 2, 1978, pp. 268–281. *JSTOR*, JSTOR, www.jstor.org/stable/3787139.

Read, Sara, 'Bleeding in Seventeenth-Century England: Guest Post by Sara Read', *The Seventeenth Century Lady,* 4 September 2013, www.andreazuvich.com/history/sara-read-menstruation-and-female-bleeding-in-seventeenth-century-england/

Robertson, Karen, 'Pocahontas at the Masque.' *Signs*, vol. 21, no. 3, 1996, pp. 551–583. *JSTOR*, www.jstor.org/stable/3175171.

Royal Museums Greenwich. 'Health in the 17th century: Nicholas Culpeper was an influential figure': https://www.rmg.co.uk/DISCOVER/EXPLORE/HEALTH-17TH-CENTURY [Accessed 27 January 2019].

Skuse, Alanna, 'One Stroak of His Razour': Tales of Self-Gelding in Early Modern England, *Social History of Medicine*, hky100, https://doi.org/10.1093/shm/hky100 [Accessed 15 December 2018].

Von Goeth, Aurora, 'Julie d'Aubigny, Mademoiselle Maupin'. http://partylike1660.com/julie-daubigny-mademoiselle-maupin/ [Accessed 30 January 2019].

Zuvich, Andrea, '12 Facts About the Stuarts', *BBC History Extra*, December 2015. https://www.historyextra.com/period/stuart/facts-about-stuarts-royals-mary-queen-scots-witchcraft/

Zuvich, Andrea, 'The Allure of the Royal Mistress', *The Huffington Post*. https://www.huffingtonpost.co.uk/endeavour-press/allure-of-the-royal-mistress_b_3414079.html

Zuvich, Andrea, 'Crossing the Line: Queen Anne and Her Favourite, Sarah Churchill'. *History of Royals Magazine*. Issue 17. Imagine Publishing, 2017.

Zuvich, Andrea, 'The Real Favourite: Sarah Churchill'. *All About History Magazine*. Future Publishing, 2019.

Zuvich, Andrea, 'Stuart Britain: What Was Life Like for Ordinary People?' *BBC History Extra*. https://www.historyextra.com/period/stuart/stuart-britain-what-was-life-like-for-ordinary-people/ July 2016.

Books:

Ackroyd, Peter, *Newton* (Vintage Books, London, 2007).

Adamson, John, *The Noble Revolt: The Overthrow of Charles I* (Weidenfeld & Nicolson, London, 2007).

Adolph, Anthony, *The King's Henchman: Henry Jermyn, Stuart Spymaster and Architect of the British Empire* (Gibson Square Books, London, 2012).

Akkerman, Nadine, *Invisible Agents: Women and Espionage in Seventeenth-Century Britain* (Oxford University Press, Oxford, 2018).

Aldersey-Williams, Hugh, *In Search of Sir Thomas Browne: The Life and Afterlife of the Seventeenth-Century's Most Inquiring Mind* (W.W. Norton & Company, New York, 2015).

Armitage, Jill, *Arbella Stuart: The Uncrowned Queen* (Amberley Publishing, Stroud, 2017).

Arnold, Catherine, *City of Sin: London and Its Vices* (Simon & Schuster, London, 2010).

Atkins, John, *Sex in Literature: The Erotic Impulse in Literature* (Grove Press Inc., New York, 1970).

Baird, Rosemary, *Mistress of the House: Great Ladies and Grand Houses, 1670–1830* (Weidenfeld & Nicolson, London, 2003).

Barbier, Patrick, *The World of the Castrati: The History of an Extraordinary Operatic Phenomenon* (Souvenir Press, London, 1996).

Barker, Hannah and Elaine Chalus (editors), *Gender in Eighteenth-Century England: Roles, Representations and Responsibilities* (Addison Wesley Longman Limited, Harlow, 1997).

Bellany, Alastair & Thomas Cogswell, *The Murder of King James I* (Yale University Press, New Haven and London, 2015).

Bell, Walter George, *The Great Plague in London* (The Folio Society, London, 2001).

Berkowitz, Eric, *Sex & Punishment: 4000 Years of Judging Desire* (The Westbourne Press, London, 2012).

Bernau, Anke, *Virgins: A Cultural* History (Granta Books, London, 2007).

Bevan, Bryan, *The Duchess Hortense: Cardinal Mazarin's Wanton Niece* (The Rubicon Press, London, 1987).

Bevan, Bryan, *King William III: Prince of Orange, the first European* (The Rubicon Press, London, 1997).

Bloch, Ivan, *Ethnological and Cultural Studies of the Sex Life in England Illustrated, As Revealed in Its Erotic and Obscene Literature and Art* (Falstaff Press Inc., New York, 1934).

Bloch, Ivan, *Sexual Life in England* (Corgi Books, London, 1958).

Bolger, Angela, *The First Field Marshal & the King's Mistress: Earl & Countess of Orkney, George Hamilton and Elizabeth Villiers* (Taplow, 2002).

Borman, Tracy, *Witches: James I and the English Witch-Hunts* (Vintage, London, 2014).

Boxer, Marilyn J., and Jean H. Quataert, *Connecting Spheres: European Women in a Globalizing World, 1500 to the Present* (Oxford University Press, New York, 2000).

Braddick, Michael, *God's Fury, England's Fire: A New History of the English Civil Wars* (Penguin, London, 2008).

Bramley, Zoe, *William Shakespeare in 100 Facts* (Amberley Publishing, Stroud, 2016).

Brandon, David, *Life in a 17th Century Coffee Shop* (The History Press, Stroud, 2007).

Brook, Timothy, *Vermeer's Hat: The Seventeenth Cenutry and the Dawn of the Global World* (Profile Books, London, 2009).

Buckley, Veronica, *Madame de Maintenon: The Secret Wife of Louis XIV* (Bloomsbury Publishing Plc, London, 2008).

Burg, B.R., *Sodomy and the Pirate Tradition: English Sea Rovers in the Seventeenth-Century Caribbean* (New York University Press, New York, 1995).

Callow, John, *James II: King in Exile* (The History Press, Stroud, 2017).

Carlton, Charles, *Royal Mistresses* (Routledge, London, 1990).

Cecil, David, *The Cecils of Hatfield House* (Constable, London, 1973).

Chalmers, Alexander, *The General Biographical Dictionary: Containing an Historical and Critical Account of the Lives and Writings of the Most Eminent Persons in Every Nation; Particularly the British and Irish, from the Earliest Accounts to the Present Time, Volume V* (J. Nichols and Son, London, 1812).

Chapman, Hester W., *Four Fine Gentlemen* (Constable and Company, Ltd, London, 1977).

Chapman, Hester W., Queen Anne's Son (Andre Deutsch Limited, London, 1954).

Chapman, Hester W., *Queen Mary II* (Jonathan Cape, London, 1953).

Clegg, Melanie, *The Life of Henrietta Anne* (Pen & Sword History, Barnsley, 2017).

Codd, Daniel J, *Crimes & Criminals of 17th Century Britain* (Pen & Sword History, Barnsley, 2018).

Cogswell, Thomas, *James I: The Pheonix King* (Allen Lane, 2017).

Cooper, Susan Margaret, *Thomas Alcock: A Biographical Account* (Kindle edition, 2017).

Crawford, Mary Caroline, *The Days of the Pilgrim Fathers* (Little, Brown, & Co, Boston, 1920).

Crawford, Patricia and Laura Gowing (ed.), *Women's Worlds in Seventeenth-Century England: A Sourcebook* (Routledge, London, 2000).

Cressy, David, *Birth, Marriage & Death: Ritual, Religion, and the Life-Cycle in Tudor and Stuart England* (Oxford University Press, Oxford, 1997).

Dabhoiwala, Faramerz, *The Origins of Sex: A History of the First Sexual Revolution* (Penguin Books, London, 2013).

Darcy, Eamon, *The World of Thomas Ward: Sex and Scandal in Late Seventeenth-Century Co. Antrim* (Four Courts Press, Dublin, 2016).

Davenport Adams, W.H, *Good Queen Anne; Or, Men and Manners, Life and Letters in England's Augustan Age* (Remington & Co. Publishers, London, 1886).

Davis, Robert C, *Christian Slaves, Muslim Masters: White Slavery in the Mediterranean, the Barbary Coast, and Italy, 1500–1800* (Palgrave MacMillan, Houndsmills, 2003).

De Lisle, Leanda, *After Elizabeth: The Death of Elizabeth and the Coming of King James* (HarperPerennial, London, 2006).

De Lisle, Leanda, *White King: Charles I: Traitor, Murderer, Martyr* (Chatto & Windus, London, 2018).

Doherty, Richard, *The Siege of Derry 1689: A Military History* (Spellmount, Stroud, 2010).

Dolman, Brett, *Beauty, Sex, and Power* (Scala Publishers/Historic Royal Palaces, London, 2012).

Dolnick, Edward, *The Clockwork Universe: Isaac Newton, the Royal Society & the Birth of the Modern World* (Harper Perennial, New York, 2011).

Durston, Christopher, *James I* (Routledge, London, 1993).

Ede, Mary, *Arts and Society in England under William and Mary* (Stainer & Bell, London, 1979).

Evenden, Doreen, *The Midwives of Seventeenth-Century London* (Cambridge University Press, Cambridge, 2000).

Fairfax, Brian, *Memoirs of the Life of George Villiers* (W. Bathoe, London, 1753).

Fagan, Brian, *The Little Ice Age: How Climate Made History, 1300–1850* (Basic Books, New York, 2000).

Fausto-Sterling, Anne, *Sexing the Body: Gender Politics and the Construction of Sexuality* (Basic Books, New York, 2000).

Field, Jacob F, *One Bloody Thing After Another: The World's Most Gruesome History* (Michael O'Mara Books Limited, London, 2012).

Field, Ophelia, *The Kit-Cat Club* (Harper Perennial, London, 2009).

Fisher, Kate and Sarah Toulalan (ed,), *Bodies, Sex and Desire from the Renaissance to the Present* (Palgrave MacMillan, Houndsmills, 2011).

Fletcher, Anthony, *Gender, Sex, & Subordination in England 1500–1800* (Yale University Press, New Haven and London, 1995).

Foucault, Michel, *The History of Sexuality: Volume I, An Introduction* (Penguin Books, London, 1978).

Fraser, Antonia, *Cromwell: Our Chief of Men* (Book Club Associates, London, 1973).

Fraser, Antonia, *King James VI of Scotland, I of England* (Weidenfeld & Nicolson, London, 1974 (1994 edition).

Fraser, Antonia, *Mary Queen of Scots: The 50th Anniversary Edition* (Weidenfeld & Nicolson Ltd, London, 1969).

Fraser, Antonia, *The Weaker Vessel: A Woman's Lot in Seventeenth-Century England* (George Weidenfeld and Nicholson, Ltd, London, 1993).

Fraser, Sarah, *The Prince Who Would Be King: The Life and Death of Henry Stuart* (William Collins, London, 2017).

Friedman, David F. *A Mind of Its Own: A Cultural History of the Penis* (Penguin Books, New York, 2001).

Geyl, Pieter, *Orange and Stuart: 1641–1672* (Pheonix Press, London, 1969).

Goldstone, Nancy, *Daughters of the Winter Queen: Four Remarkable Sisters and the Enduring Legacy of Mary, Queen of Scots* Weidenfeld & Nicolson, London, 2018).

Gore-Browne, Robert, *Gay Was The Pit: The Life and Times of Anne Oldfield, Actress* (Max Reinhardt, London, 1957).

Gowing, Laura, *Gender Relations in Early Modern England* (Pearson Education Limited, Harlow, 2012).

Graham, Elspeth, Hilary Hinds, Elaine Hobby, Helen Wilcox (eds.), *Her Own Life: Autobiographical writings by seventeenth-century Englishwomen* (Routledge, London, 1989).

Green, David, *Queen Anne* (The History Book Club, Glasgow, 1970).

Greene, Graham, *Lord Rochester's Monkey: Being the Life of John Wilmot, Second Earl of* Rochester (The Viking Press, New York, 1974).

Gregg, Edward, *Queen Anne* (Yale University Press, Yale, 2001).

Gristwood, Sarah, *Arbella: England's Lost Queen* (Bantam, London, 2004).

Hamilton, Elizabeth, *The Illustrious Lady: A Biography of Barbara Villiers, Countess of Castlemaine and Duchess of Cleveland* (Hamish Hamilton, London, 1980).

Hamilton, Elizabeth, *William's Mary: A Biography of Mary* II (Hamish Hamilton, London, 1972).

Harris, Frances, *A Passion for Government: The Life of Sarah, Duchess of Marlborough* (Clarendon Press, Oxford, 1991).

Hart, Avril and Susan North, *Seventeenth and Eighteenth-Century Fashion in Detail* (V&A Publishing, London, 1998).

Haswell, Jock, *James II: Soldier and Sailor* (Hamish Hamilton, London, 1972).

Herman, Eleanor, *The Royal Art of Poison* (St. Martin's Press, New York, 2018).

Herman, Eleanor, *Sex With Kings* (William Morrow, New York, 2004).

Herrup, Cynthia B, *A House in Gross Disorder: Sex Law, and the 2nd Earl of Castlehaven* (Oxford University Press, Oxford, 1999).

Hibbert, Christopher, *Charles I* (Corgi Books, London, 1972).

Hill, Christopher, *God's Englishman: Oliver Cromwell and the English Revolution* (Penguin Books, Harmondsworth, 1973).

Hill, C.P., *Who's Who in British History: Stuart Britain 1603–1714* (Stackpole Books, Mechanicsburg, 1988).

Hilton, Lisa, *The Real Queen of France: Athénaïs & Louis XIV* (Abacus, London, 2003).

Holden, Anthony, *William Shakespeare: His Life and Work* (Little, Brown, & Co., London, 1999).

Holmes, Frederick, *The Sickly Stuarts: The Medical Downfall of a Dynasty* (Sutton Publishing, Stroud, 2005).

Hopkins, Graham, *Constant Delights: Rakes, Rogues, and Scandal in Restoration England* (Robson Books, London, 2002).

Houston, S.J, *James I: Seminar Studies in History* (Pearson Education Limited, Harlow, 1995).

Howe, Elizabeth, *The First English Actresses: Women and Drama, 1660–1700* (Cambridge University Press, Cambridge, 1992).

Hume, David, *The History of England, Vol. II* (T. Cadell, London, 1789).

Ingram, Martin, *Church Courts, Sex and Marriage in England, 1570–1640* (Cambridge University Press, Cambridge, 1987).

Jardine, Lisa, *The Curious Life of Robert Hooke: The Man Who Measured London* (Harper Collins, London, 2003).

Jones, Robert, *The Muses Gardin for Delights* (B.H. Blackwell, Oxford, 1901).

Jordan, Don and Michael Walsh, *The King's Bed: Sex, Power, & the Court of Charles II* (Abacus, London, 2016).

Keay, Anna, *The Last Royal Rebel: The Life and Death of James, Duke of Monmouth* (Bloomsbury, London, 2017).

Keay, Anna, *The Magnificent Monarch: Charles II and the Ceremonies of Power* (Continuum Books, London, 2008).

Kenyon, J.P., *The* Stuarts (William Collins Sons & Co., Glasgow, 1970).

Lacey, Andrew, *The English Civil War in 100 Facts* (Amberley Publishing, Stroud, 2017).

Lamb, Jeremy, *So Idle A Rogue: The Life and Death of Lord Rochester* (Allison & Busby, London, 1993).

Lander Johnson, Bonnie, *Chastity in Early Stuart Literature and Culture* (Cambridge University Press, Cambridge, 2015).

Larman, Alexander, *Blazing Star: The Life and Times of John Wilmot, Earl of Rochester* (Head of Zeus, London, 2014).

Laurence, Anne, *Women in England: 1500–1760. A Social History* (Phoenix Press, London, 1996).

Laver, James, *The Ladies of Hampton Court* (William Collins, London, 1942).

License, Amy, *In Bed With The Tudors: The Sex Lives of a Dynasty from Elizabeth of York to Elizabeth I* (Amberley Publishing, Stroud, 2013).

Lincoln, Marguerite (ed.), *Samuel Pepys: Plague, Fire, Revolution* (Thames & Hudson/National Maritime Museum, 2015).

Lindley, David, *The Trials of Frances Howard* (Routledge, London, 1996).

Livingstone, Natalie, *The Mistresses of Cliveden: Three Centuries of Scandal, Power, and Intrigue* (Arrow Books, London, 2015).

London County Council, *Geffrye Museum: 17th Century Children at Home* (Waterlow & Sons, London, 1964).

Loughlin, Marie H. (editor), *Same-Sex Desire in Early Modern England, 1550–1735* (Manchester University Press, Manchester, 2014).

Marshall, Rosalind K., *Scottish Queens: The Queen and Consorts Who Shaped A Nation* (Birlinn Ltd, Edinburgh, 2019).

Massie, Alan, *The Royal Stuarts: A History of the Family that Shaped Britain* (Thomas Dunne Books, New York, 2010).

Matthews-Grieco, Sara F. (ed.), *Cuckoldry, Impotence, and Adultery in Europe (15th-17th century)* (Ashgate Publishing, Abingdon, 2014).

Matusiak, John, *James I: Scotland's King of England* (The History Press, Stroud, 2015).

McClain, Mary, *Beaufort: The Duke and his Duchess, 1657–1715* (Yale University Press, New Haven, 2001).

McLeod, Catherine, Timothy Wilks, Malcolm Smuts, Rab MacGibbon, *The Lost Prince: The Life and Death of Henry Stuart* (National Portrait Gallery, London, 2012).

Melford Hall, Suffolk: A Property of The National Trust, Home of Sir Richard Hyde Parker, Bt. (The National Trust, 1968).

Mendelson, Sara and Patricia Crawford, *Women in Early Modern England: 1550–1720* (Clarendon Press, Oxford, 1998).

Milton, Giles, *White Gold: The Extraordinary Story of Thomas Pellow and North Africa's One Million European Slaves* (Hodder & Stoughton, London, 2005).

Mitford, Nancy, *The Sun King* (Vintage Books, London, 1966).

Moore, Lucy, *Lady Fanshawe's Receipt Book: An Englishwoman's Life During the Civil War* (Atlantic Books, London, 2018).

Mondimore, Francis Mark, *A Natural History of Homosexuality* (The John Hopkins University Press, Baltimore, 1996).

Murray, Nicholas, *World Enough and Time: The Life of Andrew Marvell* (Little, Brown & Company, London, 1999).

Néret, Gilles, *Erotica 17th-18th Century* (Taschen GmbH, Koln, 2001).

O'Callaghan, Sean, *To Hell or Barbados: The Ethnic Cleansing of Ireland* (Brandon, Dingle, 2000).

Oman, Carola, *Mary of Modena* (Hodder and Stoughton, Bungay, 1962).

Page, Nick, *Lord Minimus: The Extraordinary Life of Britain's Smallest Man* (St. Martin's Press, New York, 2002).

Partridge, Eric, *Shakespeare's Bawdy* (Routledge, London, 1968).

Peters, Belinda Roberts, *Marriage in Seventeenth-Century English Political Thought* (Palgrave Macmillan, Houndmills, 2004).

Picard, Liza, *Restoration London: Everyday Life in London 1660–1670* (Phoenix, London, 2004).

Pimm, Geoffrey, *The Violent Abuse of Women in 17th and 18th Century Britain* (Pen & Sword History, Barnsley, 2019).

Plowden, Alison, *Henrietta Maria: Charles I's Indomitable Queen* (Sutton Publishing, Stroud, 2002).

Plowden, Alison, *The Stuart Princesses* (Alan Sutton Publishing Ltd, Stroud, 1996).

Porter, Linda, *Royal Renegades: The Children of Charles I and the English Civil Wars* (Pan Books, London, 2016).

Porter, Ray and Lesley Hall, *The Facts of Life: The Creation of Sexual Knowledge in Britain, 1650–1950*, (Yale University Press, New Haven and London, 1995).

Porter, Jennifer, *The Jamestown Brides: The Bartered Wives of the New World* (Atlantic Books, London, 2019).

Probert, Rebecca, *Marriage Law for Genealogists: The Definitive Guide* (Takeaway Publishing, Kenilworth, 2016).

Purkiss, Diane, *The English Civil War: A People's History* (Harper Perennial, London, 2007).

Quaife, G.R., *Wanton Wenches and Wayward Wives: Peasants and Illicit Sex in Early Seventeenth-Century England* (Croom Helm Ltd, London, 1979).

Read, Sara, *Exploring the Lives of Women, 1558–1837* (Pen & Sword History, 2018).

Read, Sara, *Maids, Wives, Widows: Exploring Early Modern Women's Lives, 1540–1740* (Pen & Sword, Barnsley, 2015).

Reynolds, Anna, *In Fine Style: The Art of Tudor and Stuart Fashions* (Royal Collection Trust, 2013).

Rowell, Christopher, *Petworth: The People and the Place* (Scala Publishers Ltd/National Trust, London and Swindon, 2012).

Royle, Trevor, *Civil War: The Wars of the Three Kingdoms, 1638–1660* (Abacus, London, 2005).

Sanders, Mary F., *Princess and Queen of England, Life of Mary II* (Stanley, Paul & Co., London, 1913).

Sanger, William W., *The History of Prostitution: Its Extent, Causes, and Effects throughout the World* (Harper & Brothers, New York, 1859).

Seward, Desmond, *The King Over The Water: A Complete History of the Jacobites* (Birlinn Limited, Edinburgh, 2019).

Scruton, Roger, *Sexual Desire: A Philosophical Investigation* (Phoenix, London, 1986 (1994 edition).

Shapiro, James, *1606: William Shakespeare and the Year of Lear* (Faber & Faber, London, 2015).

Sharpe, James, *The Bewitching of Anne Gunter: A horrible and true story of football, witchcraft, murder, and the King of England* (Profile Books, London, 1999).

Shoemaker, Robert B., *Gender in English Society 1650–1850: The Emergence of Separate Spheres?* (Routledge, Abingdon, 1998).

Smith, Captain Alexander, *A Complete History of the Highwaymen* (George Routledge & Sons, London, 1933).

Smith, Merril D. (ed.), *Sex and Sexuality in Early America* (New York University Press, New York, 1998).

Somerset, Anne, *Queen Anne: The Politics of Passion* (HarperPress, London, 2012).

Speck, W.A., *James II* (Pearson Education Limited, Harlow, 2002).

Speck, W.A., *Reluctant Revolutionaries: Englishmen and the Revolution of 1688* (Oxford University Press, Oxford, 1988).

Spencer, Charles, *Killers of the King: The Men Who Dared to Execute Charles I* (Bloomsbury, London, 2014).

Spencer, Charles, *Prince Rupert: The Last Cavalier* (Phoenix, London, 2008).

Spencer, Charles, *To Catch a King: Charles II's Great Escape* (William Collins, London, 2017).

Starkey, David, *Crown & Country: The Kings & Queens of England* (Harper Press, London, 2011).

Stone, Lawrence, *Uncertain Unions & Broken Lives* (Oxford University Press, Oxford, 1993).

Stubbs, John, *John Donne: The Reformed Soul* (W.W. Norton & Company, Inc, New York, 2007).

Tallis, Nicola, *Elizabeth's Rival: The Tumultuous Tale of Lettice Knollys, Countess of* Leinster (Michael O'Mara Books Ltd, London, 2017).

Tannahill, Reay, *Sex in History* (Scarborough House, 1992).

Thomas, Keith, *Religion and the Decline of Magic: Studies in Popular Beliefs in Sixteenth- And Seventeenth-Century England* (Penguin Books, London, 1991).

Thompson, Roger, *Unfit For Modest Ears: A study of pornographic, obscene and bawdy works written or published in England in the second half of the seventeenth century* (MacMillan Press, London, 1979).

Tinniswood, Adrian, *The Rainborowes: Pirates, Puritans and a Family's Quest for the Promised Land* (Vintage Books, London, 2014).

Toulalan, Sarah, *Imagining Sex: Pornography and Bodies in Seventeenth-Century England* (Oxford University Press, Oxford, 2007).

Traub, Valerie, *The Renaissance of Lesbianism in Early Modern England* (Cambridge University Press, Cambridge, 2002).

Trevelyan, G.M., *Illustrated English Social History: Volume Two: The Age of Shakespeare and the Stuart* Period (Penguin Books Ltd, Harmondsworth, 1964).

Uglow, Jenny, *A Gambling Man: Charles II and the Restoration* (Faber & Faber Limited, London, 2009).

Underdown, David, *A Freeborn People: Politics and the Nation in Seventeenth-Century England* (Clarendon Press, Oxford, 1996).

Walker, Garthine, *Crime, Gender and Social Order in Early Modern England* (Cambridge University Press, Cambridge, 2003).

Waller, Maureen, *1700: Scenes From London Life* (Hodder & Stoughton, London, 2000).

Waller, Maureen, *Ungrateful Daughters: The Stuart Princesses Who Stole Their Father's Crown* (Sceptre Books, London, 2002).

Waterson, Nellie M., *Mary II, Queen of England 1689–1694* (Duke University Press, Durham, 1928).

Watkins, Sarah-Beth, *The Tragic Daughters of Charles I: Mary, Elizabeth, & Henrietta Anne* (Chronos Books, Winchester, 2019).

Watkins, Susan, *Mary Queen of Scots* (Thames & Hudson, London, 2009).

Wauchope, Piers, *Patrick Sarsfield and the Williamite War* (Irish Academic Press, Dublin, 1992).

Wellicome, Lavinia and Chris Gravett, *Woburn Abbey*, (Jarrold Publishing, Norfolk, 2009).

Wells, Stanley, *Shakespeare, Sex & Love* (Oxford University Press, Oxford, 2010).

Wheatley, Dennis, *'Old Rowley': A Very Private Life of Charles II* (Arrow Books, London, 1969).

Whitaker, Katie, *A Royal Passion: The Turbulent Marriage of Charles I and Henrietta Maria* (Pheonix, London, 2011).

Whitehead, Julian, *Cromwell and His Women* (Pen & Sword History, Barnsley, 2019).

Wilkinson, Josephine, *Louis XIV: The Real King of Versailles* (Amberley Publishing, Stroud, 2019).

Wilson, Derek, *All the King's Women: Love, Sex, and Politics in the Life of Charles II* (Hutchinson, London, 2003).

Winn, James Andersen, *Queen Anne: Patroness of Arts* (Oxford University Press, Oxford, 2014).

Winsham, Willow, *England's Witchcraft Trials* (Pen & Sword History, Barnsley, 2018).

Wooley, Benjamin, *Heal Thyself: Nicholas Culpeper and the Seventeenth-Century Struggle to Bring Medicine to the People* (Harper Collins Publishers, New York, 2004).

Wright, Robert, *The Moral Animal: Why We Are The Way We Are* (Abacus, London, 1996).

Zuvich, Andrea, *The Stuarts in 100 Facts* (Amberley Publishing Ltd, Stroud, 2015).

Zuvich, Andrea, *A Year in the Life of Stuart Britain* (Amberley Publishing Ltd, Stroud, 2016).

Notes

Author's Note

1. I have not found sufficient evidence to support the idea that there was an exact equivalence in the Stuart period for what some use these terms for today, and so have omitted these terms in this book.
2. De La Rivière, Mary, *Secret Memoirs and Manners of Several Persons of Quality, of Both Sexes from the new Atalantis* (John Morphew, London, 1709), p. 172. Also, the word 'gay' as used to describe homosexuals and lesbians only became popularised in the mid-twentieth century (so we clearly can't use it to describe people in the Stuart period).
3. Mondimore, Francis Mark, *A Natural History of Homosexuality* (The John Hopkins University Press, Baltimore, 1996), p. 3.

Introduction

1. Burnet, Gilbert, *A Thanksgiving Sermon Preached before the House of Commons* (John Starkey, London, 1689), p. 1.
2. Peters, Belinda Roberts, *Marriage in Seventeenth-Century English Political Thought* (Palgrave Macmillan, Houndmills, 2004), p. 11.
3. Beard, Thomas and Thomas Taylor, *The Theatre of God's Judgements* (S.I & M.H., London, 1648).
4. Stubbs, John, *John Donne: The Reformed Soul* (W.W. Norton & Company, Inc, New York, 2007), p. 187.

PART ONE

Chapter 1: The Anatomy of a Stuart-Age Person

1. N.H., *The Ladies Dictionary, Being a General Entertainment for the Fair-Sex: A Work Never attempted before in England* (John Dunton, London, 1694), p. 284.
2. There were some writers, however, such as Charles Ancillon in his *Eunuchism Display'd*, that stated that the ancients also recognised a 'third sort of Man'—which in that case meant a man who had been made a eunuch.
3. Cawdrey, Robert, *The First English Dictionary 1604: Robert Cawdrey's A Table Alphabeticall* (Bodleian Library, Oxford, 2007), p. 91.

4. Lemnius, Levinus, *The Secret Miracles of Nature*, (Jo. Street, London, 1658).

5. Culpeper, Nicholas, *Pharmacopœia Londinensis, Or, The London Dispensatory* (Nicholas Boone, Boston, 1720), pp. A3 & A4.

6. Cockeram, Henry, *The English Dictionarie of 1623* (Huntington Press, New York, 1930), p. 120.

7. Graham, Elspeth, Hilary Hinds, Elaine Hobby, Helen Wilcox, *Her Own Life: Autobiographical writings by seventeenth-century Englishwomen* (Routledge, London, 1989), p. 152.

8. Thornton, Alice, *The Autobiography of Mrs. Alice Thornton, of East Newton, Co. York* (Andrews & Co., Durham, 1875), p. 54.

9. Zuvich, Andrea, *The Stuarts in 100 Facts*, p. 36.

10. Anonymous, *The Women's Petition Against Coffee* (London, 1674). It is still undetermined whether this pamphlet was actually written by women, or by men.

11. Sinibaldi, Giovanni Benedetto, *Rare Verities: The Cabinet of Venus Unlocked, and Her Secrets Laid Open* (P. Briggs, London, 1658), p. 21.

12. Ibid, p. 27.

13. Ibid, p. 20.

14. The word 'cock' is generally believed to have been used as a vulgar term for the penis in the late 1610s, having previously been associated with the cockerel, or rooster.

15. Sinibaldi, *The Cabinet of Venus Unlocked*, p. 38.

16. Rabelais, François, *Gargantua*, Chapter XI, 1693.

17. Bourgeois, Louise, *The Complete Midwife's Practice Enlarg'd* (O. Blagrave, London, 1680), p. 36.

18. Bartholin, Thomas & Caspar, *Bartholinus Anatomy: made from the precepts of his father, and from the observations of all modern anatomists* (Peter Cole, London, 1665), p. 54.

19. *The School of Venus, Or The Ladies Delight, Reduced into Rules of Practice, being the Translation of the French L'Escoles des filles* (London, 1680), p. 20.

20. Thompson, *Unfit for Modest Ears*, p. 148.

21. Sinibaldi, *The Cabinet of Venus Unlocked*, p. 38.

22. Ibid, p. 39.

23. Ibid, p. 40.

24. 'fourteen, at which time they are capable of conceiving', as found in *The School of Venus*, p. 30.

25. Ibid.

26. Thompson, *Unfit for Modest Ears*, p. 149.

27. Find these and many more at 'The Timeline of Slang Terms for the Vagina', created from *Green's Dictionary of Slang*, published in 2010 and written by Jonathon Green: http://timeglider.com/timeline/07f47d6b843da763 [Accessed 30 January 2020].

28. Ibid.

29. Toulalan, Sarah, *Imagining Sex: Pornography and Bodies in Seventeenth-Century England* (Oxford University Press, Oxford, 2007), p. 218.

30. Ibid.
31. Falloppio, Gabriele, *Gabrielis Falloppi Medici Mutinensis Observationes Anatomicæ* (Marcum Antonium Ulmum, Venice, 1561).
32. Yonge, James, *An Account of Balls of Hair Taken from the Uterus and Ovaria of Several Women* (Royal Society of London, London, 1753), p. 2392.
33. Crawford, Patricia and Laura Gowing, *Women's Worlds in Seventeenth-Century England*, p. 304.
34. Read, Sara, 'Bleeding in Seventeenth-Century England: Guest Post by Sara Read', *The Seventeenth Century Lady*, 4 September 2013, www.andreazuvich.com/history/sara-read-menstruation-and-female-bleeding-in-seventeenth-century-england/
35. Cockeram, *The English Dictionarie of 1623*, p. 120.
36. As quoted in Wooley, Benjamin, *Heal Thyself: Nicholas Culpeper and the Seventeenth-Century Struggle to Bring Medicine to the People* (Harper Collins Publishers, New York, 2004), p. 19.
37. Tomalin, Claire, 'Samuel Pepys, Renaissance Man', *Samuel Pepys: Plague, Fire, Revolution* (Thames & Hudson/National Maritime Museum, 2015).
38. Read, Sara, *Maids, Wives, Widows: Exploring Early Modern Women's Lives* (Pen & Sword History, Barnsley, 2015), p. 84.
39. Ibid, p. 77.
40. Bartholin, Thomas and Caspar, *Bartholinus Anatomy*, p. 77.
41. 'the *Clitoris* encreases to an over great measure...and which undergoes Erection in the Act of Venery', Barret, Robert, *A companion for midwives, child-bearing women, and nurses directing them how to perform their respective offices,* (Thomas Ax, London, 1699), p. 38. Transcribed for the Text Creation Partnership (Ann Arbor and Oxford, 2007) and published online http://name.umdl.umich.edu/A31042.0001.001
42. *Aristotle's Complete Master-Piece* (J. How, London, 1684), pp. 16 & 17.
43. Ibid, p. 23.
44. Female genital mutilation—https://www.gov.uk/government/publications/female-genital-mutilation-resource-pack/female-genital-mutilation-resource-pack
45. Cleveland, John, *The Works of Mr. John Cleveland containing his poems, orations, epistles, collected into one volume, with the life of the author* (Obadiah Blagrave, London, 1687), p. 19.
46. Loughlin, Marie H. (editor), *Same-Sex Desire in Early Modern England, 1550–1735: An Anthology of Literary Text and Contexts* (Manchester University Press, Manchester, 2014), p. 570.
47. Wallis, John, *The Doctrine of the Blessed Trinity, briefly explained in a letter to a friend* (Thomas Parkhurst, London, 1690), pp. 24–25.
48. Ibid.
49. Wallis, John, 'A Second Sermon Concerning the Trinity: To the University of Oxford, April 26, 1691', as found in *Three Sermons Concerning the Sacred Trinity* (Thomas Parkhurst, London, 1691), p. 57.

50. Fausto-Sterling, Anne, *Sexing the Body: Gender Politics and the Construction of Sexuality* (Basic Books, New York, 2000), p. 35.
51. Anonymous (OR Wilmot, John, 2nd Earl of Rochester), *The Farce of Sodom, or The Quintessance of Debauchery,* 1684, as found on *Wikisource* https://en.wikisource.org/wiki/The_Farce_of_Sodom,_or_The_Quintessence_of_Debauchery. Text is available under the Creative Commons Attribution-ShareAlike License
52. Ibid, *Dramatis Personae.*
53. What would they have made of twenty-first-century beauty salons that offer an array of waxing styles for a lady's personal topiary? If there's one thing you can say about the Stuarts, it's that they knew how to 'keep it real' when it came to body hair!
54. Thompson, Roger, *Unfit For Modest Ears: A study of pornographic, obscene and bawdy works written or published in England in the second half of the seventeenth century* (MacMillan Press, London, 1979), p. 149.
55. Fisher, Kate and Sarah Toulalan (ed.), *Bodies, Sex and Desire from the Renaissance to the Present* (Palgrave MacMillan, Houndmills, 2011), p. 136.
56. Sinibaldi, *The Cabinet of Venus Unlocked,* p. 28.
57. Olearius, Adam, *The Voyages and Travells of the Ambassadors sent by Frederick Duke of Holstein to the Great Duke of Muscovy, and the King of Persia...Containing a Compleat History of Muscovy, Tartary, Persia and other adjacent Countries* (John Starkey and Thomas Basset, London, 1669), p. 97.
58. My thanks to Dr Jonathan Healey for this information.
59. Smith, John, *The Voyages and Discoveries of Captaine John Smyth in Virginia* (Joseph Barnes, Oxford, 1612), p. 22.
60. Barbier, Patrick, *The World of the Castrati: The History of an Extraordinary Operatic Phenomenon* (Souvenir Press, London, 1996), pp. 12–13
61. Bevan, Bryan, *The Duchess Hortense: Cardinal Mazarin's Wanton Niece* (The Rubicon Press, London, 1987), p. 89.
62. Hamilton, Elizabeth, *William's Mary: A Biography of Mary II* (Hamish Hamilton, London, 1972), p. 109.
63. Ancillon, Charles, *Eunuchism Display'd: Describing all the different Sorts of Eunuchs* (E. Curll, London, 1718), title page and p. 151.
64. Zuvich, Andrea, *The Stuarts in 100 Facts* (Amberley Publishing, Stroud, 2015), p. 103.
65. London County Council, *Geffrye Museum: 17th Century Children at Home* (Waterlow & Sons, London, 1964), images 1 & 2.

Chapter 2: How To Be A Sexy Stuart!

1. Thanks to @joinLordGrey for this https://twitter.com/joinLordGrey/status/1104438125999415296
2. C 9/27/136, *Sex v Feake,* 1660, TNA.

3. Marshall, Alan (2010, September 23), Sexby, Edward (c. 1616–1658), parliamentarian army officer and conspirator, *Oxford Dictionary of National Biography,* Retrieved 18 Nov. 2019, from https://www.oxforddnb.com/view/10.1093/ref:odnb/9780198614128.001.0001/odnb-9780198614128–e-25151

4. Houle, Brian, 'How Obesity Relates to Socioeconomic Status', *Population Reference Bureau:* https://www.prb.org/obesity-socioeconomic-status/ [Accessed 11 November 2019].

5. Austin, William, *Hæc Homo,* 1639, p. 24. Contributor: Princeton Theological Seminary Library and published at https://archive.org/details/haechomowhereine00aust/page/24

6. Brémond, Gabriel de, *The Amorous Abbess: Or, Love in a Nunnery* (R. Bentley: London, 1684), p. 10. [Wing B4343, ESTC R5008.] Transcribed for the Text Creation Partnership (Ann Arbor and Oxford, 2007) and published online at http://name.umdl.umich.edu/A29288.0001.001.

7. Halifax, George Savile, Marquis of, *The Lady's New-Year's Gift: Or, Advice to a Daughter* (Matt Gillyflower, London, 1688), p. 147–148.

8. Brown, Thomas and Edward Ward, *A Comical View of London and Westminster* (Sam Briscoe, London, 1705), p. 146.

9. Shakespeare, William, *The Works of Mr William Shakespear, Vol. 1* (Jacob Tonson, London, 1709), p. 333. Discussing what makes an attractive man, Beatrice says, 'With a good leg and a good foot, Uncle, with money enough in his Purse, such a Man would win any Woman in the World, if he could get her good Will'.

10. *In Praise of a Deformed, but Virtuous, Lady; Or, A Satyr on Beauty*, p. 127.

11. Brown and Ward, *A Comical View of London and Westminster,* p. 145.

12. Wilmot, John, *The Works of John Earl of Rochester: Containing Poems on Several Occasions* (Jacob Tonson, London, 1714), p. 116.

13. Waterson, Nellie M, *Mary II, Queen of England 1689–1694* (Duke University Press, Durham, 1928), p. 194.

14. Addison, Joseph, *The Spectator*, No. 129, July 28, 1711.

15. Hammond, H. *The Whole Duty of Man* (E. Pawlet, London, 1657), p. 195.

16. 'C' & Joseph Addison, *The Spectator*, No. 129, July 28, 1711.

17. Shapiro, James, *1606: William Shakespeare and the Year of Lear* (Faber & Faber, London, 2015), pp. 285–287.

18. Mendelson, Sara and Patricia Crawford, *Women in Early Modern England: 1550–1720* (Clarendon Press, Oxford, 1998), p. 19.

19. Reynolds, Anna, *In Fine Style: The Art of Tudor and Stuart Fashions* (Royal Collection Trust, 2013), p. 261.

20. Thompson, *Unfit For Modest Ears,* p. 149.

21. Pepys, Samuel, '11 June 1666', *Diary* (George Bell & Sons, London, 1893).

22. Wood, Anthony, *Wood's Life and Times, Vol. I,* p. 509.

23. Ibid.

24. Penn, William, *Reflections and Maxims,* p. 21.

25. Ibid, pp. 21–22.

26. Coke, Edward, *The Third Part of the Institutes of the Law of England: Concerning High Treason, and other Pleas of the Crown, and Criminal Causes: The Fourth Edition* (A. Crooke, W. Leake, A. Roper, et al, London. 1669), p. 199.

27. Zuvich, *The Stuarts in 100 Facts*, p. 27.

28. Pepys, '21 May 1662', *Diary*.

29. As someone who dabbles in historical re-enactment, I find them very comfortable compared with the modern bra; they support the breasts wonderfully!

30. Hart, Avril and Susan North, *Seventeenth and Eighteenth-Century Fashion in Detail* (V&A Publishing, London, 1998), pp. 12 & 138.

31. Shakespeare, William, *The Tragicall Historie of Hamlet, Prince of Denmark.* Act III, Scene I (I.R. for N.L, London, 1604), p. 35.

32. Evelyn, John, *The Diary of John Evelyn, Vol. I* (M. Walter Dunne, Washington & London, 1901), p. 286.

33. Anonymous, song or ballad: 'A Hue and Cry after Beauty and Virtue', shelfmark C.161.f.2(83), British Library, p. 1.

34. Herman, Eleanor, *The Royal Art of Poison* (St. Martin's Press, New York, 2018), p. 33.

35. Picard, Liza, *Restoration London: Everyday Life in London 1660–1670* (Phoenix, London, 2004), p. 104.

36. Digby, Kenelm, *The Closet of Sir Kenelm Digby Knight Opened* (Philip Lee Warner, London, 1910), p. 272.

37. Read, Sara, *Exploring the Lives of Women, 1558–1837* (Pen & Sword History, 2018), p. 14.

38. Field, Ophelia, *The Kit-Cat Club* (Harper Perennial, London, 2009), pp. 60–61.

39. Hall, T., *The Queen's Royal Cookery* (S. Bates, London, 1729), shelfmark C.155.aa.7, British Library.

40. Markham, Gervase, *The English House-wife* (Nicholas Okes for John Harison, London, 1631), p. 148.

41. Pepys, '8 March 1663–1664', *Diary*.

42. Culpeper, *Pharmacopœia Londinensis,* p. 218.

43. *The Spectator: Vol. I* (S. Buckley & J. Tonson, London, 1712), p. 155.

44. Ibid.

45. Zuvich, *The Stuarts in 100 Facts*, p. 32.

46. Pepys, '31 May 1662', *Diary*. We find Pepys 'had Sarah to comb my head clean, which I found so foul with powdering and other troubles, that I am resolved to try how I can keep my head dry without powder'.

47. Pepys, '30 October 1663', *Diary*. http://www.gutenberg.org/cache/epub/3331/pg3331.html [Accessed 18 January 2019].

48. Ibid, '28 September 1668'. 'Here I also, standing by a candle that was brought for sealing a letter, do set my periwigg a-fire; which made such an odd noise nobody could tell what it was till they saw the flame, my back being to the candle'.

49. Steele, Richard, *The Spectator,* No. 17, March 20, 1711.

50. Doomed because she died aged only nineteen (some historians say twenty), and rumours of her having been poisoned persist, though it seems likely that she never really recovered from her miscarriage—a theory put forth by Anne Somerset in *The Affair of the Poisons*, p. 292.
51. Wilkinson, Josephine, *Louis XIV: The Real King of Versailles* (Amberley Publishing, Stroud), p. 195.
52. Le Clerc, Monsieur, *A Description of Bandages and Dressings* (W. Freeman, J. Walthoe, T. Newborough, J. Nicholson and R. Parker, London, 1701), p. 36.
53. *The Guardian.* Number III. Saturday, March 14, 1713. Periodical (J. Tonson, London, 1713).
54. Ward, Edward, *The London-Spy Compleat* (J. Howe, London, 1703), edited by Ben Neudorf and Allison Muri, p. 47. The Grub Street Project, text quoted here under the CC BY-SA 4.0 license. http://grubstreetproject.net/works/T119938?image=56&display=text [Accessed 23 January 2020].
55. Fagan, Brian, *The Little Ice Age* (Basic Books, New York, 2000), p. 113.
56. Evelyn, *The Diary of John Evelyn,* p. 194.
57. Ibid, p. 264.
58. Paleis Het Loo is in modern-day Apeldoorn in the Netherlands and I urge anyone who has a love of late seventeenth-century history in particular to visit this beautiful palace.
59. *The Life and Death of Damaris Page, That Great, Arch, Metropolitan (Old-Woman) of Ratcliff High-Way* (R. Burton, London, 1669), p. 6.
60. Culpeper, Nicholas, *The English Physitian Enlarged* (John Streater, London, 1669), pp. 243–244.
61. Baptista, Mantuanus, *Mantuan English'd, and Paraphras'd, Or, The Character of A Bad Woman* (London, 1679), p. 3. From the Luttrell broadsides, published by Newberry Library at https://archive.org/details/case_6a_158_no_10/page/n1.
62. Markham, *The English House-wife*, p. 149.
63. Fraser, *The Weaker Vessel*, pp. 421–422.
64. http://www.fashioningtheearlymodern.ac.uk/object-in-focus/visard-mask/ [Accessed 18 January 2019].
65. Penn, William, *Fruits of Solitude*, pp. 110–111.
66. Buckley, Veronica. *Madame de Maintenon: The Secret Wife of Louis XIV* (Bloomsbury Publishing Plc, London, 2008), p. 125.
67. Penn, William, *Reflections & Maxims,* p. 115.
68. Pepys, '12 June 1663', *Diary.*
69. Ibid, '3 February 1664–65'.
70. Brown and Ward, *A Comical View of London and Westminster,* p. 121.
71. *The Winter habit of an English Gentlewoman* (1644), The Metropolitan Museum of Art. https://www.metmuseum.org/art/collection/search/356521 [Accessed 19 January 2019].
72. Lincoln, Marguerite (ed.), *Samuel Pepys: Plague, Fire, Revolution* (Thames & Hudson/National Maritime Museum, 2015), p.116.
73. Ibid.

74. Cox, Nancy and Karin Dannehl, 'Tooth brush—Toy card', in *Dictionary of Traded Goods and Commodities 1550–1820* (Wolverhampton, 2007), *British History Online* http://www.british-history.ac.uk/no-series/traded-goods-dictionary/1550–1820/tooth-brush-toy-card [accessed 19 November 2018].
75. Markham, *The English House-wife*, p. 18.
76. Ibid.
77. Mortimer, Ian, *A Time Traveller's Guide to Restoration Britain*, p. 300.
78. Trevelyan, G.M. *Illustrated English Social History: Volume Two: The Age of Shakespeare and the Stuart Period* (Penguin Books Ltd: Harmondsworth, 1964), p. 123.
79. King James VI/I, *A Counterblaste to Tobacco* (London, 1604), p. 104.
80. 'King James VI/I, A Counterblaste to Tobacco 1604,' *Document Bank of Virginia*, accessed December 21, 2018, http://edu.lva.virginia.gov/dbva/items/show/124.
81. Bell, Walter George, *The Great Plague in London* (The Folio Society, London, 2001), p 94.
82. Pepys, '29 June 1661', *Diary*.
83. Prade, Jean Le Royer, *Histoire du tabac, ou il est traité particulierement du tabac en poudre* (M. Le Prest, Paris, 1677).
84. *The Post Boy With the Freshest Advices, Foreign and Domestick*. Periodical. Number 1238. From Tuesday November 1 to Thursday November 3, 1709.
85. Chardin, Sir John, *The Travels of Sir John Chardin* (The Argonaut Press, London, 1927), p. 142.
86. Pepys, '21 December 1666', *Diary*.
87. Laver, James, *The Ladies of Hampton Court* (William Collins, London, 1942), p. 13.
88. Pepys, '21 August 1668', *Diary*.
89. Rowell, Christopher, *Petworth: The People and the Place* (Scala Publishers Ltd/National Trust, London and Swindon, 2012), p. 27.

Chapter 3: Pornography and Erotic Literature

1. Wilmot, John, *The Farce of Sodom, or The Quintessence of Debauchery,* (London, 1689), https://en.wikisource.org/wiki/The_Farce_of_Sodom,_or_The_Quintessence_of_Debauchery (Accessed 11 January 2020) CC BY-SA 3.0.
2. Baxter, Richard, *A Treatise of Self-Denial* (Robert White, London, 1675), p. 142.
3. Cockeram, *The English Dictionarie of 1623*, p. 77.
4. Shoemaker, Robert B., *Gender in English Society 1650–1850: The Emergence of Separate Spheres?* (Routledge, Abingdon, 1998), p. 66.
5. N.H., *The Ladies Dictionary*, p. 389.
6. McClain, Mary, *Beaufort: The Duke and his Duchess, 1657–1715* (Yale University Press, New Haven, 2001), p. 10.
7. *The School of Venus*, p. 59.

8. Pepys, '13 January 1667/1668', *Diary.*
9. Pepys, '9 February 1667/68', *Diary.*
10. Ibid: 'but it did hazer my prick para stand all the while, and una vez to décharger'.
11. The two works which comprised *La Puttana Errante* were published anonymously, and there is debate as to who authored them. For some time, they were believed to have been written by Pietro Aretino (1492–1556), but now believed to be by Niccolo Franco (1515–1570).
12. These are my English translations from the 1776 French translation.
13. Thompson, Roger, *Unfit for Modest Ears,* p. 57.
14. Garfield, John, *The Wandring Whore, Continued: A Dialogue* (London, 1660),
15. Bartholin, Thomas, *Bartholinus Anatomy*, Introduction, pp. 5, 16, 44, 54.
16. Ibid, p. 161.
17. Winstanley, William, *The Lives of the Most Famous English Poets, or The Honour of Parnassus* (Samuel Manship, London, 1687), p. 207.
18. From the long-winded original title, *The Fortunate Mistress: Or, A History of the Life and Vast Variety of Fortunes of Mademoiselle de Beleau, Afterwards Call'd The Countess de Wintselsheim, in Germany, Being the Person known by the Name of the Lady Roxana, in the Time of King Charles II* (T. Warner, London, 1724).
19. Sucking, Sir John, *The Poems of Sir John Suckling* (White, Stokes, & Allen, New York, 1886), p. 87.
20. Ibid, p. 89.
21. Herrick, Robert, *Poems selected from the Hesperides by Robert Herrick* (The Elston Press, New Rochelle, 1903).
22. Thompson, Roger, *Unfit For Modest Ears,* p. 147.
23. Brémond, Gabriel de, *The Amorous Abbess, Or, Love in a Nunnery.*
24. Sorbière, Samuel, *A Journey to London, In the Year 1698* (A. Baldwin, London, 1698), p. 13.
25. Burford, EJ, *Bawds and Lodgings: A History of the London Bankside Brothels, c.100–1675* (Peter Owen, London, 1976), p. 178.
26. Ward, Edward, *The London-Spy Compleat* (J. Howe, London, 1703), edited by Ben Neudorf and Allison Muri, p. 137. The Grub Street Project, text quoted here under the CC BY-SA 4.0 license. http://grubstreetproject.net/works/T119938?image=76 [Accessed 23 January 2020].
27. 'Agostino Carracci's Erotica', *The Seventeenth Century Lady.* http://www.andreazuvich.com/art/agostino-carracci-erotica/ [Accessed 15 September 2018].
28. The work of art is *The Holy Family with Saints John the Baptist and Catherine of Alexandria*, c.1580–90, Royal Collection Trust. Although this is some debate about which Carracci actually created it, it is nevertheless presently attributed to Agostino Carracci. https://www.rct.uk/collection/search#/1/collection/407405/the-holy-family-with-saints-john-the-baptist-and-catherine-of-alexandria [Accessed 4 November 2018].

29. One theory about this painting is that it depicts a father giving his daughter a necklace—but this seems unlikely given the very intimate look the older man gives the woman, his hand tenderly brushing her breast, and her hand softly upon his. There is nothing paternalistic in this gesture, but everything to do with lovers.
30. Néret, Gilles, *Erotica 17th-18th Century* (Taschen GmbH, Koln, 2001), p. 5.
31. Dolman, Brett, *Beauty, Sex, and Power* (Scala Publishers/Historic Royal Palaces, London, 2012), p. 14.
32. Untitled print by Marcellus Laroon II, dated 1680–1700, British school, museum number 1866,0623.47, British Museum.
33. 'The Farce of Sodom' (Ref: SA:194/F1/1, reproduced here with permission of Suffok Archives) https://www.suffolkarchives.co.uk/suffolk-stories/stories-from-other-records/the-farce-of-sodom/ [Accessed 16 September 2018].
34. Gowing, Laura, 'Women in the World of Pepys', *Samuel Pepys: Plague, Fire, Revolution* (Thames & Hudson/National Maritime Museum, 2015), p. 76.
35. Williams, Gordon, *Shakespeare, Sex, and the Print Revolution* (The Athlone Press Ltd, London, 1996), p. 59.
36. Collier, James, *A Short View of the Immorality, and Profaneness of the English Stage, Together With the Sense of Antiquity upon this Argument* (S. Keble, R. Sare, and H. Hindmarsh, London, 1698), p. 74.
37. Wycherley, William, *The Country Wife: A Comedy as it is Acted at the Theatre-Royal* (C. Bathhurst, London, 1751), p. 5.
38. Ibid, p. 9.
39. De La Rivière, Mary (aka Delarivier Manley), *Secret Memoirs and Manners of Several Persons of Quality, of Both Sexes, from the new Atalantis* (John Morphew: London, 1709).
40. Winn, James Anderson, *Queen Anne – Patroness of Arts* (Oxford University Press, Oxford, 2014), p. 503.
41. Anonymous, *The Night-Walker: Or, Evening Rambles in search after Lewd Women* (J. Orme, London, 1696), p. 1.

Chapter 4: Stuart Prostitution: Or, Whoredom in Stuart Britain

1. Alice Pierce is probably Alice Perrers (1348–1400) the mistress of King Edward III of England. Jane Shore (c. 1445 – c. 1527) was the mistress of King Edward IV of England.
2. A / Prophetick LAMPOON, Made Anno 1659. / By his Grace George Duke of Buckingham: / Relating to what would happen to the GOVERNMENT / under KING CHARLES II. National Library of Scotland. Crawford.EB.1318
3. Cockeram, Henry, *The English Dictionarie of 1623* (Huntington Press, New York, 1930), p. 120.
4. The word 'punk' for 'whore' is used in Aurelian Townshend's poem, *Bacchus, Iacchus*—as found in page 191 of *Love & Drollery* by John Wardroper, 1969.

5. Adams, Thomas, *The Diuell's Banket,* (Thomas Snodham for Ralph Mab, London, 1614), p. B3.

6. As quoted in Robert Baylie's, *Errours and Induration, Are The Great Sins and the Great Judgements of the Time* (R. Raworth for Samuel Gellibrand: London, 1645), p. 18.

7. Dekker, Thomas, *Villanies discouered by lanthorne and candle-light* (Aug. Mathewes, London, 1620). Digitised by Boston Public Library and published at https://archive.org/details/villaniesdiscoue00dekk/page/n43 Chapter VII.

8. Anonymous, song, late c17: 'A Hue and Cry after Beauty and Virtue', shelfmark C.161.f.2(83), British Library, p. 2.

9. Brevint, Daniel, *The Depth and Mystery of the Roman Mass* (London, 1672), p. 185.

10. Anonymous, *The Night-Walker: Or, Evening Rambles in search after Lewd Women* (J. Orme, London, 1696), p. 3.

11. Ibid, p. 135.

12. Printed in London, for W. Thackeray, T. Passinger, and W. Whitmore (c. 1666–1679).

13. Ballad—Roud Number: V3164 http://ballads.bodleian.ox.ac.uk/view/sheet/2220) http://ballads.bodleian.ox.ac.uk/static/images/sheets/30000/25164.gif

14. Milton, John, *Paradise Lost: A Poem in Twelve Books* (S. Simmons: London, 1674), pp. 107–108.

15. Wilmot, John, *Regime de Vivre* (poem).

16. *The Life of Epicurus*, London. The Seventeenth Century Lady Archives. XXIII.

17. 15 March. 'Middlesex Sessions Rolls: 1611', in *Middlesex County Records: Volume 2, 1603–25*, ed. John Cordy Jeaffreson (London, 1887), pp. 70–78. *British History Online* http://www.british-history.ac.uk/middx-county-records/vol2/pp70–78 [accessed 4 November 2018].

18. 'Middlesex Sessions Rolls: 1647', in *Middlesex County Records: Volume 3, 1625–67*, ed. John Cordy Jeaffreson (London, 1888), pp. 98–102. *British History Online* http://www.british-history.ac.uk/middx-county-records/vol3/pp98–102 [accessed 5 January 2019].

19. Ibid.

20. Belchier, Dabridgcourt, *Hans Beer-Pot, His Invisible Comedie, Or, See me, See me not* (Bernard Alsop, London, 1618). Transcribed for the Text Creation Partnership (Ann Arbor and Oxford, 2007) and published online at http://name.umdl.umich.edu/A07637.0001.001

21. E.M.A.D.O.C. *Novembris Monstrum: Or, Rome Brought to Bed in England, with the Whores Miscarying* (John Burroughes, London, 1641). Transcribed for the Text Creation Partnership (Ann Arbor and Oxford, 2007) and published online at http://name.umdl.umich.edu/A38409.0001.001

22. *A Defence of the Missionaries Arts* (London, 1689), p. a1. There is some debate as to who actually authored this work—in some sources, the author is William Wake, in others, George Hickes.

23. Adams, Jack, *Jack Adams, His Perpetual Almanack, with Astrological Rules and Instructions* (London, 1663), p. 22.
24. Felltham, Owen, *Resolves: Divine, Moral, Political* (J.G. & T.C. Brown, Leicester, 1840), p. 232.
25. Traub, Valerie, *The Renaissance of Lesbianism in Early Modern England* (Cambridge University Press, Cambridge, 2002), p. 167.
26. Arnold, Catherine, *City of Sin: London and Its Vices* (Simon & Schuster, London, 2010), p. 59.
27. 'Middlesex Sessions Rolls: 1627', in *Middlesex County Records: Volume 3, 1625–67*, ed. John Cordy Jeaffreson (London, 1888), pp. 13–17. *British History Online* http://www.british-history.ac.uk/middx-county-records/vol3/pp13–17 [accessed 3 November 2018].
28. Dekker, Thomas, *Villanies discouered by lanthorne and candle-light* (Aug. Mathewes, London, 1620).
29. 'May 1650: An Act for suppressing the detestable sins of Incest, Adultery and Fornication.' *Acts and Ordinances of the Interregnum, 1642–1660.* Eds. C H Firth, and R S Rait. London: His Majesty's Stationery Office, 1911. 387–389. *British History Online.* Web. 1 March 2019. http://www.british-history.ac.uk/no-series/acts-ordinances-interregnum/pp387–389.
30. *The Life and Death of Damaris Page* (R. Burton, London, 1669).
31. Ibid, p. 4.
32. *The Whores Rhetorick*, 1683, ii.
33. Harris, T. (1986), The Bawdy House Riots of 1668. *The Historical Journal, 29*(3), 537–556. doi:10.1017/S0018246X00018902.
34. *The Poor-Whores Petition.*
35. Pepys, '6 April 1668', *Diary.*
36. Irish brothel in Drury Lane: 1638 (WJ/SR (NS)/50/32). http://www.london.umb.edu/index.php/doc_repository/poor_whores_petition/ [Accessed 10 November 2018].
37. 'The Parish and Vestry of St. Paul', in *Survey of London: Volume 36, Covent Garden*, ed. F H W Sheppard (London, 1970), pp. 53–63. *British History Online* http://www.british-history.ac.uk/survey-london/vol36/pp53–63 [accessed 31 March 2019].
38. Burford, EJ, *Bawds and Lodgings: A History of the London Bankside Brothels, c.100–1675* (Peter Owen, London, 1976), pp. 146 & 174.
39. Ibid, p. 175.
40. Garfield, *The Wandring Whore, No. 2,* p. 4.
41. *Old Bailey Proceedings Online* (www.oldbaileyonline.org, version 8.0, 02 December 2019), May 1693, trial of Elizabeth Elye (t16930531–45).
42. *Old Bailey Proceedings Online* (www.oldbaileyonline.org, version 8.0, 02 December 2019), May 1693 (s16930531–1).
43. Woodward, Josiah, *An Account of the Progress of the Reformation of Manners* (Joseph Downing, London, 1704), p. 26.
44. https://www.nationalarchives.gov.uk/education/civilwar/g4/key/#p2

45. Purkiss, Diane, *The English Civil War: A People's History* (Harper Perennial, London, 2007), p. 3.
46. Spencer, Charles, *Prince Rupert: The Last Cavalier* (Phoenix, London, 2008), pp. 146–147.
47. Braddick, Michael, *God's Fury, England's Fire (*Penguin, London, 2008), p. 378.
48. Purkiss, *The English Civil War*, p. 398.

Chapter 5: Stuart Players & Femmes Fatales

1. Prynne, William, *Healthes: Sicknesse* (London, 1628), p. 22.
2. Wood, Anthony, *Wood's Life and Times, Vol.,* p. 299.
3. Downes, John, *Roscius Anglicanus, Or, An Historical Review of the Stage from 1660 to 1706* (J.W. Jarvis & Son, London, 1886), p. 19.
4. Prynne, William, *Historio-Mastix: Or, The Players Scourge, Or Actors Tragedie* (E.A. and W.I. for Michael Sparke, London, 1633), p. 206.
5. Bramley, Zoe, *William Shakespeare in 100 Facts* (Amberley Publishing, Stroud, 2016), pp. 155–156.
6. Bergeron, David M, 'Court Masques about Stuart London.' *Studies in Philology*, vol. 113, no. 4, 2016, pp. 822–849. *JSTOR*, www.jstor.org/stable/44329617
7. Lindley, David, *The Trials of Frances Howard* (Routledge, London, 1996), p. 43.
8. Robertson, Karen, 'Pocahontas at the Masque.' *Signs*, vol. 21, no. 3, 1996, pp. 551–583. *JSTOR*, www.jstor.org/stable/3175171. [Accessed 24 January 2019].
9. Laurence, Anne, *Women in England, 1500–1760,* p. 142.
10. Shapiro, *1606: William Shakespeare and the Year of Lear,* p. 285.
11. Prynne, *Historio-Mastix*, pp. 376–377.
12. Hutchinson, Lucy, *Memoirs of the Life of Colonel Hutchinson, Governor of Nottingham Castle and Town* (Henry G. Bohn, London, 1863), p. 78.
13. Collier, *A Short View of the Immorality, and Profaneness of the English Stage*, p. Preface.
14. Wood, Anthony, *The Life and Times of Anthony Wood, antiquary, of Oxford, 1632–1697, described by Himself: Vol. I.* ed. Andrew Clark (Oxford Historical Society, Oxford, 1891), p. 406.
15. Mortimer, Ian, *A Time Traveller's Guide to Restoration Britain*, p. 91.
16. Wood, *The Life and Times of Anthony Wood,* p. 406.
17. Zuvich, *The Stuarts in 100 Facts*, p. 96.
18. Greene, Graham, *Lord Rochester's Monkey: Being the Life of John Wilmot, Second Earl of Rochester* (The Viking Press, New York, 1974), p. 127.
19. Gregg, Edward, *Queen Anne* (Yale University Press, Yale, 2001), p. 12.
20. Gore-Browne, Robert, *Gay Was The Pit: The Life and Times of Anne Oldfield, Actress* (Max Reinhardt, London, 1957), pp. 27–28.

21. Downes, John, *Roscius Anglicanus, Or, An Historical Review of the Stage from 1660 to 1706* (J.W. Jarvis & Son, London, 1886), p. viii.
22. Ibid, p. 30.
23. Ibid, p. 14.
24. *The Life and Posthumous Works of Arthur Maynwaring, Esq.* (A. Bell, W. Taylor, and J. Baker, London, 1715), p. 43.
25. Ede, Mary, *Arts and Society in England under William and Mary* (Stainer & Bell, London, 1979), p. 61.
26. This according to list in Appendix 2 of Elizabeth Howe's *The First English Actresses: Women and Drama, 1660–1700* (Cambridge University Press, Cambridge, 1992), pp.190–191.
27. Aemilia Lanyer's *Salve Deus Rex Judaeorum*, 1611, C.71.h.15. British Library. https://www.bl.uk/collection-items/emilia-laniers-salve-deus-rex-judaeorum-1611 [Accessed 28 December 2019].
28. Laurence, Anne, *Women in England: 1500–1760: A Social History* (Phoenix Press, London, 1996), p. 175.
29. Winstanley, *The Honour of Parnassus,* pp. 188–189.
30. Zuvich, Andrea, *A Year in the Life of Stuart Britain* (Amberley Publishing, Stroud, 2016), pp. 150–151.
31. Akkerman, Nadine, *Invisible Agents: Women and Espionage in Seventeenth-Century Britain* (Oxford University Press, Oxford, 2018), p. 112–114. My thanks to Dr Akkerman for discussing this with me further for this section.
32. Ibid.
33. Ibid, p. 25.
34. Tallis, Nicola, *Elizabeth's Rival: The Tumultuous Tale of Lettice Knollys, Countess of Leinster* (Michael O'Mara Books Ltd, London, 2017), p. 324.
35. Herman, *The Royal Art of Poison*, p. 185.
36. Plowden, Alison, *Henrietta Maria: Charles I's Indomitable Queen* (Sutton Publishing, Stroud, 2001), p. 57.
37. Hibbert, Christopher, *Charles I* (Corgi Books, London, 1972), p. 113.
38. Rowell, *Petworth: The People and the Place,* p. 34.
39. Ibid.
40. Fraser, Antonia, *The Weaker Vessel: A Woman's Lot in Seventeenth-Century England,* (George Weidenfeld and Nicholson, Ltd, London, 1993), p. 320.
41. Evelyn, '10 March 1682', *Diary*, p. 167.
42. Fraser, *The Weaker Vessel,* p. 321.

Chapter 6: Virginity & Pre-Marital Sex: Or, Fornication!

1. Baxter, *A Treatise of Self-Denial*, p. 142.
2. *Aristotle's Complete Master-Piece*, p. 32.
3. Wallis, John, *An Eighth Letter Concerning the Sacred Trinity* (Thomas Parkhurst, London, 1692), p. 12.

4. Atkins, Sir Robert, *A Defence of the Late Lord Russel's Innocency, by way of Answer of Confutation of a Libellous Pamphlet, Intituled, An Antidote Against Poyson* (Timothy Goodwin, London, 1689), p. 11.

5. N.H., *The Ladies Dictionary*, p. 285.

6. Porter, Ray and Lesley Hall, *The Facts of Life: The Creation of Sexual Knowledge in Britain, 1650–1950* (Yale University Press, New Haven and London, 1995), p. 49.

7. *Aristotle's Complete Master-Piece*, p. 36.

8. Ibid.

9. Haughton, William, *English-men, For my Money: Or, A pleasant Comedy called A Woman will have her Will* (W. White, London, 1616). Contributed by Boston Public Library and published at https://archive.org/details/englishmenformym1616haug/page/n5

10. Dekker, Thomas, *The Magnificent Entertainment* (Thomas Man the Younger, London, 1604), p. B1.

11. Shakespeare, William, *Romeo and Juliet, Act III, Scene II* (J & R Towson, London, 1753), p. 21.

12. *Aristotle's Complete Master-Piece*, p. 30.

13. Markham, *The English House-wife*, p. 38.

14. Waller, Maureen, *1700: Scenes From London Life* (Hodder & Stoughton, London, 2000), p. 25.

15. Head, Richard, *The English Rogue: Being a Complete History of the Most Eminent Cheat of Both Sexes* (London, 1650).

16. *Record of the Courts of Chester County, Pennsylvania, 1681–1697* (Colonial Society of Pennsylvania, Philadelphia, 1910), p. 288.

17. Ibid, p. 128.

18. Shurtleff, Nathaniel B. (ed), *Records of the Colony of New Plymouth in New England: printed by order of the legislature of the Commonwealth of Massachusetts* (William White, Boston, 1855).

19. *Record of the Courts of Chester County, Pennsylvania, 1681–1697*, p. 166.

20. Ibid, p. 184.

21. Ibid, p. 194.

Chapter 7: Stuart-era Gender Roles

1. Chamberlayne, Edward, *Angliæ Notitia: Or, The Present State of England, The First Part* (T.N. for J. Martin, London, c.1679), p. 254.

2. Gouge, William, *Of Domesticall Duties* (William Bladen, London, 1622), p. 270.

3. Zuvich, Andrea, 'Stuart Britain: What Was Life Like for Ordinary People?' *BBC History Extra*. https://www.historyextra.com/period/stuart/stuart-britain-what-was-life-like-for-ordinary-people/ July 2016.

4. Burton, Robert, *Anatomy of Melancholy* (Tudor Publishing Company, New York, 1927), p. 686.

5. Savile, George, *Advice to a Daughter,* p. 28.
6. Talbot, Charles, Duke of Shrewsbury, *Private and Original Correspondence of Charles Talbot, Duke of Shrewsbury, with King William, The Leaders of the Whig Party, And Other Distinguished Statesmen,* editor William Coxe (Longman, Hurst, Rees, Orme, and Brown, London, 1821), p. 85.
7. Allestree, Richard, *The Ladies Calling, In Two Parts, Part I* (James Glen, Edinburgh, 1675), p. 7.
8. Penn, William, *Reflections and Maxims,* p. 28.
9. Haughton, William, *English-men, For my Money: Or, A pleasant Comedy called A Woman will have her Will* (W. White, London, 1616). Contributed by Boston Public Library and published at https://archive.org/details/englishmenformym1616haug/page/n5
10. Osborne, Francis, *Advice to a Son* (R.D., London, 1673), p. 40.
11. Read, *Maids, Wives, Widows,* pp. 148–149.
12. Burton, *The Anatomy of Melancholy: Part 3,* p. 828.
13. Ibid.
14. Brown, Thomas, *A Legacy for the Ladies* (London, 1705), p. 13.
15. Ambrose, Isaac, *Media; The Middle Things* (Archibald Ingram, James Dechman, John Hamilton, and John Glasford, Glasgow, 1737), p. 189.
16. Ibid.
17. Ibid.
18. Stone, Lawrence, *Uncertain Unions & Broken Lives,* pp. 305–307.
19. Browne, William Hand (ed.). *Judicial and Testamentary Business of the Provincial Court 1649/50–1657* (Maryland Historical Society, Baltimore, 1891), p. 464.
20. Ibid.
21. *Consistory Court of London Deposition Book,* LMA, DL/C 218, pp. 50–2, 88. June 1608.
22. Ibid.
23. Winstanley, *The Honour of Parnassus,* pp. 98–99.
24. Chamberlayne, *The Present State of England,* p. 44.
25. *A True Relation of Four Most Barbarous and Cruel Murders Committed in Leicester-Shire by Elizabeth Ridgway* (George Croom, London, 1684), p. 4.
26. Newton, John, *The penitent recognition of Joseph's brethren a sermon occasion'd by Elizabeth Ridgeway who for the petit treason of poysoning her husband, was, on March 24, 1683/4, according to the sentence of the Right Honourable Sir Thomas Street ... burnt at Leicester* (Richard Chiswel, London, 1684).
27. *A True Relation of Four Most Barbarous and Cruel Murders Committed in Leicester-Shire by Elizabeth Ridgway* (George Croom, London, 1684), p. 5. The blood oozing out from her victim probably didn't happen, but made for a more compelling account of her wickedness!
28. Codd, Daniel J., *Crimes & Criminals of 17th Century Britain* (Pen & Sword History, Barnsley, 2018), p. 153.

29. N.H., *The Ladies Dictionary,* p. 239.

30. Speck, W.A., *James II* (Pearson Education Limited, Harlow, 2002), p. 90.

31. Lacey, *The English Civil War in 100 Facts,* pp. 116–117.

32. Plowden, *Henrietta Maria: Charles I's Indomitable Queen,* p. 96.

33. Smith, Captain Alexander, *A Complete History of the Highwaymen* (George Routledge & Sons, London, 1933), p. 282.

34. Middleton, Thomas and Thomas Dekker, *The Roaring Girl, Or, Moll Cutpurse* (Thomas Archer, London, 1611).

35. Lindley, *The Trials of Frances Howard,* p. 175.

36. 'House of Lords Journal Volume 12: 3 January 1667', in *Journal of the House of Lords: Volume 12, 1666–1675* (London, 1767–1830), pp. 60–65. *British History Online* http://www.british-history.ac.uk/lords-jrnl/vol12/pp60–65 [accessed 3 November 2018].

37. Halifax, George Savile, *The Lady's New-Year's Gift: Or, Advice to a Daughter* (Matt Gillyflower, London, 1688), p. 98.

38. Pepys, '18 August 1667', *Diary,* https://www.pepysdiary.com/diary/1667/08/18/ [Accessed 3 November 2018].

39. Marie Catherine, Baronne D'Aulnoy, 'Memoirs of the Court in England in 1675', Translated by M. H. Arthur, edited and annotated by G. D. Gilbert (London, 1927), pp. 146–148.

40. Ibid, p. 165.

41. *A True Relation of Four Most Barbarous and Cruel Murders Committed in Leicester-Shire by Elizabeth Ridgway* (George Croom, London, 1684), p. 4.

42. Pritchard, R.E., *Scandalous Liaisons: Charles II and His Court* (Amberley, Stroud, 2015), pp. 122–123.

43. Pepys, '10 July 1666', *Diary.*

44. Wood, *The Life and Times of Anthony Wood,* p. 472.

45. Ackroyd, Peter, *Newton* (Vintage Books, London, 2007), p.102.

46. Baptista, Mantuanus, *Mantuan English'd, and Paraphras'd, Or, The Character of A Bad Woman* (London, 1679), p. 4. From the Luttrell broadsides, published by Newberry Library at https://archive.org/details/case_6a_158_no_10/page/n1.

47. Beaumont, Francis and John Fletcher, *The vvoman hater As it hath beene lately acted by the Children of Paules* (Robert Raworth, London, 1607).

48. Felltham, *Resolves: Divine, Moral, Political,* p.86.

49. Davies, Owen, 'The War on Witches', *The Life and Times of The Stuarts,* BBC History Magazine, p. 68.

50. Bell, John, *Witch-Craft Proven, Arreign'd, and Condemn'd in its Professors, Profession and Marks...*Robert Sanders, Glasgow, 1697. Transcribed for the Text Creation Partnership (Ann Arbor and Oxford, 2007) and published online at http://name.umdl.umich.edu/A76359.0001.001

51. Winsham, Willow, *England's Witchcraft Trials* (Pen & Sword History, Barnsley, 2018), p. 88.

52. 'Middlesex Sessions Rolls: 1653', in *Middlesex County Records: Volume 3, 1625–67,* ed. John Cordy Jeaffreson (London, 1888), pp. 212–220.

British History Online http://www.british-history.ac.uk/middx-county-records/ vol3/pp212–220 [accessed 18 December 2019].

53. Bell, *Witch-Craft Proven, Arreign'd, and Condemn'd*, p. 5.
54. Sharpe, James, *The Bewitching of Anne Gunter* (Profile Books, London, 1999), p. xii.
55. Fraser, Antonia, *King James VI of Scotland, I of England* (Weidenfeld & Nicolson, London, 1974), p. 57.
56. James VI & I, *Dæmonologie*, (Robert Walde-Grave, 1597), p. 67.
57. Ibid.
58. Ibid.
59. 'The Information of Joane Jones, the Wife of Anthony Jones of Biddi/ford in the County aforesaid Husband/man, taken upon her Oath before us Thomas Gist Mayor, and John Da/vie Alderman, the 18th day of July Anno Dom. 1682', as found in *True and impartial relation of the informations against three witches, viz., Temperance Lloyd, Mary Trembles, and Susanna Edwards* (Freeman Collins, London, 1682), p. 31. Transcribed for the Text Creation Partnership (Ann Arbor and Oxford, 2007) and published online at http://name.umdl.umich.edu/A63409.0001.001
60. Sanger, William W., *The History of Prostitution: Its Extent, Causes, and Effects throughout the World* (Harper & Brothers, New York, 1859), p. 104.
61. Borman, Tracy, *Witches: James I and the English Witch-Hunts* (Vintage, London, 2014), p. 162.
62. 'The examination of Margaret Flower, 25th February 1618', as found in *The wonderful discouerie of the vvitchcrafts of Margaret and Phillip Flower, daughters of Ioan Flower neere Beuer Castle: executed at Lincolne, March 11. 1618 Who were specially arraigned and condemned before Sir Henry Hobart, and Sir Edward Bromley, iudges of assise, for confessing themselues actors in the destruction of Henry L. Rosse, with their damnable practises against others the children of the Right Honourable Francis Earle of Rutland. Together with the seuerall examinations and confessions of Anne Baker, Ioan Willimot, and Ellen Greene, witches in Leicestershire* (G. Eld for I. Barnes, London, 1619). Transcribed for the Text Creation Partnership (Ann Arbor and Oxford, 2007) and published online at http://name.umdl.umich.edu/a01001.0001.001
63. Hopkins, Matthew, *A Discovery of Witches: In Answer to several Queries, Lately delivery to the Judges of Assize for the County of Norfolk* (1647).
64. Winsham, *England's Witchcraft Trials*, p. 76.
65. 'The Examination of *Mary Trembles* **of** *Biddiford* in the County aforesaid Single woman, taken before *Thomas Gist* Mayor of the Burrough, Town, and Mannor of *Biddiford* aforesaid, and *John Davie* Alderman, two of his Majesties Justices of the Peace within the same Burrough, &c. the 18 day of July, Anno Dom. 1682', as found in *True and impartial relation of the informations against three witches, viz., Temperance Lloyd, Mary Trembles, and Susanna Edwards*, p. 35.

66. *A Most Certain, Strange, and true Discovery of a Witch: Being taken by some of the Parliament Forces, as she was standing on a small plank board and sayling on it over the River of Newbury: Together with the strange and true manner of her death, with the propheticall words and speeches she used at the same time* (John Hammond, 1643).

67. Field, Jacob F., *One Bloody Thing After Another: The World's Most Gruesome History* (Michael O'Mara Books Limited, London, 2012), p. 116.

68. Winsham, *England's Witchcraft Trials*, p. 76.

69. Gardiner, Ralph, *England's Grievance Discovered* (D. Akenhead and Sons, Newcastle, 1796), p. 114

70. Ady, Thomas, *A Candle in the Dark: or, A Treatise Concerning the Nature of Witches and Witchcraft: Being Advice to Judges, Sheriffes, Justices of the Peace, and Grand-Jury-men, what to do, before they passe Sentence on such as are Arraigned for their Lives as Witches* (R.I., London, 1656). Witchcraft Collection, Cornell University Library. http://ebooks.library.cornell.edu/cgi/t/text/text-idx?c=witch;cc=witch;view=toc;subview=short;idno=wit002 [Accessed 18 January 2020]

Chapter 8: Stuart Marriage: Or, Legal Sex!

1. Anonymous, *An Account of Marriage, Or The Interests of Marriage Considered and Defended against the Unjust Attacques of this Age* (B.G., London, 1672), p. 47. Transcribed for the Text Creation Partnership (Ann Arbor and Oxford, 2007) and published online at http://name.umdl.umich.edu/A24497.0001.001

2. Dugard, Samuel, *Populaidias: A Discourse Concerning the Having of Many Children. In Which the Prejudices against a Numerous Offspring Are Removed* (W. Rogers, London, 1695), p. 19. ESTC R24303, Wellcome Library, published at https://archive.org/details/b30334020/page/n11

3. Ancillon, *Eunuchism Display'd*, pp. xiv, xv.

4. Cockeram, Henry, *The English Dictionarie of 1623*, p. 112.

5. Defoe, Daniel, *A Treatise Concerning the Use and Abuse of the Marriage Bed*, p. 21.

6. Ibid, p. 26.

7. Adams, *Jack Adams, His Perpetual Almanack*, p. 20.

8. Ibid, p. xv.

9. Bentley, Thomas, *The Sixt Lampe of Virginitie*, p. 12. (Thomas Dawson, Henry Denham, William Seres, London, 1582), p. 75. Transcribed for the Text Creation Partnership (Ann Arbor and Oxford, 2007) and published online at http://name.umdl.umich.edu/A08629.0001.001

10. Fraser, *The Weaker Vessel*, p. 10.

11. Ibid.

12. Probert, Rebecca, *Marriage Law for Genealogists: The Definitive Guide* (Takeaway Publishing, Kenilworth, 2016), p. 90.

13. 'August 1653: An Act touching Marriages and the Registring thereof; and also touching Births and Burials', in *Acts and Ordinances of the Interregnum, 1642–1660*, ed. C H Firth and R S Rait (London, 1911), pp. 715–718. *British History Online* http://www.british-history.ac.uk/no-series/acts-ordinances-interregnum/pp715–718 [accessed 23 February 2019].

14. Misson, Henri, *M. Misson's Memoirs and Observations in his Travels over England* (D. Brown, London, 1719), p. 182.

15. Taylor, Denise, *17th Century Wedding Customs* (Stuart Press, Bristol, 1997), p. 33.

16. 'August 1653: An Act touching Marriages and the Registring thereof; and also touching Births and Burials', in *Acts and Ordinances of the Interregnum, 1642–1660*, ed. C H Firth and R S Rait (London, 1911), pp. 715–718. *British History Online* http://www.british-history.ac.uk/no-series/acts-ordinances-interregnum/pp715–718 [accessed 23 February 2019].

17. Misson, *M. Misson's Memoirs,* p. 184.

18. Taylor, Denise, *17th Century Wedding Customs* (Stuart Press, Bristol, 1997), p. 21.

19. Swift, Deborah, 'The Institution of Marriage in 17th Century England: A Guest Post By Deborah Swift', *The Seventeenth Century Lady*, 5 July 2018, http://www.andreazuvich.com/history/the-institution-of-marriage-in-17th-century-england-a-guest-post-by-deborah-swift/

20. Herrick, Robert, *Selections from the Poetry of Robert Herrick with Drawings by Edwin A. Abbey* (Harper & Brothers Publishers, New York, 1882), pp. 45 & 46.

21. Herrick, *Selections from the Poetry of Robert Herrick with Drawings by Edwin A. Abbey*, p. 46.

22. Evelyn, *Diary, Vol. I*, p. 241.

23. Graham, Hilary, Elaine Hobby, Helen Wilcox, *Her Own Life,* p. 152.

24. Misson, *M. Misson's Memoirs*, pp. 353–354.

25. Luttrell, Narcissus, *A Brief Relation of State Affairs, from September 1678 to April 1714: 1694* (London) p. 372.

26. Fraser, Antonia, *Cromwell: Our Chief of Men* (Book Club Associates, London, 1974), p. 204.

27. Gentles, Ian J, 'Rainborowe [Rainborow], Thomas (d. 1648), parliamentarian army officer and Leveller.' Oxford Dictionary of National Biography. January 03, 2008. Oxford University Press. Date of access 9 Mar. 2019, http://www.oxforddnb.com/view/10.1093/ref:odnb/9780198614128.001.0001/odnb-9780198614128-e-23020

28. Luttrell, *A Brief Relation of State Affairs,* p. 421.

29. Osborne, *Advice to a Son*, pp. 29–30.

30. Woolley, Hannah, *The Gentlewoman's Companion: Or, A Guide to the Female Sex*, an electronic edition (A. Maxwell for Edward Thomas, London, 1675), p. 88. Lewis H. Beck Center Emory University Atlanta, Georgia. Text available via the Emory Center for Digital Scholarship.

31. Defoe, Daniel, *A Treatise Concerning the Use and Abuse of the Marriage Bed* (T. Warner, London, 1727), pp. 230–231.
32. Ibid.
33. Felltham, *Resolves: Divine, Moral, Political*, p. 264.
34. Bentley, Thomas, *The Sixt Lampe of Virginitie* (Thomas Dawson, Henry Denham, William Seres, London, 1582), pp. 12–13. Transcribed for the Text Creation Partnership (Ann Arbor and Oxford, 2007) and published online at http://name.umdl.umich.edu/A08629.0001.001
35. Zuvich, Andrea, 'Stuart Britain: What Was Life Like for Ordinary People?' *BBC History Extra*. https://www.historyextra.com/period/stuart/stuart-britain-what-was-life-like-for-ordinary-people/
36. O'Callaghan, Sean, *To Hell or Barbados: The ethnic cleansing of Ireland.* (Brandon: Dingle, 2000), p. 50.
37. Hutchinson, *Memoirs of the Life of Colonel Hutchinson*, p. 12.
38. Kelliher, W. H. 'Denham, Sir John (1614/15–1669), poet and courtier.' Oxford Dictionary of National Biography. September 17, 2015. Oxford University Press,. Date of access May 15, 2019, https://www.oxforddnb.com/view/10.1093/ref:odnb/9780198614128.001.0001/odnb-9780198614128-e-7481
39. Ibid.
40. Sinibaldi, *The Cabinet of Venus Unlocked*, p. 19.
41. Ibid, p. 36.
42. Gouge, *Of Domesticall Duties*, pp. 181–182.
43. Wilmot, John, *The Works of John, Earl of Rochester* (Jacob Tonson, London, 1714), p. 18.
44. Hill, C.P, *Who's Who in British History: Stuart Britain 1603–1714*, pp. 19–20.
45. Norrington, Ruth, *My Dearest Minette: The Letters between Charles II and his sister Henrietta, Duchess d'Orléans* (Peter Owen, London, 1996), p. 153.
46. N.H., *The Ladies Dictionary*, p. 238.
47. Wood, *The Life and Times of Anthony Wood*, p. 196.
48. Evelyn, *Diary*, pp. 268–269.
49. Ibid, p. 201.
50. *Stephen, Leslie, ed. (1889). 'Fitzroy, George (1665–1716)', Dictionary of National Biography. 19. London: Smith, Elder & Co.*
51. Wauchope, Piers, *Patrick Sarsfield and the Williamite War,* (Irish Academic Press, Dublin, 1992), pp. 299–300.

Chapter 9: Contraception & Fertility: Or, How to Sheathe Your Sword

1. *The School of Venus*, p. 115.
2. Gowing, Laura, 'Women in the World of Pepys', *Samuel Pepys: Plague, Fire, Revolution* (Thames & Hudson/National Maritime Museum, 2015), p. 77.
3. King James Version.
4. License, Amy, *In Bed With The Tudors: The Sex Lives of a Dynasty from Elizabeth of York to Elizabeth I* (Amberley Publishing, Stroud, 2013), p. 25.

5. Bernau, Anke, *Virgins: A Cultural History* (Granta Books, London, 2007), p. 19.
6. Dalton, Michael, *The Countrey Justice: Containing The Practice, Duty and Power of The Justices of the Peace* (Henry Lintot, Savoy [London], 1746), p. 336.
7. *The Post Boy: With the Freshest Advices, Foreign and Domestick.* Number 2095. From Saturday October 16 to Tuesday October 19, 1708.
8. Dolnick, Edward, *The Clockwork Universe: Isaac Newton, the Royal Society & the Birth of the Modern World* (Harper Perennial, New York, 2011), p. 115.
9. Ibid.
10. Cockeram, Henry, *The English Dictionarie of 1623* (Huntington Press, New York, 1930), p. 169.
11. Tannahill, Reay, *Sex in History* (Scarborough House, 1992), p. 344.
12. Salmon, William, *Pharmacopaeia Londinensis: Or, The New London Dispensatory* (J. Dawks, London, 1702), p. 66.
13. Sinibaldi, *The Cabinet of Venus Unlocked*, p. 23.
14. Ambrose, *Media; The Middle Things*, p. 188.
15. Gouge, *Of Domesticall Duties*, pp. 182–183.
16. Larman, Alexander, *Blazing Star: The Life & Times of John Wilmot, Earl of Rochester* (Head of Zeus, London, 2014), p. 232.
17. Anonymous. *Quack Doctors' Advertisement 'Without Offense...'*, London, 1650. British Library shelfmark 1141.a.37.(3).
18. Garfield, *The Wandring Whore*, No. 1 (London, 1660), pp. 12–13.
19. Cummings, Megan, 'What urinating after sex does and does not prevent in women', My Med, https://www.mymed.com/health-wellness/sex-and-relationships/what-urinating-after-sex-does-and-does-not-prevent-in-women [Accessed 1 February 2020].
20. *The School of Venus*, p. 115.
21. Burford, EJ, *Bawds and Lodgings: A History of the London Bankside Brothels, c.100–1675* (Peter Owen, London, 1976), p. 174.
22. Gaimster, David, Peter Boland, Steve Linnane, & Caroline Cartwright (1996). 'The Archaeology of Private Life: the Dudley Castle Condoms'. *Post-Medieval Archaeology*, 30:1, 129–142, DOI: 10.1179/pma.1996.003 [Accessed 17 December 2018].
23. According to a BBC article from 2003, 'Antique condoms' Dutch journey', the number of condoms found was five, not ten. http://news.bbc.co.uk/1/hi/england/west_midlands/3228255.stm [Accessed 17 December 2018].
24. The Friends of Dudley Castle. http://www.dudleycastle.org.uk/history.html [Accessed 17 December 2018].
25. 'Antique condoms' Dutch journey', http://news.bbc.co.uk/1/hi/england/west_midlands/3228255.stm [Accessed 17 December 2018].

Chapter 10: Bigamy, Widowhood, & Remarriage
1. Gouge, *Of Domesticall Duties*, p. 205.
2. Stubbs, *John Donne: The Reformed Soul*, pp. 156, 159.

3. Ibid, pp. 164 & 165.
4. Duffy, Maureen, *Henry Purcell* (Fourth Estate, London, 1994), p. 63.
5. Pickering, Danby, *The Statutes at Large, From the First Year of K. William and Q. Mary, to the Eighth Year of K. William III, Vol. IX* (Charles Bathurst, Cambridge, 1764), p. 499.
6. Ibid.
7. Bentley, Thomas, *The Sixt Lampe of Virginitie*, p. 12 (Thomas Dawson, Henry Denham, William Seres: London, 1582). Transcribed for the Text Creation Partnership (Ann Arbor and Oxford, 2007) and published online at http://name.umdl.umich.edu/A08629.0001.001
8. Misson, *M. Misson's Memoirs and Observations in his Travels over England*, p. 184.
9. Zuvich, *A Year in the Life of Stuart Britain*, p. 215.
10. Hearne, Thomas, *Remarks and Collections, Vol. I*, p. 306.
11. Bentley, Thomas, *The Sixt Lampe of Virginitie* (Thomas Dawson, Henry Denham, William Seres, London, 1582), p. 75. Transcribed for the Text Creation Partnership (Ann Arbor and Oxford, 2007) and published online at http://name.umdl.umich.edu/A08629.0001.001
12. Donne, John, *A Collection of Letters Made by Sr Tobie Mathews*, (J. Donne, London, 1692), [Wing/M1321], and published by EEBO Editions/ProQuest.
13. Holland, Nick, *The Real Guy Fawkes* (Pen & Sword History, Barnsley, 2017).
14. *Melford Hall, Suffolk: A Property of The National Trust, Home of Sir Richard Hyde Parker, Bt.* (The National Trust, 1968), p. 6.
15. *A Table of Statutes: Publick and Private*, (London, 1698).
16. Chamberlayne, *The Present State of England*, p. 298.
17. Dolman, Brett, David Souden and Olivia Fryman, *Beauty, Sex, and Power.* (Scala/Historic Royal Palaces), p. 82.
18. Ibid.
19. Keay, Anna, *The Last Royal Rebel: The Life and Death of James, Duke of Monmouth* (Bloomsbury, London, 2017), p. 384.

Chapter 11: Deviant Sexual Practices, Part I: Same-Sex Relations

1. Cockeram, Henry, *The English Dictionarie of 1623*, p. 138.
2. Ibid, p. 156.
3. Ibid, p. 27.
4. Ward, Edward, *The London-Spy Compleat*, (J. Howe, London, 1703), edited by Ben Neudorf and Allison Muri, p. 66. The Grub Street Project, text quoted here under the CC BY-SA 4.0 license. http://grubstreetproject.net/works/T119938?image=76 [Accessed 23 January 2020].
5. Partridge, Eric, *Shakespeare's Bawdy* (Routledge, London, 1968), p. 12.
6. Stubbs, *John Donne: The Reformed Soul*, p. 187.
7. 'State Papers, 1654: September (3 of 5)', in *A Collection of the State Papers of John Thurloe, Volume 2, 1654*, ed. Thomas Birch (London, 1742), pp. 606–618.

British History Online http://www.british-history.ac.uk/thurloe-papers/vol2/ pp606–618 [Accessed 13 October 2018].

8. Lithgow, William, *The Totall Discourse of the Rare Adventures & Painefull Peregrinations of Long Nineteen Yeares Travayles from Scotland to the Most Famous Kingdomes in Europe, Asia and Affrica,* Glasgow University Press: Glasgow, 1906), p. 38.
9. Ibid, pp. 146 & 147.
10. John Rushworth, 'Historical Collections: 1631', in *Historical Collections of Private Passages of State: Volume 2, 1629–38* (London, 1721), pp. 83–138. *British History Online* http://www.british-history.ac.uk/rushworth-papers/ vol2/pp83–138 [accessed 13 October 2018].
11. Evelyn, *Diary*, p. 6.
12. The Castlehaven episode is becoming a more popular subject due to the intricacies and variety of topics touching upon sexuality, gender, class, and more. 'Early Stuart Libels: an edition of poetry from manuscript sources.' Ed. Alastair Bellany and Andrew McRae. Early Modern Literary Studies Text Series I (2005). http://purl.oclc.org/emls/texts/libels/
13. *Old Bailey Proceedings Online* (www.oldbaileyonline.org, version 8.0, 02 December 2019), May 1694, trial of Mustapha Pochowachett (t16940524–20).
14. *Old Bailey Proceedings Online* (www.oldbaileyonline.org, version 8.0, 02 December 2019), May 1694 (s16940524–1).
15. 'Charles II, 1661: An Act for the Establishing Articles and Orders for the regulateing and better Government of His Majesties Navies Ships of Warr & Forces by Sea.', in *Statutes of the Realm: Volume 5, 1628–80*, ed. John Raithby (s.l, 1819), pp. 311–314. *British History Online* http://www.british-history. ac.uk/statutes-realm/vol5/pp311–314 [accessed 13 October 2018].
16. ADM 106/414/316, TNA.
17. Ibid.
18. Ibid.
19. My thanks to Dr Steve Murdoch for bringing this case to my attention. *Register of the Privy Council of Scotland, 2nd Series VIII*, pp. 419–20; G. Lind, Danish Data Archive 1573; T. Riis, Should Auld Acquaintance Be Forgot (Odense, 1988), II, p. 139.
20. 'Charles II: September 1684', in *Calendar of State Papers Domestic: Charles II, 1684–5*, ed. F H Blackburne Daniell and Francis Bickley (London, 1938), pp. 132–160. *British History Online* http://www.british-history.ac.uk/cal-state-papers/domestic/chas2/1684–5/pp132–160 [accessed 13 October 2018].
21. Berkowitz, Eric, *Sex & Punishment: 4000 Years of Judging Desire* (The Westbourne Press, London, 2012), p. 289.
22. 'America and West Indies: January 1679', in *Calendar of State Papers Colonial, America and West Indies: Volume 10, 1677–1680*, ed. W Noel Sainsbury and J W Fortescue (London, 1896), pp. 313–321. *British History Online* http://www.british-history.ac.uk/cal-state-papers/colonial/america-west-indies/vol10/pp313–321 [accessed 13 October 2018].

23. 'Charles I—volume 428: September 1–20, 1639', in *Calendar of State Papers Domestic: Charles I, 1639*, ed. William Douglas Hamilton (London, 1873), pp. 471–513. *British History Online* http://www.british-history.ac.uk/cal-state-papers/domestic/chas1/1639/pp471–513 [accessed 13 October 2018].

24. 'America and West Indies: February 1679', in *Calendar of State Papers Colonial, America and West Indies: Volume 10, 1677–1680*, ed. W Noel Sainsbury and J W Fortescue (London, 1896), pp. 321–334. *British History Online* http://www.british-history.ac.uk/cal-state-papers/colonial/america-west-indies/vol10/pp321–334 [accessed 13 October 2018]. This is interesting, as it shows how race trumps the crime in this case: were they not white men, they would certainly have been executed.

25. 'William III: December 1698', in *Calendar of State Papers Domestic: William III, 1698*, ed. Edward Bateson (London, 1933), pp. 423–441. *British History Online* http://www.british-history.ac.uk/cal-state-papers/domestic/will-mary/1698/pp423–441 [accessed 13 October 2018].

26. ADM 106/427/196, TNA.

27. Burg, B.R., *Sodomy and the Pirate Tradition: English Sea Rovers in the Seventeenth-Century Caribbean* (New York University Press, New York, 1995), pp. 128–129.

28. Ibid, p. 129.

29. 'Sessions, 1613: 18 and 19 May', in *County of Middlesex. Calendar To the Sessions Records: New Series, Volume 1, 1612–14*, ed. William Le Hardy (London, 1935), pp. 87–116. *British History Online* http://www.british-history.ac.uk/middx-sessions/vol1/pp87–116 [accessed 13 October 2018].

30. 'The fourth Parliament of Charles II: First session (5 of 5)—begins 23/12/1680', in *The History and Proceedings of the House of Commons: Volume 2, 1680–1695* (London, 1742), pp. 48–101. *British History Online* http://www.british-history.ac.uk/commons-hist-proceedings/vol2/pp48–101 [accessed 13 October 2018].

31. STAC 8/49/21, TNA.

32. Clarke, Aidan, 'Atherton, John (1598–1640), Church of Ireland bishop of Waterford and Lismore.' Oxford Dictionary of National Biography, January 03, 2008, Oxford University Press. Date of access 13 May 2019, https://www.oxforddnb.com/view/10.1093/ref:odnb/9780198614128.001.0001/odnb-9780198614128-e-835

33. It is difficult to understand what Childe's motivations for this could have been; for in accusing Atherton, he condemned himself as well.

34. Loughlin, *Same-Sex Desire in Early Modern England,* p. 69.

35. *The Life and Death of John Atherton* (J. Barker, London, 1641).

36. 'State Papers, 1654: February-March', in *A Collection of the State Papers of John Thurloe, Volume 2, 1654*, ed. Thomas Birch (London, 1742), pp. 106–127. *British History Online* http://www.british-history.ac.uk/thurloe-papers/vol2/pp106–127 [accessed 13 October 2018].

37. De Lisle, Leanda, *White King: Charles I: Traitor, Murderer, Martyr* (Chatto & Windus, London, 2018), p. 90.

38. Barnes, Barnabe, *The Devil's Charter* (Louvain University, Louvain, 1904), p. 34.

39. Loughlin, *Same-Sex Desire in Early Modern England, 1550–1735,* p. 61.

40. Ibid, p. 59.

41. Carlton, *Royal Mistresses*, p. 74.

42. Jordan, Don and Michael Walsh, *The King's Bed: Sex, Power, & the Court of Charles II* (Little, Brown, London, 2015), p. 247.

43. Von Goeth, Aurora, 'Julie d'Aubigny, Mademoiselle Maupin', *Party Like 1660:*   http://partylike1660.com/julie-daubigny-mademoiselle-maupin/ [Accessed 30 January 2019].

44. Johnson, Charles, *A History of the Pyrates, from their first rise and settlement in the Island of Providence, to the present time. With the remarkable actions and adventures of the two female pyrates Mary Read and Anne Bonny* (T. Warner, London, 1724), pp. 157–173.

45. Anonymous, *Comical NEWS from BLOOMSBURY. / THE / FEMALE CAPTAIN: / OR, THE /Counterfit Bridegroom: / Giving a Full and True Relation how one Madam-Mary Plunket, alias, Williams; / a young Woman of eighteen Years of Age, who put on Man's Apparel, assum'd the Name of / Capt. Charles Fairfax...*Printed for J. Butcher, at the Sign of the Hartichoak, near Lud-gate, 1690–1701, Pepys Ballads 5.424, Pepys Library, Magdalene College Cambridge.

46. Mendelson, Sara H. 'Hunt, Arabella (1662–1705), singer and musician.' Oxford Dictionary of National Biography. January 03, 2008. Oxford University Press. Date of access 15 May 2019, https://www.oxforddnb.com/view/10.1093/ref:odnb/9780198614128.001.0001/odnb-9780198614128-e-14190

47. Crowne, John, *Calisto: Or, The Chaste Nymph, The late Masque at Court, as it was frequently presented there, by Several Persons of Quality* (Magnes & Bentley, London, 1675).

48. Joannis Meursii Elegantiae Latini sermonis. Aloisi Author: Meursius, Joannes, the Younger / 1690. Source/Shelfmark: P.C.30.i.10, plate 24. 'Two naked women in a bedroom'. BL3279264, British Library.

49. Arnold, Catherine, *City of Sin: London and Its Vices* (Simon & Shuster, London, 2010), p. 149. See also: 'Venus Reply', a poem from the late Stuart era.

50. Prynne, *Histrio-Mastix*, p. 169.

51. Ibid, p. 204.

52. Hilton, Lisa, *The Real Queen of France: Athénaïs & Louis XIV* (Abacus, London, 2003), p. 99.

53. 'Portrait of an Unidentified Woman', *New York Historical Society,* object no. 1952.80.   https://www.nyhistory.org/exhibit/portrait-unidentified-woman-2 [Accessed 7 February 2020].

54. Haswell, Jock, *James II: Soldier and Sailor* (Hamish Hamilton, London, 1972), pp. 35–37.

55. Watkins, Sarah-Beth, *The Tragic Daughters of Charles I: Mary, Elizabeth, & Henrietta Anne* (Chronos Books, Winchester, 2019), p. 31.

56. Seward, Desmond, *The King Over The Water: A Complete History of the Jacobites* (Birlinn Limited, Edinburgh, 2019), p. 156.

57. Pepys, *Diary*, 6 December, 1667.

Chapter 12: Deviant Sexual Practices, Part II: Incest, Bestiality, & Flagellation

1. 'May 1650: An Act for suppressing the detestable sins of Incest, Adultery and Fornication.', in *Acts and Ordinances of the Interregnum, 1642–1660*, ed. C H Firth and R S Rait (London, 1911), pp. 387–389. *British History Online* http://www.british-history.ac.uk/no-series/acts-ordinances-interregnum/pp387–389 [accessed 1 March 2019].

2. Gregg, Edward, *Queen Anne* (Yale University Press: Yale, 2001), p. 124.

3. Clegg, Melanie, *The Life of Henrietta Anne* (Pen & Sword History, Barnsley, 2017), p. 93.

4. 'Charles I—volume 261: February 1634', in *Calendar of State Papers Domestic: Charles I, 1633–4*, ed. John Bruce (London, 1863), pp. 479–481. *British History Online* http://www.british-history.ac.uk/cal-state-papers/domestic/chas1/1633–4/pp479–481 [accessed 23 October 2018].

5. LB/14/800, Shropshire Archives.

6. Bloch, Ivan, *Sexual Life in England* (Corgi Books, London, 1958), p. 381.

7. 'Early Stuart Libels: an edition of poetry from manuscript sources.' Ed. Alastair Bellany and Andrew McRae. Early Modern Literary Studies Text Series I (2005). http://www.earlystuartlibels.net/htdocs/lake_roos_section/J0.html

8. Luthman, Johanna, *Love, Madness, & Scandal: The Life of Frances Coke Villiers, Viscountess Purbeck* (Oxford University Press, Oxford, 2017), pp. 48–49.

9. 'Cecil Papers: January-June 1618', in *Calendar of the Cecil Papers in Hatfield House: Volume 22, 1612–1668*, ed. G Dyfnallt Owen (London, 1971), pp. 56–77. *British History Online* http://www.british-history.ac.uk/cal-cecil-papers/vol22/pp56–77 [accessed 12 May 2019].

10. Jardine, Lisa, *The Curious Life of Robert Hooke: The Man Who Measured London* (Harper Collins, London, 2003), pp. 255–257.

11. First cousins, child of one's aunt or uncle.

12. Dugard, Samuel (attributed), *The Marriages of Cousin Germans*, (Hen Hall, Oxford, 1673), p. 83.

13. Quaife, G.R., *Wanton Wenches and Wayward Wives* (Croom Helm, London, 1979), pp. 175–176.

14. *A Complete Collection of State-Trials and Proceedings Upon High Treason, Volume 3*. London, 1730. Google Play Books, [Accessed 21 October 2018), p. 516.

15. Behn, Aphra, *Love Letters Between a Nobleman and His Sister,* (London, 1684).
16. The idea that these historical persons were the inspiration for Behn's work is also put forward by Maureen Duffy in her biography, *Aphra Behn.*
17. 'James 1 - volume 80: February 1615', in *Calendar of State Papers Domestic: James I, 1611–18*, ed. Mary Anne Everett Green (London, 1858), pp. 271–276. *British History Online* http://www.british-history.ac.uk/cal-state-papers/domestic/jas1/1611–18/pp271–276 [accessed 27 December 2019].
18. Oaks, Robert F. "Things Fearful to Name': Sodomy and Buggery in Seventeenth-Century New England.' *Journal of Social History*, vol. 12, no. 2, 1978, pp. 268–281. *JSTOR*, JSTOR, www.jstor.org/stable/3787139.
19. Leviticus 20:15.
20. Tannahill, *Sex in History,* p. 329.
21. Shurtleff (ed.), *Records of the colony of New Plymouth in New England*, p. 51.
22. *Correspondance complète de madame duchesse d'Orléans née Princesse Palatine, mère du régent; traduction entièrement nouvelle par G. Brunet, accompagnée d'uné annotation historique, biographique et littéraire du traducteur* (Paris, 1855).
23. Zuvich, Andrea, *A Year in the Life of Stuart Britain* (Amberley Publishing, Stroud, 2016), pp. 139–140.
24. *Old Bailey Proceedings Online* (www.oldbaileyonline.org, version 8.0, 02 December 2019), July 1677, trial of married woman (t16770711–1).
25. Cleveland, *The Works of Mr. John Cleveland*, p. 337. Transcribed for the Text Creation Partnership (Ann Arbor and Oxford, 2007) and published online at http://name.umdl.umich.edu/A33421.0001.001 [Accessed 29 January 2020].
26. Sinibaldi, *The Cabinet of Venus Unlocked,* p. 14.
27. Aristotle's *Masterpiece* (1684).
28. Burford, EJ, *Bawds and Lodgings: A History of the London Bankside Brothels, c.100–1675* (Peter Owen, London, 1976), p. 145.
29. Ibid, p. 175.
30. Quaife, *Wanton Wenches and Wayward Wives*, p. 174.
31. Dalton, *The Countrey Justice*, p. 367.
32. *Old Bailey Proceedings Online* (www.oldbaileyonline.org, version 8.0, 02 December 2019), May 1676, trial of Schoolmaster (t16760510–7).
33. *Old Bailey Proceedings Online* (www.oldbaileyonline.org, version 8.0, 03 December 2019), July 1678, trial of young fellow (t16780703–3).
34. Wilmot, John, *The Farce of Sodom, or The Quintessance of Debauchery,* 1684.
35. Rabelais, *Gargantua*, Chapter XI.
36. Shadwell, Thomas, *The Virtuoso: A Comedy, Acted at the Duke's Theatre,* (T.N. for Henry Herringman, London, 1676), p. 42.
37. Butler, Samuel, *Hudibras,* (D. Appleton & Co, New York, 1864), p. 320.
38. Joannis Meursii Elegantiae Latini sermonis. (Aloisiae Sigeae ... Satyrae Sotadicae ... Pars altera.) British Library BL3285722, Shelfmark: PC.30.I.10 pullout 26.

39. https://www.gordsellar.com/2016/04/20/street-mobs-and-cyber-mobs/amp/ [Accessed 26 November 2018].
40. Wilmot, John, 'Signior Dildo'.
41. *The Farce of Sodom, or The Quintessence of Debauchery,* Actus Quartus.
42. As quoted in Roger Thompson's *Unfit for Modest Ears*, p. 184.
43. Bodleian, MS. Firth C.15, fol. 257.
44. Johnson, Charles, *A History of the Pyrates, from their first rise and settlement in the Island of Providence, to the present time. With the remarkable actions and adventures of the two female pyrates Mary Read and Anne Bonny* (T. Warner, London, 1724), pp. 75–76.
45. Ibid.

Chapter 13: Reproduction: Or, Ye Natural Consequences of Hanky Panky

1. Miscarriage (NHS). https://www.nhs.uk/conditions/Miscarriage/ [Accessed 28 September 2019].
2. Astell, Mary, *An Essay in Defence of the Female Sex* (A. Roper, E. Wilkinson, London, 1698), A2.
3. Hutchinson, *Memoirs of the Life of Colonel Hutchinson*, p. 254.
4. Thornton, *The Autobiography of Mrs. Alice Thornton,* p. 86.
5. Ibid.
6. Read, *Maids, Wives, Widows*, p. 101.
7. Culpeper, *Pharmacopœia Londinenseis*, p. 1.
8. Moore, Lucy, *Lady Fanshawe's Receipt Book: An Englishwoman's Life During the Civil War* (Atlantic Books, London, 2018), pp. 152–153.
9. Markham, *The English House-wife*, pp. 39–40.
10. Thornton, *The Autobiography of Mrs. Alice Thornton,* p. 116.
11. Boursier, *The Complete Midwife's Practice Enlarg'd*, Contents pages.
12. Culpeper, *Pharmacopœia Londinenseis*, p. 1.
13. Boxer, Marilyn J., and Jean H. Quataert, *Connecting Spheres: European Women in a Globalizing World, 1500 to the Present* (Oxford University Press, New York, 2000), p. 48.
14. Ibid.
15. Evenden, Doreen, *The Midwives of Seventeenth-Century London* (Cambridge University Press, Cambridge, 2000), p. 1.
16. That being said, Willughby's *Observations in Midwifery* tended to downplay and disparage the expertise and knowledge of the female midwives of the time, which led to the belief that these women were not very capable. More recent studies, such as that by Doreen Evenden, show that this was quite possibly mistaken. Indeed, Willughby wrote in his introduction that his aim was 'to inform the ignorant common midwives'.
17. Willughby, Percival, *Observations in Midwifery, as also The Countrey Midwifes Opsculum, or Vade Mecum* (Shakespeare Print Press, Warwick, 1863), p. 10. Willughby refers to her here as 'a poor foole'.

18. Ibid, p. 51.
19. Yonge, *An Account of Balls of Hair oTaken from the Uterus and Ovaria of Several Women*, p. 2387.
20. Ibid.
21. *A Collection of Letters, Made by Sr Tobie Mathews, Kt.* (Tho. Horne, Tho. Bennet, and Francis Saunders, London, 1692), p. 94.
22. Graham, Hinds, Hobby, Wilcox (eds.), *Her Own Life: Autobiographical writings by seventeenth-century Englishwomen* (Routledge, London, 1989), p. 152.
23. McCafferty, John (jdmccafferty), '14 Dec 1599: Richard Boyle's (future Earl of #Cork) first wife Joan Apsley d. in childbirth #otd (NPG - identified as him, as we don't have a pic of her)'. https://twitter.com/jdmccafferty/status/1205793513872543745?s=20 10:15 AM—Dec 14, 2019. Tweet.
24. Barret, Robert, *A companion for midwives, child-bearing women, and nurses directing them how to perform their respective offices* (Thomas Ax, London, 1699), pp. 35 & 36.
25. Cressy, David, *Birth, Marriage & Death: Ritual, Religion, and the Life-Cycle in Tudor and Stuart England* (Oxford University Press, Oxford, 1997), p. 81.
26. 'The Importance of Skin to Skin for Parents and Baby' https://www.royalwolverhampton.nhs.uk/services/service-directory-a-z/infant-feeding/skin-to-skin-contact/ [Accessed 5 November 2019].
27. Cressy, *Birth, Marriage & Death*, p. 87.
28. Ibid, p. 88.
29. Coleworts—a kind of cabbage.
30. Markham, *The English House-wife*, p. 39.
31. Ibid.
32. Le Doare, Kirsty et al. 'Mother's Milk: A Purposeful Contribution to the Development of the Infant Microbiota and Immunity.' *Frontiers in immunology* vol. 9 361. 28 Feb. 2018, doi:10.3389/fimmu.2018.00361 [Accessed 5 November 2019].
33. Sharp, Jane, *The Midwives Book, Or: The Whole Art of Midwifery Discovered* (Oxford University Press, Oxford, 1999), p. 259.
34. Moore, *Lady Fanshawe's Receipt Book*, p. 92.
35. Clinton, Elizabeth Knevet, *The Countesse of Lincolnes Nurserie*, an electronic edition. http://pid.emory.edu/ark:/25593/17bfb [Accessed 4 November 2019]. Lewis H. Beck Center Emory University Atlanta, Georgia. Text available via the Emory Center for Digital Scholarship.
36. Tinniswood, Adrian, *The Rainborowes: Pirates, Puritans and a Family's Quest for the Promised Land* (Vintage Books, London, 2014), p. 17.
37. Newcome, Henry, *The Compleat Mother, Or An Earnest Perswasive to all Mothers (especially those of Rank and Quality) to Nurse their own Children* (J. Wyat, London, 1695), p. 3.
38. Cressy, *Birth, Marriage & Death*, p. 88.

39. Shakespeare, William, *Romeo & Juliet, Act I, Scene II, The Works of Mr. William Shakespear, Volume the Fifth* (Jacob Tomson, London, 1709), p. 2084.

40. Sinibaldi, *The Cabinet of Venus Unlocked*, p. 22.

41. Anyone who has had their breasts engorged with milk following childbirth and are unwilling or unable to breastfeed knows how painful this can be if the milk isn't removed.

42. Markham, *The English House-wife*, p. 39.

43. Again, we have Shakespeare's fictional 'Nurse' stating that she remembers applying wormwood to her nipples to make them bitter-tasting—a tactic sometimes used to start weaning a child off milk and onto solid food.

44. Evelyn, *Diary, Vol. I*, pp. 319–322.

45. Ibid, p. 372.

46. *A Collection of Letters, Made by Sr Tobie Mathews, Kt.* (Tho. Horne, Tho. Bennet, and Francis Saunders, London, 1692), Page 102.

47. Aldersey-Williams, Hugh, *In Search of Sir Thomas Browne* (W.W. Norton & Company, New York, 2015), p. 33.

48. Lacey, Andrew, *The English Civil War in 100 Facts* (Amberley Publishing, Stroud, 2017), pp. 70–71.

49. Jonson, Ben, *Plays and Poems by Ben Jonson* (George Routledge & Sons, London, 1895), p. 315.

50. Ibid.

51. Duffy, *Henry Purcell*, p. 63.

52. Schreiber, Roy E, 'Hay [née Percy], Lucy, countess of Carlisle (1599–1660), courtier.' Oxford Dictionary of National Biography. January 03, 2008. Oxford University Press. Date of access 18 Feb. 2019, http://www.oxforddnb.com/view/10.1093/ref:odnb/9780198614128.001.0001/odnb-9780198614128-e-12733

53. 'Aemilia Lanyer', *Poetry Foundation*, https://www.poetryfoundation.org/poets/aemilia-lanyer [Accessed 20 February 2029}

54. Bell, Walter George, *The Great Plague in London* (The Folio Society, London, 2001), p. 95.

55. Purkiss, *The English Civil War*, p. 483.

56. Charmian Mansell and Mark Hailwood, editors, 'Bastardy', *Court Depositions of South West England, 1500–1700*, University of Exeter, http://humanities-research.exeter.ac.uk/womenswork/courtdepositions/#credits [Accessed 9 December 2018]

57. Chamie, Joseph, 'Out-of-Wedlock Births Rise Worldwide', YaleGlobal, Yale University, March 16, 2017. https://yaleglobal.yale.edu/content/out-wedlock-births-rise-worldwide [Accessed 12 January 2020].

58. Baillie, Robert, *The Letters and Journals of Robert Baillie, 1637–1662*, p. 31.

59. Shurtleff (ed.), *Records of the colony of New Plymouth in New England*, p. 93.

60. *Record of the Courts of Chester County, Pennsylvania, 1681–1697*, p. 276.

61. Ibid, p. 277.

62. Winthrop, John, *Winthrop Papers, Volume III: 1631–1637* (The Merrymount Press, Boston, 1943), p. 386.

63. Geyl, Pieter, *Orange and Stuart: 1641–1672* Phoenix Press, London, 1969), p. 131.
64. Holden, Anthony, *William Shakespeare: His Life and Work* (Little, Brown, & Co., London, 1999), p. 242.
65. Winstanley, *The Honour of Parnassus*, pp. 185–186.
66. Quigley, Laura, *The Devil Comes to Dartmoor: The Haunting True Story of Mary Howard, Devon's 'Demon Bride'* (The History Press, Stroud, 2011), timeline.

Chapter 14: Rape, Abortion, & Infanticide

1. C 7/451/88, TNA.
2. An example of this can be found on page 12 of *Relations and Observations, Historical and Politick, upon the Parliament begun Anno Dom. 1640* by Clement Walker from 1648, 'Children are ravished from their parents' arms, and shipped away'.
3. Thornton, *The Autobiography of Mrs. Alice Thornton*, p. 347.
4. Ibid, p. 47.
5. Dalton, *The Countrey Justice*, p. 366.
6. Ibid.
7. Ibid.
8. SP 34/38/42, Folio 62, TNA.
9. Royle, Trevor, *Civil War: The Wars of the Three Kingdoms, 1638–1660* (Abacus, London, 2005), p. 604.
10. Cressy, *Birth, Marriage & Death*, pp. 49–50.
11. Markham, *The English House-wife*, p. 148.
12. Salmon, *Pharmacopœia Londinensis*, p. 19.
13. Newcome, *The Compleat Mother*, p. 6.
14. Hambleton, Else L., 'The Regulation of Sex in Seventeenth-Century Massachussetts: The Quarterly Court of Essex County vs. Priscilla Willson and Mr. Samuel Appleton', in *Sex and Sexuality in Early America*, ed. Merril D. Smith, (New York University Press, New York, 1998), p. 89.
15. Gowing, Laura, *Gender Relations in Early Modern England*, p. 117.
16. N.H., *The Ladies Dictionary*, p. 239.
17. Dalton, *The Countrey Justice*, p. 367.
18. Codd, Daniel J, *Crimes & Criminals of 17th Century Britain* (Pen & Sword History, Barnsley, 2018), pp. 145–146.
19. Pimm, Geoffrey, *The Violent Abuse of Women in 17th and 18th Century Britain* (Pen & Sword History, Barnsley, 2019), p. 22.
20. *A True Relation of the Most Horrid and Barbarous murders committed by Abigall Hill of St. Olaves Southwark, on the persons of foure Infants* (F. Coles, London, 1658).
21. Shurtleff, *Records of the colony of New Plymouth in New England. Court Orders: Vol. I, 1633–1640* (William White, Boston, 1855), pp. 133–134.
22. Tinniswood, Adrian, *The Rainborowes: Pirates, Puritans and a Family's Quest for the Promised Land* (Vintage Books, London, 2014), p. 204.

23. *Old Bailey Proceedings Online* (www.oldbaileyonline.org, version 8.0, 03 December 2019), July 1679, trial of Katherine Tumince (t16790716–2).

24. *Old Bailey Proceedings Online* (www.oldbaileyonline.org, version 8.0, 03 December 2019), January 1683, trial of Elizabeth Neal (t16830117–2).

25. *Old Bailey Proceedings Online* (www.oldbaileyonline.org, version 8.0, 03 December 2019), October 1685, trial of Katharine Brown (t16851014–27).

26. *Old Bailey Proceedings Online* (www.oldbaileyonline.org, version 8.0, 12 December 2019), October 1695, trial of Frances Boddyman (t16951014–3).

Chapter 15: Sexually Transmitted Diseases: Or, Ye Curse Upon Fornicators!

1. Larman, Alexander, *Blazing Star,* p. 263.
2. Wiseman, Richard, *Eight Chirurgical Treatises,* p. 468.
3. Phil-Porney, *A Modest Defence of Publick Stews, Or, An Essay Upon Whoring* (T. Read, London, 1740), p. 3.
4. Gonorrhoea: Overview. NHS. https://www.nhs.uk/conditions/gonorrhoea/ [Accessed 16 March 2019].
5. Wiseman, *Eight Chirurgical Treatises*, p. 469.
6. Gonorrhea: Basic Fact Sheet. CDC: Centers for Disease Control, https://www.cdc.gov/std/gonorrhea/stdfact-gonorrhea.htm [Accessed 16 March 2019]
7. 'Gonorrhoea: Complications', UK National Health Service (NHS), https://www.nhs.uk/conditions/gonorrhoea/complications/ [Accessed 2 February 2020].
8. Salmon, *Pharmacopœia Londinensis*, p. 66.
9. Wilmot, John, *Regime de Vivre* (poem).
10. Ibid. 'And missing my whore, I bugger my page.'
11. Sayre, Gordon, 'Native American Sexuality', *Sex and Sexuality in Early America,* edited by Merril D. Smith (New York University Press, New York, 1998), p. 47.
12. Ibid, p. 316.
13. Syphilis symptoms (NHS). https://www.nhs.uk/conditions/syphilis/symptoms/ [Accessed 24 January].
14. Wallis, Jennifer, 'Looking back: This fascinating and fatal disease'. British Psychological Society. https://thepsychologist.bps.org.uk/volume-25/edition-10/looking-back-fascinating-and-fatal-disease [Accessed 24 January 2019]. This 'insanity' is often a result of untreated syphilis, which has been allowed to continue into a tertiary phase, aka neurosyphilis.
15. Aubrey, 'Elizabeth Broughton', *Brief Lives, Vol. 1* (The Clarendon Press, Oxford, 1898), eBook.
16. It is not absolutely certain how a prosthetic nose was applied to face. 'Artificial nose, Europe, 1601–1800'. Credit: Science Museum, London. https://wellcomecollection.org/works/vwkeypvj [Accessed 25 November 2019].
17. Page, Nick, *Lord Minimus: The Extraordinary Life of Britain's Smallest Man* (St. Martin's Press, New York, 2002), pp. 78–79.

18. 'Genital Herpes', CDC: Centers for Disease Control and Prevention. https://www.cdc.gov/std/herpes/stdfact-herpes.htm [Accessed 26 February 2019].
19. Anderson, A. L., & Chaney, E., (2009), Pubic lice (Pthirus pubis): history, biology and treatment vs. knowledge and beliefs of US college students, *International journal of environmental research and public health*, 6(2), 592–600, [Accessed 26 February 2019].
20. http://www.rsc.org/periodic-table/element/80/mercury [Accessed 29 September 2018]
21. Markham, *The English House-wife*, p. 51.
22. Wiseman, *Eight Chirurgical Treatises*, pp. 471, 473.
23. Ibid, p. 479.
24. Queen Anne's Revenge Project. https://www.qaronline.org/conservation/artifacts/tools-and-instruments/urethral-syringe [Accessed 27 September 2019].

Chapter 16: Libido & Masturbation: Or, Ye Art of Self-Pleasuring

1. Sinibaldi, *The Cabinet of Venus Unlocked,* p. 22.
2. Ibid, p. 23.
3. Floyer, John, *Psychrolousia, Or, the History of Cold Bathing*, (London, 1715), Dedication.
4. Culpeper, *Pharmacopœia Londinenseis*, Advertisement, opposite page 1.
5. Dufour, Philippe Sylvestre, *The Manner of Making of Coffee, Tea, and Chocolate* (William Crook, London, 1685). Transcribed for the Text Creation Partnership (Ann Arbor and Oxford, 2007) and published online at http://name.umdl.umich.edu/A36763.0001.001
6. Garfield, *The Wandring Whore,* p. A2.
7. Byrd II, William, *Letters of William Byrd II, and Sir Hans Sloane Relative to Plants and Minerals of Virginia,* p. 195.
8. Markham, *The English House-wife*, p. 148.
9. Culpeper, *Pharmacopœia Londinensis*, p. 43.
10. Vaginal dryness, https://www.nhs.uk/conditions/vaginal-dryness/ [Accessed 28 November 2018]
11. *The School of Venus*, p. 69.
12. Matthews-Grieco, Sara, *Cuckoldry, Impotence, and Adultery in Europe*, pp. 63–64.
13. Ibid, p. 64.
14. Thomas, Keith, *Religion and the Decline of Magic: Studies in Popular Beliefs in Sixteenth- And Seventeenth-Century England* (Penguin Books, London, 1991), p. 519.
15. 'A Rare new Ballad Entituled / My Husband has no Courage / in Him, National Library of Scotland – Rosebery, Ry.III.a.10(53).
16. '*The Quaker's Wives Lamentation For the LOSS of Her Husband's Jewels, Who Gelded Himself (in Petticoat-Lane,) to Vex His Wife*' (London, James Bissel, 1684–1700), Pepys Library, Magdalene College

Cambridge. Pepys Library Ballads 3, p. 302. <http://ebba.english.ucsb.edu/ballad/21317> [Accessed 15 December 2018].

17. Sinibaldi, *The Cabinet of Venus Unlocked,* p. 25.
18. Culpeper, Nicholas, *Culpeper's Directory for Midwives: Or, A Guide for Women* (Peter Cole, London, 1662), p. 117.
19. Pepys, '9 February 1667/68', *Diary.*
20. Dolnick, *The Clockwork Universe,* p. 116.
21. *The School of Venus,* p. 98.
22. Osborne, *Advice to a Son,* p. 18.
23. Pepys, Samuel, *Diary*, Vol. VIII: 'But here I did make myself to do *la cosa* by mere imagination, *mirando a jolie mosa* and with my eyes open, which I never did before—and God forgive me for it, it being in the Chapel'.
24. Bartholin, Thomas & Caspar, *Bartholinus Anatomy,* (Peter Cole, London, 1665), p. 77.
25. Wilmot, 'Signior Dildo'.
26. Baptista, *The Character of A Bad Woman*, p. 3.
27. As quoted in Jeremy Lamb's *So Idle A Rogue: The Life and Death of Lord Rochester* (Allison & Busby, London, 1993), p. 128.

Chapter 17: Stuart Love, Or Ye Heart's Delighte & Torment

1. Osborne, *Advice to a Son*, p. 27.
2. Ambrose, *Media; The Middle Things*, p. 195.
3. McLeod, Catherine, Timothy Wilks, Malcolm Smuts, Rab MacGibbon, *The Lost Prince: The Life and Death of Henry Stuart* (National Portrait Gallery, London, 2012), p. 169.
4. Zuvich, *The Stuarts in 100 Facts*, pp. 191 & 192.
5. Chapman, Hester, *Four Fine Gentlemen* (Constable and Company, Ltd, London, 1977), p. 96.
6. Bacon, Sir Francis, *The Works of Francis Bacon: Baron of Verulam, Viscount St. Albans and Lord High Chancellor of England, In Five Volumes. Volume I,* (A. Millar, London, 1765), p. 342.
7. Wellicome, Lavinia and Chris Gravett, *Woburn Abbey* (Jarrold Publishing, Norfolk, 2009), p. 4.
8. This painting is in the care of the Metropolitan Museum of Art, New York City.
9. This painting is in the care of the Musée du Louvre, Paris.
10. Charmian Mansell and Mark Hailwood, editors. *Court Depositions of South West England, 1500–1700*, University of Exeter, http://humanities-research.exeter.ac.uk/womenswork/courtdepositions. Accessed 6 December 2018.
11. Berwick-upon-Tweed, Northumberland, England.
12. The bridge mentioned here is probably Berwick Bridge, constructed during the Stuart period between 1611–1624.
13. Kirk, Thomas, 'An Account of a Tour in Scotland', *Tours in Scotland, 1677–1681* (David Douglas, Edinburgh, 1892), p. 7.
14. Wood, *The Life and Times of Anthony Wood, Vol. I.* p. 199.

15. Ibid.
16. Shakespeare, William, *A Midsummer Night's Dream*, Act 1, Scene 1.
17. Armitage, Jill, *Arbella Stuart: The Uncrowned Queen* (Amberley Publishing, Stroud, 2017), p. 215.
18. Gristwood, Sarah, *Arbella: England's Lost Queen* (Bantam, London, 2004), p.346.
19. Ibid, p. 18.
20. Gristwood, *Arbella: England's Lost Queen*, p. 212.
21. Ibid, p. 434.
22. Armitage, *Arbella Stuart: The Uncrowned Queen*, p. 252.
23. N.H., *The Ladies Dictionary*, p. 335.

Chapter 18: Adultery & Divorce in Stuart Britain: Or, O Lamentable Sinne!

1. Gowing, Laura, 'Women in the World of Pepys', *Samuel Pepys: Plague, Fire, Revolution* (Thames & Hudson/National Maritime Museum, 2015), p. 75.
2. https://www.british-history.ac.uk/no-series/acts-ordinances-interregnum/pp387–389#p11 [ACCESSED 12 AUGUST 2018]
3. 'March 1649: An Act for the Abolishing the House of Peers.' *Acts and Ordinances of the Interregnum, 1642–1660.* Eds. C H Firth, and R S Rait. London: His Majesty's Stationery Office, 1911. 24. *British History Online.* Web. 1 March 2019. http://www.british-history.ac.uk/no-series/acts-ordinances-interregnum/p24.
4. Ibid.
5. Penn, William, *Reflections and Maxims*, pp. 22–23.
6. Marmaduke, thanks to Prof. Laurie Johnson and Dr. Jacqueline Reiter for confirming (though it's still unclear as to whether it is Marmadux or Marmaduci).
7. ARR/1/2/17a, Folio 2. Lancashire Record Office.
8. Ambrose, *Media; The Middle Things*, p. 37.
9. Behn, Aphra, *The Town-Fopp, Or, Sir Timothy Tawdrey: A Comedy* (Roger L'Estrange: London, 1677). Transcribed for the Text Creation Partnership (Ann Arbor and Oxford, 2007) and published online at http://name.umdl.umich.edu/A27328.0001.001
10. Blount, Charles, 'Defense of his Marriage with Lady Penelope Rich (1606?)' British Library, Additional MS 11600, ff. 56v-64v via *Manuscript Pamphleteering in Early Stuart England* https://mpese.ac.uk/t/BlountMarriageLadyRich1606.html [Accessed 26 January 2019].
11. Maginn, Christopher, 'Blount, Charles, eighth Baron Mountjoy and earl of Devonshire (1563–1606), soldier and administrator,' Oxford Dictionary of National Biography. January 03, 2008. Oxford University Press. Date of access 19 May. 2019, https://www.oxforddnb.com/view/10.1093/ref:odnb/9780198614128.001.0001/odnb-9780198614128-e-2683
12. Adams, *Jack Adams, His Perpetual Almanack*, pp. 19 & 20.
13. Pepys, 'December 7 1661', *Diary.*

14. Ibid.
15. Beddard, R. A. P. J. 'Palmer, Roger, earl of Castlemaine (1634–1705), diplomatist and Roman Catholic apologist.' Oxford Dictionary of National Biography. January 03, 2008. Oxford University Press, Date of access 28 Jan. 2019, http://www.oxforddnb.com/view/10.1093/ref:odnb/9780198614128.001.0001/odnb-9780198614128-e-21209
16. Osborne, *Advice to a Son*, p. 24.
17. Hammond, *The Whole Duty of Man*, p. 217.
18. Austin, William, *Haec Homo: Wherein the excellency of the creation of woman is described,* (R.O. for R.M. and C.G., London, 1639), p. 25.
19. '*The Pennyless Parliament of Thread-bare Poets: Or, All Mirth and witty Conceits (1608)*' as found in *The Harleian Miscellany, Vol. I,* (T. Osborne, London, 1744), p. 181. Shelfmark RB.23.a.38840.(2), British Library.
20. Shurtleff, *Records of the Colony of New Plymouth*, p. 98.
21. Crawford, Mary Caroline, *The Days of the Pilgrim Fathers* (Little, Brown, & Co, Boston, 1920), p. 194.
22. Tinniswood, Adrian, *The Rainborowes: Pirates, Puritans and a Family's Quest for the Promised Land* (Vintage Books, London, 2014), p.164.
23. Tinniswood, *The Rainborowes*, p.164.
24. Fraser, *The Weaker Vessel*, p. 13.
25. Womack, Pamela J., 'The Reluctant Bride: A Jacobean Tragedy', *The Seventeenth Century Lady*. (http://www.andreazuvich.com/history/the-reluctant-bride-a-jacobean-tragedy-a-guest-post-by-pamela-j-womack/#content)
26. Behn, Aphra, *Young Jemmy, Or, The Princely Shepherd*, P. Brooksby, London. Transcribed for the Text Creation Partnership (Ann Arbor and Oxford, 2007) and published online at http://name.umdl.umich.edu/B01555.0001.001
27. Wood, *The Life and Times of Anthony Wood, Vol. I*, p. 472.
28. Keay, Anna, *The Last Royal Rebel: The Life and Death of James, Duke of Monmouth* (Bloomsbury, London, 2017), p. 240.
29. Winstanley, *The Honour of Parnassus*, pp. 74–75.
30. Greene, Robert, *Greene's Groatsworth of Wit, Bought With a Million of Repentance: Describing the Folly of Youth, the Falshood of Make-shift Flatterers, the Miserie of the negligent, and mischiefes of deceiving Curtezans* (Henry Bell, London, 1629). No page number.
31. Probert, *Marriage Law for Genealogists*, p. 48.
32. Rainolds, John, *A defence of the iudgment of the Reformed churches,* (George Walters, Dordrecht, 1609), *[STC 20607.]* p. 3. *Transcribed for the Text Creation Partnership (Ann Arbor and Oxford, 2007).* Copy from Henry E. Huntington Library and Art Gallery (reel 726:8a) and Boston Public Library (reel 2340:8a).
33. Ibid.
34. Probert, *Marriage Law for Genealogists*, p. 76.
35. Zuvich, Andrea, 'Stuart Britain: What Was Life Like for Ordinary People?' *BBC History Extra*. https://www.historyextra.com/period/stuart/stuart-britain-what-was-life-like-for-ordinary-people/

Chapter 19: Rakes & Rogues: Or, The Stuart Libertine

1. Baxter, *A Treatise of Self-Denial*, p. 160.
2. Cockeram, Henry, *The English Dictionarie of 1623,* p. 112.
3. Beard Thomas and Thomas Taylor, *The Theatre of God's Judgements* (S.I & M.H., London, 1648), p. A2.
4. Burnet, *History of His Own Time, Vol. I,* p. 264.
5. Ibid.
6. Cooper, Susan Margaret, *Thomas Alcock: A Biographical Account,* (2017), ebook location 992.
7. Keay, *The Last Royal Rebel,* pp. 76–77.
8. Cooper, *Thomas Alcock,* ebook location 992.
9. Burnet, *History of His Own Time, Vol. I,* p. 265.
10. Fairfax, *Memoirs of the Life of George Villiers,* p. 31.
11. Zuvich, *The Stuarts in 100 Facts,* p. 114.
12. Ibid, pp. 38 & 39.
13. Bevan, Bryan, *King William III: Prince of Orange, the first European* (The Rubicon Press, London, 1997), p. 12.
14. Pritchard, *Scandalous Liaisons,* p. 61.
15. Pepys, '29 July 1667', *Diary.*
16. Evelyn, '13 June 1673', *Diary,* p. 89.
17. Pritchard, *Scandalous Liaisons,* p. 9.
18. Pepys, '1 July 1663', *Diary.*
19. Picard, *Restoration London,* p. 162.
20. Pepys, '13 July 1667', *Diary.*
21. Wilson, Derek, *All the King's Women: Love, Sex, and Politics in the Life of Charles II* (Hutchinson, London, 2003), p. 238.
22. Burnet, *History of His Own Time, Vol. I,* p. 266.
23. Seward, *The King Over The Water,* p. 113.
24. St. John Bolingbroke, Henry & Dr Goldsmith, *The Works of the Late Right Honourable Henry St. John, Lord Viscount Bolingbroke: Volume 1, With the Life of Lord Bolingbroke by Dr Goldsmith* (J. Johnson, Otridge & Son, Foulder & Son, T. Payne, Wilkie & Robinson, et al, London, 1809), p. vi.
25. Zuvich, *A Year in the Life of Stuart Britain,* p. 102.
26. Ibid, p. 212.
27. Spencer, *Prince Rupert: The Last Cavalier,* p. 41.
28. Aubrey, 'Henry Martin', *Brief Lives, Vol. 2,* eBook.
29. Ibid.
30. Ibid.
31. Lithgow, *The Totall Discourse of the Rare Adventures & Painefull Peregrinations,* p. 33.
32. Darcy, Eamon, *The World of Thomas Ward: Sex and Scandal in Late Seventeenth-Century Co. Antrim* (Four Courts Press, Dublin, 2016), pp. 48–49.
33. Ary de Vois: Portrait of Adriaan Beverland (1650–1716), c. 1676. Amsterdam, Rijksmuseum. inv./cat.nr. SK-A-3237. https://rkd.nl/nl/explore/images/16361 [Accessed 2 March 2019].

34. Chalmers, Alexander, *The General Biographical Dictionary* (J. Nichols and Son, London, 1812), pp. 201–202.
35. Swift, Jonathan, *The Journal to Stella* (Methuen & Co., London, 1901), p. 533.
36. Unknown, *Lettre d'un Marchand a Un de Ses Amis Sur l'Eppouvantable Tremblement de Terre, qui est arrivé au Port-Royal de la Jamaïque, Isle d'Angleterre, le 17 Juin 1692,* (Paris, 1692), p. 1.
37. Ward, Edward, *A Trip to Jamaica: With a True Character of the People and Island* (London, 1698), p. 16, edited by David Oakleaf for The Grub Street Project http://grubstreetproject.net/works/R905?func=intro&display=text
38. Penn, *Reflections and Maxims,* pp. 104–105.
39. Chapman, Hester, *Queen Mary II* (Jonathan Cape, London, 1953), p. 107.
40. Hamilton, Elizabeth, *William's Mary: A Biography of Mary II* (Hamish Hamilton, London, 1972), pp. 109–110.
41. Luttrell, *A Brief Relation of State Affairs,* p. 467.
42. Lambeth Palace Court of Arches MSS (LPCA, D. 134). Also: Stone, Lawrence, *Uncertain Unions & Broken Lives* (Oxford University Press, Oxford, 1995), pp. 116–124.

Chapter 20: Interracial & Interethnic Unions: Or, Exotick Sex

1. Peacham, Henry, *Minerva Britanna: Or, A Garden of Heroical Devices, Furnish'd, and adorned with Emblems and Impresa's of sundry nature* (Wa. Dight, London, 1612), p. 37.
2. Indeed, your humble author is a product of these unions: a recent DNA test indicated that I am approximately 42% Native South American (Araucanian/ Chilean Mapuche), and 58% European (Spain, Croatia, France, and the British Isles).
3. Lithgow, *The Totall Discourse of the Rare Adventures & Painefull Peregrinations,* p. 8.
4. Laurence, *Women in England,* p. 20.
5. Seraglios are the women's living quarters, or apartments, in a harem.
6. *The New Atlas: Or, Travels and Voyages in Europe, Asia, Africa, and America, Thro' the most Renowned Parts of the World* (J. Cleave and A. Roper, London, 1698), pp. 18–23
7. Olearius, Adam, *The Voyages and Travells of the Ambassadors sent by Frederick Duke of Holstein to the Great Duke of Muscovy, and the King of Persia...Containing a Compleat History of Muscovy, Tartary, Persia and other adjacent Countries* (John Starkey and Thomas Basset, London, 1669), p. 97.
8. Psalmaanazaar, George, *A Historical and Geographical Description of Formosa.* Dan. Brown, London, 1704), p. 165.
9. Duffy, *Henry Purcell,* p. 213.
10. Chardin, Sir John, *Travels of Sir John Chardin into Persia and Ye East Indies* (Moses Pitt, London, 1686), p. 89.

11. Ibid, p. 190.
12. Sherley, Sir Antony, *Sir Antony Sherley: His Relation of his Travels into Persia, etc.* (Nathaniel Butter and Joseph Bagset, London, 1613), p. 128.
13. Raiswell, Richard, 'Shirley, Sir Robert, Count Shirley in the papal nobility (c. 1581–1628), diplomat.' Oxford Dictionary of National Biography. September 23, 2004. Oxford University Press, Date of access: 26 Feb. 2019, http://www.oxforddnb.com/view/10.1093/ref:odnb/9780198614128.001.0001/odnb-9780198614128-e-25433
14. Ibid.
15. Laurence, Anne, *Women in England: 1500–1760. A Social History* (Phoenix Press, London, 1996), p. 21.
16. Vaughan, A, (2017, September 01), Pocahontas [Matoaka, Amonute; married name Rebecca Rolfe] (c. 1596–1617), Algonquian Indian princess, *Oxford Dictionary of National Biography.* Ed. Retrieved 27 Mar. 2019, from http://www.oxforddnb.com/view/10.1093/ref:odnb/9780198614128.001.0001/odnb-9780198614128-e-22418.
17. Winstanley, *The Honour of Parnassus,* p. 152.
18. Wear, Andrew, 'Medicine and Health in the Age of European Colonialism', *The Healing Arts: Health, Disease and Society in Europe 1500–1800,* Elmer, Peter (ed.). p. 321.
19. Smith, *The Voyages and Discoveries of Captaine John Smyth in Virginia,* p. 5.
20. Porter, Jennifer, *The Jamestown Brides: The Bartered Wives of the New World* (Atlantic Books, London, 2019), p. 106.
21. Olearius, *The Voyages and Travells of the Ambassadors sent by Frederick Duke of Holstein to the Great Duke of Muscovy,* p. 185.
22. Ibid.
23. Spencer, *Prince Rupert: The Last Cavalier,* p. 275.
24. Berkowitz, *Sex & Punishment: 4000 Years of Judging Desire,* p. 269.
25. Ibid, p. 270.
26. Hooke, Robert, *Micrographia* (Royal Society, London, 1665).
27. Cleveland, *The Works of Mr. John Cleveland,* p. 17. Transcribed for the Text Creation Partnership (Ann Arbor and Oxford, 2007) and published online at http://name.umdl.umich.edu/A33421.0001.001 [Accessed 29 January 2020].
28. Shakespeare, *Othello,* Act I, Scene I, *The Works of Mr. William Shakespear, Volume the Fifth* (Jacob Tomson, London, 1709), p. 2557.
29. Ibid, p. 2556.
30. Burg, B.R., *Sodomy and the Pirate Tradition: English Sea Rovers in the Seventeenth-Century Caribbean* (New York University Press, New York, 1995), p. 116.
31. Ibid.
32. *Record of the Courts of Chester County, Pennsylvania, 1681–1697,* p. 288.
33. Winthrop, *Winthrop Papers, Volume III: 1631–1637,* p. 501.
34. Crawford, *The Days of the Pilgrim Fathers,* pp. 193–194.

35. Brook, Timothy, *Vermeer's Hat: The Seventeenth Century and the Dawn of the Global World* (Profile Books, London, 2009), p. 187.
36. Wiseman, *Eight Chirurgical Treatises*, p. 468.
37. C., T., *The New Atlas: Or, Travels and Voyages in Europe, Asia, Africa, and America, Thro' the most Renowned Parts of the World* (J. Cleave and A. Roper, London, 1698), p. 205.
38. Ibid. Although the author has written, 'Mollotos' (which we now spell as 'Mulatto'), which is the term for a cross between European and African, the correct term for a cross between European and Native American would be 'Mestizo'.
39. Ibid, p. 206.
40. Davis, Robert C, *Christian Slaves, Muslim Masters* (Palgrave MacMillan, Houndsmills, 2003), p. 125.
41. Milton, Giles, *White Gold: The Extraordinary Story of Thomas Pellow and North Africa's One Million European Slaves* (Hodder & Stoughton, London, 2005), pp. 6 & 121.
42. Louvois, Marquis de, *Testament Politique du Marquis de Louvois, Premier Ministre D'Etar sous le regne de Louis XIV, Roy de France* (Cologne, 1695), pp. 269–271.
43. SP44/335/202; Garside, 112; as found in Cruickshanks, Eveline, Jones, 'John (c.1610–92), of Lothbury, London and Hampton, Mdx', *The History of Parliament: the House of Commons 1660–1690*, ed. B.D. Henning, 1983. http://www.histparl.ac.uk/volume/1660–1690/member/jones-john-1610–92
44. Milton, *White Gold*, p. 219.
45. Ibid, p. 128.
46. Ibid, p. 121.

PART TWO

Chapter 21: James VI & I: Swinging Both Ways?

1. Popular saying during the early 1600s, as quoted in Burford, *Bawds and Lodgings,* p. 164.
2. Watkins, Susan, *Mary Queen of Scots* (Thames & Hudson, London, 2009), p. 82.
3. Massie, Alan, *The Royal Stuarts: A History of the Family that Shaped Britain* (Thomas Dunne Books, New York, 2010), p. 116.
4. Fraser, Antonia, *Mary Queen of Scots: The 50th Anniversary Edition* (Weidenfeld & Nicolson Ltd, London, 1969), p. 278.
5. Watkins, *Mary Queen of Scots,* p. 121.
6. Fraser, *Mary Queen of Scots: The 50th Anniversary Edition,* pp. 273–274.
7. Matusiak, John, *James I: Scotland's King of England* (The History Press, Stroud, 2015), p. 51. The causes of and agents involved in Henry, Lord Darnley's death at Kirk o' Field was a rumour-riddled topic. Although there was an explosion, his body showed signs of having been strangled.

8. 'The Scottish Reformation': http://www.bbc.co.uk/scotland/history/articles/ scottish_reformation/ [Accessed 18 November 2018].
9. Sketch of Mary Queen of Scots, c. June 1567, (SP 52/13 f.60). TNA.
10. De Lisle, Leanda, *After Elizabeth: The Death of Elizabeth and the coming of King James* (HarperPerennial, London, 2006), p. 54.
11. Fraser, Sarah, *The Prince Who Would Be King* (William Collins, London, 2017), p. 10.
12. Cogswell, Thomas, *James I: The Phoenix King* (Allen Lane, 2017), p. 14.
13. Fraser, Antonia, *King James VI of Scotland, I of England* (Weidenfeld and Nicolson, London, 1994), p. 53.
14. Marshall, Rosalind K., *Scottish Queens: The Queen and Consorts Who Shaped A Nation* (Birlinn Ltd, Edinburgh, 2019), p. 147.
15. Burford, *Bawds and Lodgings: A History of the London Bankside Brothels*, p. 175.
16. SP 14/6 f. 21r, TNA.
17. Cogswell, *James I: The Phoenix King,* pp. 6–7.
18. Whitaker, Katie, *A Royal Passion: The Turbulent Marriage of Charles I and Henrietta Maria* (Phoenix, London, 2011), p. 27.
19. Hutchinson, *Memoirs of the Life of Colonel Hutchinson*, p. 78. My emphasis.
20. Ibid, again my emphasis.
21. Cecil, David, *The Cecils of Hatfield House* (Constable, London, 1973), p. 153.
22. Houston, S.J, *James I: Seminar Studies in History* (Pearson Education Limited, Harlow, 1995), p. 45.
23. Fraser, *King James VI of Scotland I of England,* p. 141.
24. Durston, Christopher, *James I* (Routledge, London, 1993), p. 21.
25. Fraser, *King James VI of Scotland I of England,* p. 168.
26. Bellany, Alastair & Thomas Cogswell, *The Murder of King James I,* (Yale University Press, New Haven and London, 2015), p. 12.
27. Marshall, *Scottish Queens,* p. 151.
28. Fraser, *King James VI of Scotland I of England,* p. 168.
29. Durston, *James I,* p. 21.
30. Fraser, *King James VI of Scotland I of England,* p. 165.
31. Hill, C.P., *Who's Who in British History: Stuart Britain 1603–1714,* p. 16.
32. Borman, *Witches: James I and the English Witch-Hunts*, p. 125.
33. Fairfax, Brian, *Memoirs of the Life of George Villiers* (Bathoe, London, 1753), p. 24.
34. Bellany & Cogswell, *The Murder of King James I,* pp. 11 & 12.
35. Fraser, *The Weaker Vessel*, p. 9.
36. Evelyn, *The Diary of John Evelyn*, p. 307.

Chapter 22: Charles I: Lusty but Loyal

1. Fraser, *The Prince Who Would Be King*, p. 80.
2. Ibid, p. 191.
3. Whitaker, Katie, *A Royal Passion: The Turbulent Marriage of Charles I and Henrietta Maria* (Phoenix, London, 2011), p. 26.

4. James VI/I, King, *The Workes of the Most High and Mightie Prince, James, by the grace of God, King of Great Britain and Ireland* (James, Bishop of Winton, London, 1616).

5. Peña, Juan Antonio de la, Relacion de las fiestas reales... (Juan Gonzalez, Madrid, 1623). BL, 9930.gg.33. *El juego de cañas* was an equestrian entertainment popular in the sixteenth and seventeenth centuries which was usually performed by noblemen mounted on horseback in great public squares.

6. *A Continuation of a former Relation concerning the Entertainment given to the Prince His Highnesse by the King of Spaine in his Court at Madrid* (John Haviland for William Barret, London, 1623).

7. Ibid, p. 9.

8. Pearce, Dominic, *Henrietta Maria: The Betrayed Queen* (Amberley Publishing, Stroud, 2015), p. 48.

9. In order to avoid any confusion with her granddaughter Queen Mary II, or with the Tudor Queen Mary, we will refer to her as Henrietta Maria henceforth as well.

10. Dauncey, John, *The History of the Thrice-Illustrious Princess Henrietta Bourbon, Queen of England* (E.C. for Philip Chetwind, London, 1660), p. 24.

11. Stubbs, *John Donne: The Reformed Soul,* p. 421.

12. Pearce, *Henrietta Maria,* p. 64.

13. Ibid, p. 67.

14. Porter, Linda, *Royal Renegades: The Children of Charles I and the English Civil Wars* (Pan Books, London, 2016), p. 7.

15. Clegg, Melanie, *The Life of Henrietta Anne* (Pen & Sword History, Barnsley, 2017).

16. Whitaker, *A Royal Passion,* p. 81.

17. Pearce, *Henrietta Maria,* p. 88.

18. I say 'wonderfully fertile' because it was a good thing for a queen to be at this time, and certainly hushed any negative talk about her being too physically small to bear children.

19. Porter, *Royal Renegades,* pp. 21–22.

20. De Lisle, *White King,* p. 83.

21. Plowden, Alison, *The Stuart Princesses* (Alan Sutton Publishing Ltd, Stroud, 1996), p. 61.

22. Porter, *Royal Renegades,* p. 110.

23. Whitaker, *A Royal Passion,* p. 131.

24. Hibbert, Christopher, *Charles I* (Corgi Books, London, 1972), pp. 79–80.

25. Adamson, John, *The Noble Revolt: The Overthrow of Charles I* (Weidenfeld & Nicolson, London, 2007), p. 136.

26. As found in *Letters of Queen Henrietta Maria,* edited by Mary Anne Everett Green (Richard Bentley, London, 1857).

27. Ibid, pp. 141–142.

28. Hibbert, *Charles I,* p. 116.

29. Purkiss, *The English Civil War*, p. 63.

30. De Lisle, *White King,* p. 248.
31. Ibid, p. 138.
32. Spencer, Charles, *To Catch a King: Charles II's Great Escape* (William Collins, London, 2017), p. 43.
33. Adolph, Anthony, *The King's Henchman: Henry Jermyn, Stuart Spymaster and Architect of the British Empire* (Gibson Square Books, London, 2012), pp. 284 & 285.

Chapter 23: Interregnum Intimacies

1. Originally a derogatory term that has since become the main word to describe the strict religious nature of some Protestants, who sought to live in a holier, purer way.
2. Lacey, *The English Civil War in 100 Facts,* p. 19.
3. Gentles, Ian J. 'Montagu, Edward, second earl of Manchester (1602–1671), politician and parliamentarian army officer.' Oxford Dictionary of National Biography. January 03, 2008. Oxford University Press, Date of access 30 Mar. 2019, http://www.oxforddnb.com/view/10.1093/ref:odnb/9780198614128.001.0001/odnb-9780198614128-e-19009
4. Murray, Nicholas, *World Enough and Time: The Life of Andrew Marvell* (Little, Brown & Company, London, 1999), pp. 296–9.
5. Hill, C.P., *Who's Who in British History: Stuart Britain 1603–1714,* p. 138.
6. Spencer, Charles, *Killers of the King: The Men Who Dared to Execute Charles I* (Bloomsbury, London, 2014), p. 114.
7. Evelyn, '14 October 1660', *Diary.*
8. Aubrey, 'Henry Martin', *Brief Lives, Vol. 2,* eBook.
9. Marten, Henry, 'Letter 41' in *Coll. Henry Marten's Familiar Letters to his Lady of Delight* (Edmund Gayton, Oxford, 1663), p. 36.
10. Ibid, 'Letter 37', p. 33.
11. Spencer, *Killers of the King,* p. 298.
12. Hill, Christopher, *God's Englishman: Oliver Cromwell and the English Revolution* (Penguin Books, Harmondsworth, 1973), p. 204.
13. Underdown, David, *A Freeborn People: Politics and the Nation in Seventeenth-Century England,* (Clarendon Press, Oxford, 1996), p. 93.
14. Fraser, *The Weaker Vessel,* p. 252.
15. Clarkson, Laurence, *The Lost Sheep Found: Or, The Prodigal Returned to his Fathers house* (Laurence Clarkson, London, 1660).
16. Hutchinson, *Memoirs of the Life of Colonel Hutchinson,* pp. 127–128.
17. Ibid.
18. Whitehead, Julian, *Cromwell and His Women* (Pen & Sword History, Barnsley, 2019),
19. Ibid, p. 13.
20. Fraser, Antonia, *Cromwell: Our Chief of Men* (Book Club Associates, London, 1974), pp. 478–479.

21. Whitehead, *Cromwell and His Women* p. 114.
22. Spencer, *Killers of the King,* p. 220.
23. Hutchinson, *Memoirs of the Life of Colonel Hutchinson,* p. 370.
24. Trevelyan, G.M., *Illustrated English Social History: Volume Two: The Age of Shakespeare and the Stuart Period* (Penguin Books Ltd, Harmondsworth, 1964), p. 214.

Chapter 24: Charles II & The Sexually Ravenous Restoration

1. Spencer, *To Catch a King: Charles II's Great Escape*, p. 6.
2. 'Lucy Walter (c.1630–1658)', Scolton Manor Museum, Pembrokeshire County Council's Museums Service, https://artuk.org/discover/artworks/lucy-walter-c-16301658–181611 [Accessed 12 January 2020].
3. Evelyn, *Diary,* p. 249.
4. Keay, Anna, *The Magnificent Monarch: Charles II and the Ceremonies of Power,* p. 77.
5. Keay, *The Last Royal Rebel,* p. 21.
6. As quoted in James Laver's *The Ladies of Hampton Court,* p. 5.
7. Hamilton, Elizabeth, *The Illustrious Lady: A Biography of Barbara Villiers, Countess of Castlemaine and Duchess of Cleveland* (Hamish Hamilton, London, 1980), p. 142.
8. *The Present State of England*, 1675, p. 266.
9. Evelyn, *Diary*, p. 358.
10. Pepys, '31 May 1662', *Diary*.
11. Pritchard, *Scandalous Liaisons,* p. 55.
12. Norrington, Ruth, *My Dearest Minette: The Letters between Charles II and his sister Henrietta, Duchess d'Orléans* (Peter Owen, London, 1996), p. 64.
13. Ibid, p. 151.
14. Hume, David, *The History of England, Vol. II* (T. Cadell, London, 1789), pp. 379–380.
15. Jordan, Don and Michael Walsh, *The King's Bed: Sex, Power, & the Court of Charles II* (Abacus, London, 2016), p. 134.
16. Pepys, '9 November 1663', *Diary*.
17. Hamilton, Count Anthony, *Memoirs of Count Grammont* (A.H. Bullen, London, 1903) p. 136.
18. Pepys, '26 April 1667', *Diary*.
19. Hamilton, *Memoirs of Count Grammont*, p. 136.
20. Laver, *The Ladies of Hampton Court*, p. 8.
21. Jordan and Walsh, *The King's Bed*, pp. 244–245.
22. Ibid, p. 249.
23. Ibid, p. 164.
24. Uglow, Jenny, *A Gambling Man* (Faber & Faber Limited, London, 2009), p. 323.
25. Hopkins, Graham, *Constant Delights: Rakes, Rogues, and Scandal in Restoration England* (Robson Books, London, 2002), p. 177.

26. Jordan and Walsh, *The King's Bed*, p. 184.
27. Ibid, p. 192.
28. Wheatley, Dennis, *'Old Rowley': A Very Private Life of Charles II* (Arrow Books, London, 1969), p. 151.
29. Wilson, *All the King's Women*, p. 264.
30. Ibid, p. 272.
31. Sevigne, Madame de, *Letters of Madame de Rabutin Chantal, Marchioness de Sevigne, to the Countess de Grignan, Her Daughter. In Two Volumes. Translated from the French* (J Hinton, 1745), p. 73.
32. Thompson, *Unfit for Modest Ears,* p. 133.
33. *Kings of the Sea: Charles II, James II & the Royal Navy* (2018) by J.D. Davies is a wonderfully fresh look at Charles and James and their interest in naval matters—which was something previously considered a 'dilettante' interest at best.
34. Holmes, Frederick, *The Sickly Stuarts: The Medical Downfall of a Dynasty* (Sutton Publishing, Stroud, 2005), p. 132.
35. Evelyn, *Diary, Vol. II*, p. 206.
36. Herman, Eleanor, *Sex With Kings* (William Morrow, New York, 2004), p. 202.
37. Petre, Edward, *Three Letters* (London, 1688), p. 3.

Chapter 25: James II: Or, 'The Most Unguarded Ogler of His Time'

1. As quoted in Picard, Liza, *Restoration London,* p. 127.
2. Burnet, *History of His Own Time, Vol. I,* p. 168.
3. Hamilton, *Memoirs of Count Grammont*, p. 173.
4. Haswell, Jock, *James II: Soldier and Sailor* (Hamish Hamilton, London, 1972), p. 134.
5. Evelyn, *Diary*, p. 337.
6. Pepys, '7 October 1660', *Diary*.
7. Ibid.
8. Miller, James, *Yale English Monarchs: James II* (Yale University Press, New Haven & London, 2000), p. 45.
9. Holmes, *The Sickly Stuarts,* p. 255.
10. Burnet, *History of His Own Time, Vol. I,* p. 169.
11. Hamilton, *Memoirs of Count Grammont*, p. 180.
12. Ibid, p. 171.
13. Doherty, Richard, *The Siege of Derry 1689: A Military History* (Spellmount, Stroud, 2010).
14. Callow, John, *James II, King in Exile* (The History Press, Stroud, 2017), p. 261.
15. Carlton, Charles, *Royal Mistresses* (Routledge, London, 1990), p. 86.
16. Kenyon, J.P., *The Stuarts* (William Collins Sons & Co., Glasgow, 1970), p. 146.
17. See the portrait of Mary of Modena by Simon Pietersz Verelst from 1680.

18. Hume, *The History of England, Vol. II,* p. 511.
19. Oman, Carola, *Mary of Modena* (Hodder and Stoughton, Bungay, 1962), p. 30.
20. Ibid, p. 31.
21. Bloch, *Sexual Life in England,* p. 280.
22. Oman, *Mary of Modena,* p. 49.
23. Ibid, p. 256.
24. Ibid, p. 51.
25. Speck, W.A., *James II* (Pearson Education Limited, Harlow, 2002), p. 25.
26. Winn, *Queen Anne*, p. 80.
27. Oman, *Mary of Modena*, p. 256.
28. Holmes, *The Sickly Stuarts,* p. 156.
29. Evelyn, '19 January 1686', *Diary*, p. 247.
30. Zuvich, *The Stuarts in 100 Facts,* pp. 189–190.
31. Starkey, David, *Crown & Country: The Kings & Queens of England* (Harper Press, London, 2011), p. 389.
32. Oman, *Mary of Modena*, p. 170.
33. Callow, *James II,* p. 440.
34. Holmes, *The Sickly Stuarts*, p. 255.
35. Ibid, p. 256.
36. Ibid.
37. Castelow, Ellen, 'The Battle of Culloden', *Historic UK,* https://www. historic-uk.com/HistoryMagazine/DestinationsUK/The-Battle-of-Culloden/ [Accessed 10 February 2020].

Chapter 26: William & Mary: Or, Marriage between First Cousins

1. Dalrymple, Sir John, *Memoirs of Great Britain and Ireland, Vol. III, from the Dissolution of the last Parliament of Charles II until the sea-battle off La Hogue* (W. Strahan and T. Cadell, London, 1771), p. 74.
2. Zuvich, *The Stuarts in 100 Facts,* pp. 131–132.
3. Geyl, Pieter, *Orange and Stuart: 1641–1672* (Phoenix Press, London, 1969), p. 7.
4. Watkins, Sarah-Beth, *The Tragic Daughters of Charles I: Mary, Elizabeth, & Henrietta Anne* (Chronos Books, Winchester, 2019), p. 17.
5. De Lisle, *White King,* p. 218.
6. Watkins, *The Tragic Daughters of Charles I,* p. 48.
7. Bevan, *King William III: Prince of Orange, the first European,* p. 5.
8. Ibid, p. 6.
9. Watkins, *The Tragic Daughters of Charles I,* pp. 50 & 63.
10. Speck, W.A, *Reluctant Revolutionaries: Englishmen and the Revolution of 1688* (Oxford University Press, Oxford, 1988), p. 75.
11. Bevan, *King William III,* p. 160.
12. Pepys, 'May 1, 1662', *Diary.*

13. Wake, William, *Sermon Preached before the Honourable Society of Grayes-Inn: Upon the Occasion of the Death of our late Royal Sovereign Queen Mary* (R. Sare, London, 1695), pp. 30, 31, & 34.

14. McClain, Molly, 'Love, Friendship, and Power: Queen Mary II's Letters to Frances Apsley'. *Journal of British Studies*, vol. 47, no. 3, 2008, pp. 505–527. doi:10.1086/587720.

15. Chapman, Hester W., *Queen Mary II*, p. 80.

16. Wake, *Sermon Preached before the Honourable Society of Grayes-Inn*, p. C2.

17. Courtenay, Thomas Peregrine, *Memoirs of The Life, Works, and Correspondence of William Temple* (London, 1836), pp. 503–4.

18. Courtenay, *Memoirs of The Life, Works, and Correspondence of William Temple*, p. 504.

19. Chapman, Hester W., *Queen Mary II*, p. 67.

20. Ibid, p. 80.

21. Ibid, p. 92.

22. Letter 'April 19, 1678', as found in Dalrymple, *Memoirs, Vol. I*, p. 209.

23. Waterson, *Mary II, Queen of England 1689–1694*, p. 16.

24. Swift, *Journal to Stella*, p. 466.

25. Ibid.

26. Waller, Maureen, *Ungrateful Daughters: The Stuart Princesses Who Stole Their Father's Crown* (Sceptre Books, London, 2002), p. 111.

27. Ibid, p. 112.

28. Dalrymple, *Memoirs of Great Britain and Ireland, Vol. III*, pp. 68–76.

29. Letter of 'July 27/17, 1690': 'Every hour makes me more impatient to hear from you', as found in Dalrymple, Vol. III, p. 102.

30. Burnet, *History of His Own Time, Vol. II*, p. 224.

31. McCaffrey, Steven (2008, July 28), *Gay activist's 'King Billy was a homosexual' claim sparks furore*. Belfast Telegraph Digital. Retrieved from https://www.belfasttelegraph.co.uk/news/gay-activists-king-billy-was-a-homosexual-claim-sparks-furore-28767397.html on 16 December 2018.

32. I have to disagree with Nancy Mitford's assessment of this topic in *The Sun King*. After researching this subject for over a decade, I am convinced that William was a heterosexual with a low sex drive due to his chronic ill health.

33. Oman, *Mary of Modena*, p. 52.

34. When visiting William III's State Apartments in Hampton Court Palace in the early 2010s, I happened to overhear another visitor very assertively tell her (tour?) group that 'van Keppel was William's boyfriend and only he had the key to get in and out of William's apartments.' Such a privilege as having that key, she failed to mention, was part of the job description of the Groom of the Stool.

35. Burnet, *History of His Own Time, Vol. II*, p. 224.

36. Dalrymple, *Memoirs of Great Britain and Ireland, Vol. III*, p. 88.

37. Waterson, *Mary II, Queen of England 1689–1694*, p. 195.

38. Burnet, *History of His Own Time, Vol. II*, p. 137.

39. Luttrell, *A Brief Relation of State Affairs*, p. 418.
40. Whiston, William, *Memoirs of the life and writings of Mr. William Whiston* (J. Whiston and B. White, London, 1753), p. 100. Contributor: University of California Libraries and published at https://archive.org/details/memoirsoflifewri01whisiala/page/100
41. Bevan, *King William III*, p. 148.
42. 'Character of K. William', British Library, Sloane MSS 4224, fol. 87.
43. Winn, *Queen Anne*, p. 158.
44. Bevan, *King William III*, p. 160.
45. As quoted in Bevan's *King William III: Prince of Orange, the first European* (The Rubicon Press, London, 1997), p. 160.
46. Reports vary, but some (Bryan Bevan, *King William III*, p. 149) state it was hanging from a necklace around his neck, others- such as Dalrymple, believe it hung around his arm on a band (pp. 230–231). I think the former is more likely.
47. Cliveden House, near Taplow, Berkshire, England, which later became notorious after being associated with the Profumo Scandal of the early 1960s.
48. Swift, *Journal to Stella*, p. 456.

Chapter 27: Queen Anne Probably Wasn't a Lesbian

1. Or, at least, it was until the highly-acclaimed film *The Favourite* was released in 2018, which took the rumour of Queen Anne's lesbianism and ran with it (and almost completely left out any mention of Anne's beloved husband of many years, Prince George of Denmark!).
2. Waterson, *Mary II, Queen of England 1689–1694*, p. 184.
3. Green, David, *Queen Anne* (The History Book Club, Glasgow, 1970), pp. 23–33.
4. Harris, Frances, *A Passion for Government: The Life of Sarah, Duchess of Marlborough* (Clarendon Press, Oxford, 1991), p. 11.
5. Anonymous, 'Verses Upon the Late Duchess of Marlborough' (T. Webb, London, 1746), p. 4. British Library.
6. Winn, *Queen Anne*, p. 65.
7. Sanders, Mary F, *Princess and Queen of England, Life of Mary II* (Stanley, Paul & Co, London, 1913), p. 105.
8. Somerset, Anne, *Queen Anne: The Politics of Passion* (HarperPress, London, 2012), p. 36.
9. Goldstone, Nancy, *Daughters of the Winter Queen* (Weidenfeld & Nicolson, London, 2018), pp. 412–416.
10. Somerset, *Queen Anne*, pp. 40–43.
11. Evelyn, '25 July 1683', *Diary, Vol. II*.
12. Kenyon, *The Stuarts*, p. 186. Kenyon's sentence, 'George's impenetrable stupidity was confirmed by his inability to express himself idiomatically in the English language after twenty years' residence' is far too harsh, in my

opinion. An individual's lack of mastery of a foreign language after puberty is fairly common, and some people simply do not do well with languages—this should not be taken as a marker of their intelligence.

13. Petre, Edward, *Three Letters* (London, 1688), p. 3.
14. Winn, *Queen Anne,* p. 153.
15. Ibid.
16. 'James, Duke of York, by Henri Gascar', Royal Museums Greenwich, https://www.rmg.co.uk/see-do/we-recommend/attractions/james-duke-york-henri-gascar [Accessed 17 January 2020].
17. Banks, John, *The History of John, Duke of Marlborough* (James Hodges, London, 1755), p. 342.
18. Winn, *Queen Anne,* p. 62.
19. Somerset, *Queen Anne,* p. 52.
20. Starkey, *Crown & Country*, p. 407.
21. Buckley, Veronica, *Madame de Maintenon: The Secret Wife of Louis XIV* (Bloomsbury Publishing Plc, London, 2008), p. 337.
22. Hearne, *Remarks, Vol. I*, p. 287.
23. Chapman, Hester W., Queen Anne's Son (Andre Deutsch Limited, London, 1954), p. 142.
24. Evelyn, *Diary, Vol. II*, p. 298.
25. Harris, *A Passion for Government,* p. 214.
26. Ibid, p. 213.
27. Fraser, *The Weaker Vessel,* p. 354.
28. Somerset, *Queen Anne,* p. 326.
29. Ibid, p. 327.
30. Harris, *A Passion for Government,* p. 148.
31. Somerset, *Queen Anne,* p. 370.
32. Ibid, p. 371.
33. Ibid, p. 372.
34. Ibid.
35. Seward, *The King Over The Water*, p. 112.
36. Anonymous, *A New Ballad. To the tune of Fair Rosamond [A satire upon Mrs. Masham]* (London?, 1710?), shelfmark C.161.f.2.(44), British Library.
37. Ibid.
38. Ibid.
39. Dunton, John, *King-Abigail: or, The secret reign of the she-favourite,* (John Dunton, London, 1715). Shelfmark G.14047.(5.), British Library.
40. Anonymous, *Sarah's Farewell to Court, Or, A Trip from St. James's to St. Albans,* (London, 1710). Shelfmark C.161.f.2(31)/18, British Library.
41. Ibid.
42. Harris, *A Passion for Government,* p. 178.
43. Swift, '1 December 1711', *Journal to Stella*, p. 355.
44. Anonymous, *The Queen's and the Duke of Ormond's New Toast* (London, 1712). Shelfmark C.161.f.2 (38)/23, British Library.

45. Livingstone, Natalie, *The Mistresses of Cliveden: Three Centuries of Scandal, Power, and Intrigue* (Arrow Books, London, 2015), p. 159.

46. Indeed, I have to disagree with some writers who argue that just because there is no explicit proof of a sexual relationship between Anne and Sarah, that doesn't mean there wasn't one. I would argue that it is the context of a given relationship that renders something probable or not.

47. Swift, '9 October 1712', *The Journal to Stella,* p. 459.

48. DD MS 61450—Letters from Mary Montagu (1689—1751) to Sarah, 1703/04. My thanks to Antonia Keaney at Blenheim Palace for this information.

49. 'The Love Letters of the 6th Duke of Somerset', Petworth House, National Trust, https://www.nationaltrust.org.uk/petworth-house-and-park/features/the-love-letters-of-the-6th-duke-of-somerset [Accessed 11 January 2020]

50. Anonymous, 'Verses Upon the Late Duchess of Marlborough' (T. Webb, London, 1746), p. 4. British Library.

CONCLUSION

Chapter 28: Or, 'Parting is such sweet sorrow'

1. Jones, Robert, *The Muses Gardin for Delights* (B.H. Blackwell, Oxford, 1901), p. 3.

2. As quoted in Dennis Wheatley's 'Old Rowley' (p. 173).

3. Hobbes, Thomas, *The English Works of Thomas Hobbes of Malmesbury* (J. Bonn, London, 1839), p. 113.

Index